Contents

Contributors

Heather Attoe
Quality Facilitator, Mental Health
Services for the Elderly, Chichester
Priority Care Services, Chichester,
West Sussex

Pamela Brereton
formerly Dietetic Services Manager,
Northwick Park Hospital, Harrow,
Middlesex

John Brocklehurst
Associate Director, Research Unit,
Royal College of Physicians,
London

Maria Cox
Consultant Physician in Care of the
Elderly, Watford General Hospital,
Watford, Hertfordshire

Anne Davis
Partner, Anne Davis Associates
Training Consultancy, Birmingham

Michael J. Denham
Consultant Physician in Geriatric
Medicine, Northwick Park Hospital,
Harrow, Middlesex

Edward Dickinson
Associate Director, Research Unit,
Royal College of Physicians,
London

Andrew Hart
Manager for Elderly Services,
Watford General Hospital, Watford

Margaret Hastings
Superintendent Physiotherapist,
Vale of Leven District General
Hospital, Alexandria,
Dumbartonshire

Stuart Haywood
Chairman of the Management ·
Committee, The Retreat, York

Marion Hildick-Smith
Consultant Physician in Geriatric
Medicine, Kent and Canterbury
Hospital, Canterbury, Kent

Sidney Jones
Chartered Psychologist, Edgware,
Middlesex

Paul Kist
Senior Registrar, St George's
Hospital Medical School, London

William Laing
Director, Laing & Buisson, London

D.M. Langley
Tutor in Dramatherapy and
Psychodrama, South Devon
College, Torquay, Devon

G.E. Langley
Consultant Psychiatrist (retired),
Kenton, Exeter, Devon

Carolyn Mansell
Partner, Anne Davis Associates
Training Consultancy, Birmingham

Andrée le May
Principal Lecturer in Nursing,
Department of Health Studies,
Brunel University, Isleworth,
Middlesex

Peter H. Millard
Eleanor Peel Professor of Geriatric
Medicine, St George's Hospital
Medical School, London

Graham P. Mulley
Professor of Geriatric Medicine, St
James's University Hospital, Leeds,
West Yorkshire

Helen Odell-Miller
Senior Lecturer and Clinician in
Music Therapy, Anglia Polytechnic
University and Addenbrookes NHS
Trust, Cambridge

Joan Palmer
Director of Quality, Mount Vernon
and Watford General Hospitals,
Watford

Tom Penman
Chief Speech and Language
Therapist, Northwick Park and St
Mark's NHS Trust, Harrow,
Middlesex

Jackie Pool
State Registered Occupational
Therapist, Dementia Care Services,
Bishops Waltham, Hampshire

Sylvia Poulden
Author and Consultant in Art
Education and Intergenerational
Studies, London

John Rosser
Service Manager, Mental Health
Services for the Elderly, Chichester
Priority Care Services, Chichester,
West Sussex

Ruth Sander
Senior Lecturer, Elderly Care,
University of Portsmouth,
Hampshire

Brian Scott
Director of Continuing Care
Services, The Retreat, York

Jef Smith
General Manager, Counsel and
Care, London

Sylvia Taylor-Goh
Head of Speech and Language
Therapy Service, Northwick Park
and St Mark's NHS Trust, Harrow,
Middlesex

Ian Turner
Proprietor, Risby Hall Nursing
Home, Bury St Edmunds, Suffolk,
and Director, Registered Nursing
Home Association, Birmingham

Charles Twining
The Psychology Department,
Whitchurch Hospital, Cardiff

Norman Vetter
Reader in Epidemiology, Honorary
Consultant in Public Health
Medicine and Non-Executive
Director for Gwent Community
Mental Health Trust, University of
Wales College of Medicine, Cardiff

Christina R. Victor
Senior Lecturer in Health Services
Research, Department of Public
Health Science, St George's
Hospital Medical School, London

Adrian Wagg
Senior Registrar and Honorary
Lecturer in Geriatric Medicine,
University College Hospitals,
London

Preface

Many changes affecting frail older people have occurred since the second edition of *Care of the Long-Stay Elderly Patient* which was published in 1991, hence the need for a new, updated and renamed edition. Many of the present contributors have undertaken major revision of their chapters, which in some cases have been entirely rewritten in the light of developments and previous comments. Some chapters have been deleted, but the contents absorbed within others. Many chapters take account of changes within community care, and the expansion of the private sector. Consequently, there are new chapters on the mixed economy in long-term care, choices and rights of residents in homes, community care, specific standards of care, medical ethics, and the achievements within the private and voluntary sectors. Once again there are specific examples of good practice across the public and private sectors.

Introduction: setting the scene

Three major changes have occurred since publication of the second edition of *Care of the Long-Stay Elderly Patient* in 1991. Firstly, the ageing of the population in the UK has become more pronounced and the trend will continue into the next century. By the year 2010, there will be 7 million people over the age of 70, with 80-year-olds numbering 2.8 million. Currently, Her Majesty the Queen sends congratulatory telegrams to more than 2700 new centenarians annually, compared with less than one-tenth of that number sent out by the king in 1950. In 1990, half a million older people were in institutional care within the public, private or voluntary sectors. In 1992, nearly a quarter of a million people required long-term nursing care. However, to put matters into context, it must be remembered that 94% of the older population live in their own homes, and that many remain very active well into old age: Queen Elizabeth the Queen Mother is an obvious outstanding example.

A second change has been the Community Care Act (1990) which aims, amongst other features, to enable older people to stay at home with as much community care and support as necessary. Appropriate services are tailored to the person's individual requirements, although this can sometimes be limited by availability of funds. Overall, the schemes have proved most successful, even if sometimes they have proved more expensive than the cost of a residential home place. On occasion, relatives remain apprehensive about just how well the older person will cope, even with the extra support provided, and may prefer their older relative to be in the 'safety' of a home.

A third change during the past few years has been the extensive withdrawal of NHS hospitals from the provision of long-stay care. In some parts of the country, this appears to be almost total, and in consequence a huge caring workload has been thrown on general practitioners, some of whom will have limited knowledge, expertise, or interest in this client group. However, it can certainly be argued that the increased availability of accommodation within the private sector has increased patient choice. Another consequence of the change is that fewer and fewer consultant geriatricians will have expertise in the special care needs of this very fragile group of people, which must also be a cause for concern. Some wonder whether the wheel is about to turn full circle, and the events so well described by Dr Marjorie Warren in the 1930s and 1940s may be about to re-develop (Warren, 1946).

It is with all the above changes and developments in mind that this new, renamed edition of the book considers policy issues, standards, and the ways in which good quality of life for continuing care residents can be successfully achieved.

REFERENCE

Warren, M.W. (1946) Care of the chronic aged sick. *Lancet*, **i**, 841–3.

PART ONE
Preventing institutionalization: policy issues

The first chapters consider the vital importance of quality standards and ethical issues in maintaining or better still improving the care of older people in continuing care. The application of such studies is of course of considerable importance to intending purchasers of care whether in public or private sectors, which themselves have undergone dramatic changes in the last decade.

Quality issues for older people in continuing care accommodation

1

INTRODUCTION

Given a choice, the majority of frail older people would prefer to live in their own homes despite their disabilities, loneliness, problems of care and being 'at risk'. By doing so they retain their privacy, familiarity of surroundings, and, to a greater or lesser extent, control over their own lives. Such people would view a move to the 'comforts' of institutional care as a loss of independence, privacy, autonomy and responsibility for their own lives.

The position regarding NHS long-stay hospital accommodation has changed dramatically in recent years. Financial pressures have led many health authorities to withdraw from long-stay provision and to purchase it from the private sector. In some cases, these developments took place too precipitately and without due consideration to the consequences. Of course, the development of the private sector has greatly enlarged the choice of accommodation for patients, and, until NHS nursing homes were developed, NHS long-stay accommodation often left much to be desired.

What this chapter aims to do is set the scene with respect to long-stay care in the light of current changes. Some of the problems of care in recent years in both the private and public sectors are described. Some of the potential solutions are described in general terms.

INSTITUTIONALIZATION

The ideal residence for very dependent people is a complex phenomenon involving not only the building but also the environment, the atmosphere, the staff, their attitudes and standards of care. Furthermore, what may satisfy and please one resident or relative may not suit another. Unfortunately, however well the building is designed and however hard the staff try, institutionalization can develop all too easily. This can result in impoverishment of feelings, thoughts, initiative and social activity resulting in dependence, or acceptance of the institution and adaptation to the environment (Wing and Brown, 1970; Liberakis, 1981).

It is worthwhile detailing some of the features of institutionalization, as, once understood, avoiding or remedial action can be attempted. Four factors may cause institutionalization (King and Raynes, 1968):

1. de-personalization, which occurs when residents have limited personal possessions or finance;
2. social distance, which occurs when staff live off the site and do not join in socially oriented activities;
3. block activities when all activities are organized at group level with little or no variation allowed for personal preference, e.g. rigidity in getting up/going to bed/meal times;
4. lack of variety in daily routine when everybody is treated the same way no matter how much they differ from each other.

In many institutions, the activities of daily life such as sleep and work take place under one roof governed by one authority. Each phase of a person's daily routine is rigidly fixed and is carried out in the company of others, who are all treated alike. Enforced activities are part of an overall plan designed to fulfil the official aims of that institution. Inmates, who have restricted access to the world outside, are, on admission, stripped of 'habitual' supports, such as personal possessions, and 'self' is systematically, if unintentionally, mortified (Goffman, 1960). It takes little thought to realize how well homes or hospitals providing continuing care can fit this pattern.

The nature of the buildings themselves can influence institutionalization. Important factors are the appearance, size and structure of the accommodation, the furnishings and the atmosphere. Gaunt Victorian edifices may rapidly induce gloom and despondency on those who come to live there, while a well-designed, bright, attractive modern building can have quite the opposite effect. There seems to be no agreement as to the optimal or most appropriate size of a continuing care unit, since the desire to provide the personal domestic-like features of a small establishment has to be balanced against economic factors. Several studies suggest that small is beautiful, with small units tending to have better staffing, toileting facilities and freedom of choice (Townsend, 1962; Greenwald and Linn, 1971). However, in America, economic considerations have resulted in nursing homes increasing steadily in size to 300 or 400 residents.

REPORTED DEFICIENCES IN INSTITUTIONAL CARE

While the majority of care in long-stay accommodation is satisfactory, deficiencies in that care in both the public and private sectors unfortunately still occur and make newspaper headlines. Some of the worst public scandals (Martin, 1984) caused the Secretary of State for Health in 1969, Mr Richard Crossman, to establish the NHS Health Advisory Service, which is best thought of as a form of peer review. Many problems relate to 'offhand' attitudes and lack of communication and thoughtfulness by the caring staff. It is worthwhile detailing some of the more recent failures of care so that, hopefully, lessons will be learnt and not forgotten.

GENERAL FAILURES

A series of reports of care within the public and private sectors during the past 15 years have highlighted a variety of problems, many of which relate to less than satisfactory attitudes to older people.

The 1987 Annual Report of the NHS Health Advisory Service reviewed 12 consecutive reports on older people in long-stay hospital accommodation. Long-stay wards consistently failed to provide privacy, homely surroundings and personal space for belongings. None of the 12 health districts had a comprehensive personalized laundry service and half lacked effective management of incontinence. Catering was often provided according to the needs of the institution rather than the patients. Privacy was widely neglected, especially with regard to toileting, washing and dressing.

Day et al. (1988) and Denham and Lubel (1990) reviewed between them 65 Health Advisory Service reports issued between 1985 and 1989 (Table 1.1). The reports showed evidence in the majority of units of marked overcrowding, inadequate personal clothing, and poor sanitary conditions. Worse still there was widespread evidence of poor communication

Table 1.1 Percentage of reports from the NHS Health Advisory Service identified as highlighting various problems in long-term care of elderly patients

	Pecentage of reports	
	Day et al.	Denham/Lubel
Poor sanitary conditions	77	73
Overcrowding in wards	60	53
Inadequate provision of day care	37	40
Use of restraints	74	57
Inadequate personal clothing	65	53
Poor communication among and within professions	83	73

between and within the professions concerned with patient care. Individual reports mentioned patients being put on commodes in full view of others and toilets without doors or curtains. In one ward, patients were encouraged to stay in night clothes all day so that they could be easily identified if or when they 'escaped' from the ward. On another long-stay ward, patients were locked out of their bedrooms because 'they might go to sleep there during the day'.

An assessment of patients' satisfaction with life in long-stay wards of a large psychiatric hospital in London showed failure to treat patients as individuals, feelings of apathy and loneliness despite being in a crowd, loss of autonomy/status, lack of privacy (unable to bathe in private due to two baths in one room), and unpleasant physical surroundings (MacDonald *et al.*, 1988).

The United Kingdom Central Council for Nursing, Midwifery and Health Visiting (1994) reported that the percentage of complaints dealt with by the Council originating from private nursing homes is small compared with the large and increasing numbers of registered practitioners working full or part-time in the area. However, this sector is now the largest single source of complaints to the Council. Problems identified included physical and verbal abuse, inadequate systems of drug administration, ineffective management systems, mismanagement of patient monies, lack of systematic care planning and effective record keeping, and almost no induction or in-service training.

Two studies of private nursing homes in Weston-super-Mare identified several problems, which mainly related to poor communication between the general practitioner and the hospital, and a lack of guidance on common issues which arise in long-term care. There were, for example, no clear policies for managing pressure sores or maintaining continence with respect to urine. Lack of training of care attendants was noted and the use of sedation was common, with nearly half of the patients being prescribed a major tranquillizer or benzodiazepines (Hepple *et al.*, 1989; Pearson *et al.*, 1990).

Many patients do not have a contract with the home in which they are resident. For the sensible older person, this must be a source of unease and disquiet, since there is always the chance of being displaced into another home. A similar situation applies to NHS long-stay accommodation (Consumers' Association, 1992).

Local authority regulatory teams, which have the task of ensuring standards of care in local homes, have had their own problems. A recent Social Service Inspectorate report (1995) indicates that many teams/units fail to carry out the statutory number of visits each year, employ staff who lack experience or qualifications, and place too much emphasis on process and structure rather than outcome. Some teams had yet to agree standards.

DIETETIC ARRANGEMENTS

Attractive dining rooms and pleasing meals may be one of the few remaining pleasures for older people in continuing care. Unfortunately, these are not always the case, and once again, unthinking attitudes of the caring staff may be the cause.

In 1980, patients in a psychogeriatric ward in a large South London psychiatric hospital were found to have low vitamin C blood levels. Consequently they were encouraged to have vitamin C-enriched drinks. However, three years later, a clinical case of scurvy occurred, and three years later still, one-third of the patients were still vitamin C-deficient (Fenton, 1989). Examples of the dining room table from the ward concerned are shown in Figure 1.1 – anything more likely to switch off the gastric juices is hard to imagine. It requires little expense and imagination to make these tables more attractive (Figure 1.2) but it does need a major change in attitudes at all levels – nursing, management and medical. It is sad to report that the layout of tables shown in Figure 1.1 was seen in another long-stay psychiatric hospital only about four years ago.

Several studies of hospital meals provided to continuing care residents have shown the cooked food to be deficient in fibre, vitamin D, folate, vitamin C and calories (Kirk, 1990; Prior, 1992). A healthy eating policy for patients in such units can improve the nutritional content of food, resulting in less waste and fewer prescriptions for laxatives, resulting in an overall cost saving (Beveridge, 1986).

The provision of meals in NHS hospitals is not always good. Meals may be dried up during regeneration, meal items may be missing, no provision may be made for portion size, timing of meals may be inappropriate (e.g. lunch arriving 2 hours after breakfast), holding times may be long, and food wastage excessive. The catering staff themselves may have to work in cramped, old and inadequate accommodation with resulting problems in staffing. In some health districts, no nutritional or dietetic advice is available to long-stay units mainly because the need is not recognized by health authorities (M.J. Denham, unpublished data from NHS Health Advisory Service Reviews 1989–1991).

DRUG THERAPY

Modern drug therapy has brought many benefits to older people, but medication needs to be given sensibly and unnecessary prescriptions withdrawn to avoid problems with side-effects. Surveys of elderly patients in public or private institutional care have shown that nine out of ten residents are on medication, with three or four drugs on average being prescribed. However, as many as 10–12 different drugs may be given to an individual patient (Primrose et al., 1987; Nolan and O'Malley, 1989).

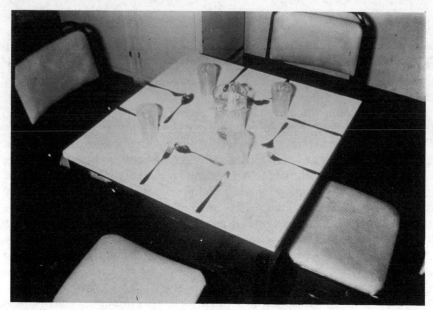

Figure 1.1 Dining room table in a long-stay psychogeriatric unit before 'enlightenment'.

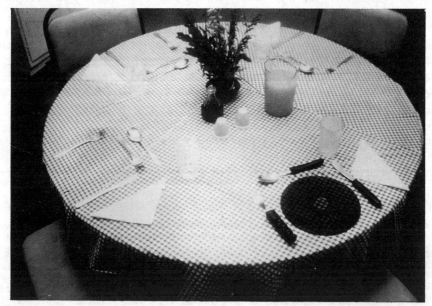

Figure 1.2 Dining room table in a long-stay psychogeriatric unit after 'enlightenment'.

Prescribing patterns vary between homes with similar clienteles, suggesting different prescribing patterns by the general practitioners. Many drugs are prescribed inappropriately and/or may be potentially hazardous. Drugs may be prescribed for a particular symptom without taking account of the patient's other clinical problems, e.g. a beta-blocker may be given to a patient for hypertension but without considering their peripheral vascular disease (Adams *et al.*, 1987; Gosney *et al.*, 1989; Lindley *et al.*, 1992).

It is alarming that the use of sedation is still widespread: nearly one in two residents in one study and approximately two in three in another were prescribed a major tranquillizer or benzodiazepines. To compound the situation, many patients were not receiving a regular medical review. It is greatly to be feared that these powerful drugs are being given to 'switch the patient off with the lights' as has been reported in the USA (Ray *et al.*, 1980; Waxman *et al.*, 1985).

THE INSTITUTION ITSELF

The institution and the attitudes of the staff can have a considerable effect on the residents. There are homes which induce conformity by a system of authority, adhering to well-established patterns of caring without question, discouraging complaining, and introducing disciplinary procedures with privilege and sanction systems. These approaches to care are likely to produce severe institutionalization. Furthermore, if staff are not adequately trained to cope with the social, psychological, psychiatric and/or physical problems of the patients, then they, the carers, are likely to suffer stress which, in turn, will make them less receptive to ideas and concepts of changes in care. Finally, the general environment of such facilities can make them less attractive places to work in and therefore make it difficult to attract high-calibre staff, leading to high turnover of staff and loss of drive, initiative and morale. It is very disconcerting for relatives to see different caring staff each time a visit is made.

ABUSE

Those who first described the problem of abuse in the 1970s were vilified by others who denied its existence. However, it is now accepted that abuse does occur, as exemplified by reports, national conferences and research on both sides of the Atlantic. Abuse may be physical, verbal, emotional or financial, or may involve neglect or inappropriate use of sedation (Social Services Inspectorate, 1992). Clues to its existence may be obtained from the patient's history, from stress becoming evident in the carer, or from recurring falls, bruises or finger marks on the older person which are not appropriately explained. However, there is often little concrete evidence to point to the diagnosis. The older person will usually not complain and consequently a high index of suspicion is required. Because of these difficulties, it is difficult to assess just how frequently the problem occurs (Eastman, 1994).

Several predisposing factors to abuse have been described, which can develop in the person's own home or that of a relative:

1. the elderly relative may move to stay with carers where the atmosphere is initially happy, but relationships may become strained when the older person or the carer becomes physically or mentally ill;
2. the relative may not have been taken in willingly, so that a potential stress situation is there from the beginning;
3. the family atmosphere may already be violent when the older person moves in and this situation may be exacerbated if there is a history of alcohol abuse by the carer;
4. the carer may be immature or unable to cope with the situation and/or provide the necessary care;
5. stress in relationships as described above may be exacerbated if the carer has had to give up paid work in order to take on the new role.

In the residential or nursing home situation, whether within the public or the private sector, residents may be subjected to physical abuse, such as the use of restraints, or they may be locked in rooms, have their legs and/ or arms tied to chairs or commodes, or tables may be placed in front of chairs to prevent the person getting up. Of course, there are grey areas when a patient or resident becomes really aggressive or restless, when restraint will be needed to prevent falls or the risk of litigation. Sedatives may be used inappropriately as indicated before to 'switch the patient out with the lights'. Abuse may be financial. Relatives may hold the pension book and be reluctant to provide 'pocket money' for the resident, while on occasion managers of homes have been accused of financial abuse of their residents.

QUALITY ISSUES: POTENTIAL SOLUTIONS

The dangers and effects of institutionalization have been detailed above but preventing them is not easy. Perhaps most important is the attitude of the caring staff. Senior medical and nursing staff may take the view that everything that can be done for the patient has already been done and it is difficult to measure changes in outcome. Consequently, they may 'switch off' and attempt nothing more than basic care. Secondly, the older types of NHS accommodation are often most unsuitable for long-stay patients from the point of view of current concepts of accommodation design, and nursing and toileting facilities may be of poor quality, badly sited and lack privacy. The physical outlook may be depressing, while bedding, chairs and other equipment may be old and unsuitable for older infirm people. Thirdly, the patient's day may be arranged to fit the nursing schedule rather than the patient's benefit. Patients may still be woken up at 5:00 a.m. and put to bed at 2:00 p.m. In addition, they may not have their own clothing but be provided with obvious institutional clothing. The opportunity for the patient to make the smallest decision may be taken away. However, it is possible to provide a high quality of life for patients in long-stay care. The potential approaches are detailed in the following sections.

ASSESSMENT OF THE ATTITUDES OF CARING STAFF

Attitudes, job satisfaction and morale amongst the caring staff are all important factors in providing high-quality care. These need to be assessed and change effected as necessary. This can be fruitful, effective and does not necessarily cost money. Staff in a high-quality home pay particular attention to the individual physical and mental capabilities of each resident and place considerable emphasis on informal contact with residents. An audit of staff attitudes to care can be quite beneficial (Harwood and Ebrahim, 1994).

IMPROVEMENT IN STAFF TRAINING

Improvements in training are essential (BGS *et al.* 1993; UKCC 1994). If the increasing numbers of older people are to be adequately cared for in public and private sectors, then more student nurses should receive experience of this form of care and the existing staff should have their current skills updated. This requires leadership from general and nursing managers. Indeed, managers at all levels should take an active and regular interest in these all too often neglected 'Cinderella' units.

PREVENTION OF ABUSE

Prevention of abuse within residential or nursing homes is not easy. It requires managers to select staff sensibly, and arrange proper induction and in-house training as well as adequate and enlightened supervision. Training should consider those values which form part of a good quality of life for residents. Managers must take care not to appoint staff who have been involved in abuse in previous employment. Sensible and open explicit care plans with clear codes of conduct should be drawn up and monitored by visiting regulatory authorities who, in turn, should be well resourced and be knowledgeable about the problem. Senior staff and visiting doctors need to be on the alert to recognize subtle clues. Residents themselves should have easy accessibility to independent advocates or telephone helplines, otherwise they are in a difficult position if they observe abuse but fear reprisals if they report what they see or hear (Bright, 1995).

ASSESSMENT OF THE RESIDENT'S VIEW OF CARE

It is not always as easy as it might seem to assess what the patient thinks of the care. Residents may be apathetic, have low expectations and/or be reluctant to make critical comments. Questionnaires such as that by Raphael and Mandeville (1979) can be applied to patients, relatives and staff. In their survey of 377 patients, relatives and staff, they found that patients preferred small rooms, while the staff preferred large; that day areas served many functions and that it was better to have two such areas; that patients and nurses liked cot sides but doctors did not; and that all groups deplored noise, lack of privacy in toileting arrangements and the lack of diversional activities. Both patients and staff criticized the poor quality of the physical environment while patients also criticized the organization of their day. Similarly, in a study of quality of life issues, Philp *et al.* (1991a) showed that patients and staff may differ quite widely on what each considers to be best for the other and that ward practice bore little resemblance to the preferences of staff and/or patients.

INTRODUCTION OF A PROGRAMME TO IMPROVE QUALITY OF CARE

The development of, and adherence to, a philosophy of care is a start. This should not be a nominal exercise. The philosophy used in the code of practice 'A Better Home Life' (Centre for Policy on Ageing, 1996), although originally designed for local authority care, has much to commend it: 'a conviction that those who live in residential care should do so with dignity, that they should have the respect of those who support them, should live with no reduction in their rights as citizens and should be entitled to live as full and active a life as their physical and mental condition allows'.

The Canterbury and Thanet Health Authority (1985), in considering the problem of quality of care, stated that 'patients should live in comfortable, clean and safe surroundings, and be treated with respect and sensitivity to their individual needs and abilities. All patients should be encouraged to enjoy as normal and as full a life as possible, and this should include the opportunity to make decisions about their life style. There should be a planned programme of care for each person which should be agreed with the patient and the medical practitioners'.

These philosophies can be usefully supported by check lists which incidentally illustrate the fact that there are no universally agreed and accepted standards of care, particularly of outcome. Examples of guide-lines include: 'Living in Hospital' (Elliott, 1982), 'Towards Good Practice in Small Hospitals' (NAHAT 1988), 'Caring for Quality'(SSI, 1990), 'Achievable standards for care for the elderly patient ...' (City and Hackney Health Authority, 1987), and 'High quality long-term care for elderly patients' (Royal College of Physicians, 1992).

ADDITION OF EXTRA ACTIVITIES TO THE PATIENT'S DAY

Addition of extra activities is well illustrated by Chapters 17–20 in this book (also McCormack and Whitehead, 1981). One of the few remaining pleasures of life for the resident or patient may be the main meal of the day. Therefore, meals should be both attractive and nutritious. If necessary, advice should be sought from the district dietitian (see Chapter 15).

IMPROVEMENT IN THE QUALITY OF THE CONTINUING CARE ACCOMMODATION

Health authorities should insist on high-quality accommodation which provides a stimulating and pleasant social environment (Vetter, 1992). The patients ought to be able to feel that they are no longer in hospital, have a good lifestyle and be able to bring in some of their own furniture and clothing, factors that are considered important by the patients (Bond et al., 1989). Many homes now try to provide attractive furnish-ings, perhaps 'tuned' to local events, places or persons. Institutional furniture is avoided. Colour coding of rooms can be introduced, thus providing cues for residents. Innovative building designs for the private sector have been developed by the Royal Surgical Aid Society, the Abbeyfield and Brendoncare organizations. Unfortunately, NHS nursing homes have not been developed further despite excellent reports of the pilot schemes.

Designers for homes for patients with dementia need to pay particular attention to the 'design for orientation'. Ten principles of design have been described including the size of the unit, providing cues, designing different rooms for different functions, controlling stimuli, providing space to move about, and good facilities for staff (Marshall, 1992). However, it must be emphasized that where care is delivered is less important than how it is delivered (Philp et al., 1991b). A good physical environment may not necessarily result in improved outcome (Bowling et al., 1991; Harwood and Ebrahim, 1992), although the quality of life in nursing homes is generally better than on wards (Bond et al., 1989; Bowling et al., 1991).

REGULAR INDEPENDENT INSPECTIONS

All long-stay nursing facilities, both public and private, should have thorough repeated inspections using nationally agreed standards of structure, process and outcome. The pharmacist member of the team should encourage sensible prescribing. Unfortunately, some inspection authorities have so many homes to visit that only the most basic of assessments can be made. This is a pity since standards can change rapidly in a home if the person in charge leaves and a less able person arrives.

CONCLUSION

Older patients who are about to enter long-stay accommodation now have a wide range of facilities to choose from. Wherever they eventually decide to settle down, they should be entitled to high-quality care. However, much depends on the vital factor of the attitudes of the caring staff, associated with sensible enlightened leadership from managers.

ACKNOWLEDGEMENTS

I thank Professor Peter Millard for permission to use Figures 1.1 and 1.2.

REFERENCES

Adams, K.R.M., Al Hamouz, S., Edmunds, E. *et al.* (1987) Inappropriate prescribing for the elderly. *J.R.Coll. Physicians Lond.*, **21**, 39–41.
Beveridge, C. (1986) Catering for health can save money. *Health Service J.*, **96**, 1110.
Bond, J., Gregson, B.A. and Atkinson, A. (1989) Measurement of outcome within a multicentre randomised controlled trial in the evaluation of experimental NHS nursing homes. *Age Ageing*, **18**, 292–302.
Bowling, A., Formby, J., Grant, K. and Ebrahim, S. (1991) A randomised controlled trial of nursing homes and long stay geriatric ward care for elderly people. *Age Ageing*, **20**, 316–24.
Bright, B. (1995) *Care Betrayed*, Counsel and Care, London.
British Geriatrics Society, Royal College of Psychiatrists and Royal College of Nursing (1993) *Working with Older People*, Royal College of Nursing, London.
Canterbury and Thanet Health Authority, (1985) *Nursing Home Registration and Inspection Handbook.* Canterbury and Thanet Health Authority, Ramsgate.
Centre for Policy on Ageing (1996) *A Better Home Life. A Code of Good Practice for Residential and Nursing Home Care: Report of an Advisory Group.* Centre for Policy on Ageing, London.
City and Hackney Health Authority (1987) *Achievable standards of care for the elderly, patient care for an acute assessment ward, continuing care wards, nursing homes and day hospitals within the City and Hackney Health Authority*, King's Fund Centre, London.
Consumers' Association (1992) *Contracting for Residential Care: a Policy Paper*, Consumers' Association London.

Day, P., Klein, R. and Tupping, S. (1988) *Inspecting for Quality*, University of Bath Centre for the Analysis of Social Policy, Bath.

Denham, M.J. and Lubel, D. (1990) Peer review and services for the elderly patients. *BMJ*, **i**, 635–6.

Eastman, M. (1994) *Old Age Abuse*, Chapman & Hall, London.

Elliott, J. (1982) *Living in Hospital*, 2nd edn, King Edward's Hospital Fund, London.

Fenton, J. (1989) Some food for thought. *Health Service J.*, **99**, 666–7.

Goffman, E. (1960) Characteristics of total institutions, in *Identity and Anxiety* (eds M.R. Stein, A. Vidick and D.N. Whit), Free Press of Glencoe, Illinois.

Gosney, M., Tallis, R.C. and Edmund, E. (1989) Inappropriate prescribing in Part III residential homes. *Health Trends*, **20**, 129–31.

Greenwald, S.R. and Linn, M.W. (1971) Intercorrelation of data on nursing homes. *Gerontologist* **11**, 337–40.

Harwood, R.H. and Ebrahim, S. (1992) Long term institutional residents – does the environment affect outcome? *J. R. Coll. Physicians Lond.*, **26**, 134–8.

Harwood, R.H. and Ebrahim, S. (1994) Assessing the effectiveness of audit in long stay hospital care for elderly people. *Age Ageing*, **23**, 287–92.

Hepple, J., Bowler, I. and Bowman, C.E. (1989) A survey of private nursing home residents in Weston Super Mare. *Age Ageing*, **18**, 61–3.

King, R.D. and Raynes, N.W. (1968) An operational measure of inmate management in residential institutions. *Soc. Sci. Med.*, **2**, 41–53.

Kirk, S.F.L. (1990) Adequacy of meals served and consumed at a long stay hospital for the elderly. *Care of the Elderly J.*, **2**, 77–80.

Liberakis, E.A. (1981) Factors predisposing to institutionalisation. *Acta Psychiatr. Scand.*, **63**, 356.

Lindley, C.M., Tully, M.P., Paramsothy, V. and Tallis, R.C. (1992) Inappropriate medication is a major cause of adverse drug reactions in elderly patients. *Age Ageing*, **20**, 294–300.

McCormack, D. and Whitehead, A. (1981) The effect of providing recreational activities on the engagement level of long stay geriatric patients. *Age Ageing*, **10**, 287–91.

MacDonald, L., Subbald, B. and Hoarce, C. (1988) Measuring patient satisfaction with life in a long stay psychiatric hospital. *Int. J. Soc. Psychiatr.*, **34**, 292–304.

Marshall, M. (1992) Designing for confused old people, in *Recent Advances in Psychogeriatrics* (ed. T. Arie), Churchill Livingstone, Edinburgh.

Martin, J.P. (1984) *Hospitals in Trouble*, Blackwell, Oxford.

National Association of Health Authorities Trusts (1988) *Towards good practice in small hospitals*, National Association of Health Authorities Trusts, Birmingham.

National Health Service Health Advisory Service Annual Report (1987), National Health Service Health Advisory Service, Sutton.

Nolan, L. and O'Malley, K. (1989) The need for a more rational approach to drug prescribing for elderly people in nursing homes. *Age Ageing*, **18**, 52–6.

Pearson, J., Challis, L. and Bowman, C.E. (1990) Problems of care in a private nursing home. *BMJ*, **301**, 371–2.

Philp, I., Mawhinney, S., Mutch, W.J. (1991a) Setting standards for long term care of the elderly in hospital. *BMJ*, **302**, 1056.

Philp, I., Mutch, W.J., Bellinger, B.R. and Boyd, L. (1991b) A comparison of care in private nursing homes, geriatric and psychogeriatric hospitals. *Int. J. Geriatr. Psychiatr.*, **6**, 253–8.

Primrose, W.R., Campbell, A.E., Simpson, G.K. and Smith, R.G. (1987) Prescribing patterns observed in registered nursing homes and long stay geriatric wards. *Age Ageing*, **16**, 25–8.

Prior, J. (1992) A project to assess and improve nutritional provision at a care of the elderly unit. *Care of the Elderly J.*, **6**, 2, 44–8.

Raphael, W. and Mandeville, J. (1979) *Old People in Hospital*, King Edward's Hospital Fund for London, London.

Ray, W.A., Federspiel, C.F. and Schaffner, W. (1980) A study of antipsychotic drug use in nursing homes. Epidemiological evidence suggesting misuse. *Am. J. Public Health*, **70**, 485–91.

Royal College of Physicians (1992) *High quality long-term care for elderly people*, Royal College of Physicians, London.

Social Services Inspectorate (1990) *Caring for Quality*, Department of Health, London.

Social Services Inspectorate (1992) *Confronting Elder Abuse*, HMSO, London.

Social Services Inspectorate (1995) *Inspection Units*, 3rd overview, HMSO, London.

Townsend, P. (1962) *The Last Refuge*, Routledge & Kegan Paul, London.

United Kingdom Central Council for Nursing, Midwifery and Health Visiting (1994) *Professional conduct. Occasional report on standards of nursing in nursing homes*, United Kingdom Central Council for Nursing, Midwifery and Health Visiting, London.

Vetter, N. (1992) Purchasing long term health care for elderly people, in *Long Term Care for Elderly People: Purchasing, Providing and Quality*, HMSO, London.

Waxman, H.W., Klein, M. and Carner, E.A. (1985) Drug misuse in nursing homes: an institutional addition. *Hosp. Community Psychiatr.*, **36**, 886–7.

Wing, J. and Brown, G. (1970) *Institutionalisation and Schizophrenia*, Cambridge University Press, Cambridge.

Standards of institutional care for older people

2

This chapter considers two aspects of standard setting: the content and nature of standards and the process of monitoring them. Both are problematic. Despite increasing emphasis on quality within the National Health Service (NHS) and nursing homes, concern about standards of care for older patients in institutions rightly persists.

Day and Klein (1987) impishly suggested that 'the only sure way of avoiding scandals in institutions is to close them down'. However, the increasing numbers of very old and frail people, combined with professional aspirations to care and treat, preclude such a development. Older people will continue to be major users of acute hospital and community health services, with a sizeable number spending their last years of life in some type of institution. Even when deterrents to admission were introduced in the 19th century, older people found their way into workhouses, and the experience of community care suggests that history is being repeated in the 1990s.

COMMUNITY CARE

INSTITUTION OR HOME?

The proposals of the NHS and Community Care Act 1990 to care for people in their own homes or in 'homely settings' were widely supported as a move to reduce the number of people receiving long-term care in institutions. However, strong fears were raised among professionals. The Royal College of Nursing (RCN) felt that the changes would lead to increasing numbers of very sick and frail older people becoming dependent for nursing services on the already stretched NHS community nursing services. A survey of nurses working with elderly people (RCN, 1992) stated that 'the RCN is extremely concerned that the nursing needs of people living in both residential and nursing homes are in many instances unmet, and that the changes due to be introduced in 1993 will not rectify this situation.' Highlighting the increasing numbers of highly dependent older people living in residential institutions, the RCN stated that it fears that 'a scandal of major proportions is inevitable'.

An increase in the age and dependency of patients and residents is evident in both nursing homes and residential care homes, and the standard of nursing care is already being questioned. We cannot feel confident that all the changes have been for the better. The United Kingdom Central Council for Nursing, Midwifery and Health Visiting (UKCC) in its occasional report on standards of nursing in nursing homes (1994) drew ominous conclusions: 'Whilst the complaints reveal serious professional misconduct such as physical and verbal abuse, they also identify wholly inadequate systems of drug administration, ineffective record keeping and almost non-existent induction or in-service training.' The number of professional conduct cases relating to nursing homes considered by the Professional Conduct Committee rose from 8% in 1990 to 26% in 1994 (UKCC, 1994). The number of nursing homes increased during this time and this trend seems likely to continue, contrary to the policy intentions of the NHS and Community Care Act 1990 which aimed to reduce the numbers of people in residential care by up to a third.

Indeed, forecasts show that there is every likelihood of the increase in institutional care continuing into the 21st century. It has been estimated that 1% of the 65–74-year-old population live in some form of institutional setting, but that, for people aged 85 and over, the proportion may reach 27%. 'Other things being equal, another 68 000 institutional places will be needed between the year 1993 and the turn of the century in order to keep pace with demographic pressure.' (Laing, 1994). Since 1981, the trend has been strongly upwards. The private sector provided an additional 20 000 nursing home beds in the UK between 1985 and 1987, and a further increase of 110 000 private and 6700 voluntary nursing home beds between 1987 and 1993.

There has been a sharp decline in the numbers of NHS long-stay beds as a result of government policies and funding, leaving some district health authorities with no long-stay NHS geriatric beds. However, there were still 155 400 public-sector long-stay places for older and chronically ill people in 1993, and there were almost 400 000 private and voluntary residential and nursing home beds. The pace of increase is now considerably greater in the nursing home sector, which includes many places in former residential care homes which are becoming 'dual registered' with both health and social service authorities, or converting completely to nursing homes to allow their frail older clients to stay in the same home as their need for nursing care increases.

Sadly, there is evidence that pressures following the reduction in the numbers of NHS beds has produced worsening, and sometimes intolerable, conditions for patients. Mixed-sex wards have become commonplace in the NHS, reducing privacy and dignity for men and women of all ages, and stories of long waits on trolleys by older and terminally ill patients continue to hit the headlines. The new Patients' Charter includes the right of patients to be informed if they cannot be accommodated in single-sex bays. To date, NHS contracts have failed to shift the emphasis towards higher patient outcome standards in both the NHS and the independent sector.

The size and design of nursing homes built by some large companies, with concentrations of 150 or more beds on one site, is contrary to the spirit of providing community care in 'homely' settings. However, contracts with large-scale providers are being made by health authorities, facilitating the wholesale transfer of patients from free care in NHS wards into the means-tested private sector. Public reaction to the loss of free NHS care for older people, the use of personal assets to pay for care, and two cases of murder by discharged psychiatric hospital patients prompted a slowing down of closures of NHS long-stay wards in 1995.

However, the shift has already transformed the distribution of care of long-stay patients and it is predicted that well over half a million frail older people will be cared for in institutions at the turn of the century (Laing, 1994). Therefore, the issue of standards in institutions will remain an important factor in the quality of life of older people.

CHANGES IN MONITORING STANDARDS OF CARE

Arrangements for the monitoring of public and private provision of care also have many critics, partly because they have not rooted out poor standards. Inspectors of this multi-million pound industry are themselves worried about the variations in ratios of inspecting officers to homes, and differing methods of audit of standards across authorities. The RCN Special Interest Group has called on health authorities to 'take more seriously the responsibility to regulate the independent health care sector' (RCN, 1994).

There was some optimism during the 1980s that standards of care were improving, with the RCN reporting progress in the NHS (RCN, 1987, para 1.16), and Day and Klein (1987) stating that standards in the private sector have also been improving. However, few observers would now deny a widespread concern with general standards. NHS professionals and the media frequently direct attention to the failings of private nursing homes (BBC *Panorama* 20 January 1992). Some homes have been closed and reports of Registered Homes Tribunals record instances of abuse, neglect and incompetence (Bevan Ashford/Anne Davis Associates, 1996).

Concern about standards of care in local authority homes led to their being monitored by the new inspection units established in 1991 as part of the community care changes (DHSS, 1990) but no similar provision was made for inspectors to scrutinize and report on standards in NHS wards. Here, the patients' Charter initiative and the introduction of competition through the 'contract culture' of the NHS and Community Care Act 1990 were intended to give impetus to improvements in quality.

Local authority contracts have placed emphasis on quality assurance systems and the quality of life of residents, but little monitoring seems to be done, and many homes continue to provide basic rather than quality care. Humberside County Council offers financial incentives of up to £20 per placement per week to homes that meet specific quality standards. Larger nursing home companies provide modern accommodation and usually have quality assurance systems. Local authority contracts are helping to reduce multiple-occupancy rooms in more traditional nursing homes.

Legal challenges to higher contract standards have met with rebuff. It was held in the High Court by Justice Auld that there was 'no reason in law why an authority should not impose a stricter contractual regime on the operators as long as the standards are reasonable and do not curtail the rights of owners under the 1984 Registered Homes Act.' Justice Auld also held that, where a local authority had a statutory duty to provide services and to fund them in part or in whole out of monies provided by its taxpayers, it had to balance its duty to provide statutory services with its fiduciary duty not to waste the money of those paying for them. An insistence on high contractual standards coupled with firm and economical means of enforcing them is an essential means of achieving such a balance (Bevan Ashford/Anne Davis Associates, 1996).

Mounting pressure for more openness and clarity about standards of care has prompted the government to review public regulation of residential and nursing homes. Providing a higher quality of life for older people in institutions requires dramatic improvements on past performance. The literature abounds with pleas for higher standards and more effective arrangements to reinforce them. Quality is improved by more attention to the outcomes of care, in which quality of life and patient preferences are accorded centre stage.

STANDARDS

WHAT STANDARDS?

The debate on existing standards has not been very well informed; there are no agreed health standards of good practice to which all would subscribe or data on which to base general judgements. DHSS statistics on nursing homes are confined to capacity: the number of hospitals and homes, facilities and beds. Performance indicators for NHS older patient services focus mainly on the adequacy of inputs and the efficiency with which facilities are used, rather than quality of care. While the NHS considers length of stay as an efficiency criterion, for patients the outcome is all too often a hastening of death, as evident from very high patient death rates in the days or weeks, rather than months, following NHS discharge.

Similarly, the Registered Homes Act does not require a nursing home to state its aims and objectives, have written policies or a complaints procedure. The Act includes these requirements for residential care and regulations demand that the welfare of the resident is paramount. Nursing homes rely on UKCC codes to regulate nursing practice. The difference is reflected in guidance for regulators (Centre for Policy on Ageing, 1984; NAHAT, 1985).

THE BOOKLET 'HOME LIFE'

'Home Life' was the first comprehensive statement of the principle of care for long-stay elderly people: surely an indicator of the low value placed on the care of older people until very recently. The booklet opens with a statement on the principles of care, referring to the 'conviction' which underlies the recommendations and requirements set out in the code: 'those who live in residential care should do so with dignity; they should have the respect of those who support them; should live with no reduction of their rights as citizens . . . and should be entitled to live as full and active a life as their physical and mental condition will allow' (para 1.1).

Personal fulfilment, dignity, autonomy, individuality, esteem, quality of experience, emotional needs and risk and choice are covered in a discussion of residents' rights (standards 1–7). The section on physical features refers to official guidance which is followed by a discussion of suitable locations, capacity, accommodation, and space and arrangements for own rooms. The latter is intended to reinforce the general message of individuality and respect: 'special reasons will be expected where there are more than two people to a room'. People should be able to bring their own furniture to bed-sitting rooms, and private wash basins should ensure privacy.

NAHAT GUIDELINES 1995

The NAHAT guidelines have two sections. One offers advice to health authorities; the second suggests model guidelines which follow this advice closely. The tone is quite different to that of Home Life, even allowing for the wider remit of the guidelines: they also cover private acute hospitals.

While there are brief references to the 'importance of flexibility and individual care' and 'sensitivity to the changing needs' of older people, and a
recommendation of regular occupational and leisure activities (para 1.3),
there is no equivalent to Home Life's statement of philosophy. Rather, the
NAHAT publication, in its own words, 'continually refers to legislation
and associated regulations concerned with the physical standards of
nursing homes and the qualifications and suitability of staff. The working
party has emphasised statutory requirements as it considers that a good
understanding and compliance with these requirements together with
vigilance on the part of registering authorities will lead to higher
standards of care' (para 1.2).

A supplement to the handbook (1988) moves NAHAT guidance a little
in the direction taken by Home Life. There is a discussion of qualitative
factors in sections on the patient relationship, including the right to
privacy and full information, and relations between staff and patients (pp.
2–5). However, most of the supplement is taken up with other topics
which reflect an administrative/professional concern with inputs rather
than quality of life. Discussions of management and staffing issues (pp. 6–
11) remain pre-occupied with qualifications and staffing ratios.

Is what is lost by this relative neglect of outcome considerations, true of
most health services? It could be argued that the systems ensure adequate
premises, space, staff, qualifications, high-standard nursing and medical
practices and prerequisites of quality. Maybe, but not all the soulless and
joyless units described in Health Advisory Service reports and reports of
Registered Homes Tribunals were deprived in these respects. Something
else was missing which can only be captured by a concern with outcomes.
Also, structural and process standards reflect professional judgements
which are not necessarily synonymous with the priorities of patients and
their families.

STRUCTURE, PROCESS, OUTPUT AND OUTCOME

The difficulties in standard setting still stem from legitimate different
perceptions of what is good quality care and the facts that should inform
judgements. Unacceptable standards may be relatively easy to identify,
but most residents are hopefully living out their time in hospitals and
homes much better than this. There is no agreement among professionals
and regulators on whether the plethora of norms and guidelines cover
and give due weight to the most important aspects of care.

One way of imposing some discipline on ideas about the content and
measurement of quality is the one suggested by Donabedian (1980). He
distinguishes between structure (number and calibre of personnel, quality
of buildings, equipment etc.) process (the way the resources are used) and
outcomes (the benefits to the patient). Output has been added to distin-

guish between substantive measures of quality of care, e.g. staff turnover, number of accidents, deaths, outbreaks of infection or skin care, and the less tangible assessments of satisfaction, comfort and well-being. Standards of good practice should include aspects of all four elements.

SOCIAL SERVICES INSPECTORATE STANDARDS

The Department of Health Social Services Inspectorate (SSI) advocated the Donabedian approach towards monitoring local authority and independent residential care homes in 'Inspecting for Quality' (DHSS, 1991). 'Inspecting for Quality' instructs local authority inspectors to evaluate the service by examining:

- the resources devoted to provision of the service;
- the processes involved in providing the service;
- the quality and quantity of service provision;
- the quality of life of users

against previously agreed aims and objectives, including standards, which may be set at 'good enough' or preferred levels.

Since 1989, a series of documents from the SSI has detailed the standards used to assess the quality of care for elderly people, people with physical disability and people with specific mental health needs. 'Homes are for Living In', a model for evaluating the quality of care provided and the quality of life experienced in residential homes for older people, details more than 400 points for consideration. Quality is defined under six headings: dignity, privacy, independence, fulfilment, rights and choice. Each has a statement of the standard: for example, 'independence' is 'Opportunities to act and think without reference to another person, including a willingness to incur a degree of calculated risk' (DHSS, 1989).

The SSI guidance on practice refers in passing to NHS inspectors, but to date little attention has been paid by government to standards in nursing homes. The NHS remains preoccupied with consideration of structures and processes in healthcare quality assessment, despite acknowledgements of the importance of outcome measures. Because the Registered Homes Act 1984 is about inputs into nursing homes (the only references to processes relate to record-keeping and informing the health authority of deaths, absences of persons-in-charge etc.), no qualitative requirements are acknowledged beyond the minimum of 'adequacy'. Inspectors are anxious to extend the scope of monitoring and many health authorities have produced qualitative monitoring tools, with the emphasis on individuality and quality of life as well as examining the quality of nursing practice.

MAKING OUTPUTS AND OUTCOMES MATTER MORE

One explanation for the continuing NHS preoccupation with inputs and process considerations is not ignorance, but that it reflects NHS beliefs. The aim is to have more professionals and facilities available. From this viewpoint, provision of services is an end in itself, evident in a concern to ensure equal access and the public outcry against closure of hospital beds. Nor is this imbalance automatically corrected by implementing one of the many quality assurance schemes now on offer.

Energies are sometimes directed to choice and implementation of systems rather than outcome measures and appropriate standards. Outputs such as continence, mobility, accidents, mental alertness, physical care (such as absence of pressure sores) and independence need to be key measures in professional audit as they impinge directly on the quality of life a patient will be able to enjoy.

OUTCOMES: CONSUMER PREFERENCES

Consumer preferences are useful as a starting point for assessments of quality and how to improve it. They provide an antidote to an obsession with the adequacy of staffing and accommodation. Consumerism also has the advantage of consistency with the self-image of NHS personnel and is less threatening to NHS personnel than 'attacks' on professionals, since the outcomes of professional procedures are not subjected to rigorous scrutiny by patients who usually focus on the 'kindness' of nurses.

The more obvious difficulty is finding a practical way of ensuring that patients' wishes are given priority in assessing quality of care. For example, who are the consumers, and how does one measure the quality of life of a person who is mentally confused? Also, a basic ingredient of satisfaction is missing for the many older people who did not want to go into a home or hospital in the first place. One way around these problems is to require providers to focus on pro-active care planning to meet individual wishes and preferences through discussion with patients and their relatives or carers. This is the basic principle of the SSI approach to inspection and assessment of services described above and is the key to real quality services when the plans are used.

PATIENTS' RIGHTS

A variant of the above approach of outcomes and consumer preference is to start from the notion of a charter of rights for patients. The protection and enhancement of patients' rights and values is central to assessment of the quality of outcomes: they are the things that matter most to the beneficiary. It is not merely an 'add-on' to input and process considerations: it transforms them, directing attention to different considerations when setting standards for care. The following list is a charter of rights used by social services departments in registering residential homes. Patients in a private home shall have the right:

1. to retain their personal dignity and independence irrespective of the severity of their physical or mental infirmity.
2. to have skilled sensitive care to enable them to achieve the highest possible quality of life.
3. to have their social, emotional, religious, cultural, political and sexual needs accepted and respected.
4. to have their personal privacy respected.
5. to be consulted about daily living arrangements in the home, and to participate in discussions about any proposed changes to those arrangements.
6. to be fully involved in and fully informed about their individual assessment of need.
7. to make informed choices about their future personal care plans.
8. to undergo a regular review of their individual circumstances, at which they have the right to be present.
9. to be fully informed about the services provided by the home and the department.
10. to choose their own medical practitioner and dentist, and to consult them in private.
11. to be responsible for their own medication and to make decisions about their medical treatment, whenever possible.
12. to manage their own financial and personal affairs.
13. to have the same access to facilities and services in the community as any other citizen.
14. not to be moved without consultation.
15. to have access to a formal complaints procedure, and to be represented by a friend and adviser if they so wish.

The only restrictions are the legal ones necessary to provide the level of care that the resident needs, and to protect the health and safety of the resident. A similar set of rights is contained in the supplement to the NAHAT guidelines (1988). In the USA, basic rights similar to those above are an integral part of the legal framework which governs publicly funded institutional care.

STANDARDS: STRUCTURE AND PROCESS

The emphasis in this chapter has been on giving practical expression to a widespread wish to give more weight to output and outcome considerations in assessments of quality of service. The purpose is not to deny the importance of structural and process considerations but to put them into context. However, they are not unaffected by the argument regarding the overriding importance of patient preferences and rights. For example, there is a conflict, recognized in 'Home Life', between freedom of choice and taking every safeguard against injury: 'Responsible risk taking should be regarded as normal, and residents should not be discouraged from undertaking certain activities solely on the grounds that there is an element of risk. Excessive paternalism and concern with safety may lead to infringement of personal rights. Those who are competent to judge the risk to themselves should be free to make their own decisions so long as they do not threaten the safety of others' (Centre for Policy on Ageing, 1984, para 2.8). 'The Right to Take Risks' (Counsel and Care, 1993) is one of a series of helpful booklets which focus on quality of care and provides model policies to implement Home Life principles.

Sadly, many of the bad practices learned in the NHS have been transferred by nursing staff to the homes they operate in the independent sector. Indeed, there is a danger of these smaller establishments being left behind in terms of modern standards and quality aspects. Conversely, other nurses have left the NHS to provide high-quality individualized nursing care: adding life to years as well as years to life.

STRUCTURE, PROCESS, OUTPUT AND OUTCOME: A BALANCE

Quality was the 'buzz word' of the early 1990s: patient surveys, audit, performance management abounded. Great strides were being made to identify significant inputs, processes and output measures. However, the slimming-down of health authority staff has removed many quality officer posts.

Training and staff supervision are fundamental to achieving a balance and changing systems. It is perhaps self-evident that the quality of leadership and management, and their ability to recruit and retain well-motivated staff are key to a good service. Training of nurses and care staff has not been a priority within either the public or private sector, and the RCN is sounding warnings of shortages. Individual performance targets and review have been introduced into many hospitals, but are often viewed with suspicion as a management tool to put pressure on staff rather than an opportunity for personal development and training. Financial pressures too often mean that training, a key to quality, is the first casualty of cutbacks: are we going into retreat, or will the work to change attitudes be sustained?

MONITORING

The development of appropriate standards is only the first step in the process of improving the quality of care in institutions. The next step is producing the conditions which encourage and sustain their application. There are two elements in more effective monitoring: the tools to do the job, and the promotion and enforcement of high standards. The technology for effective monitoring is increasingly available in the surfeit of 'systems' (official, home-grown and commercial) used to evaluate services. Managerial responsibility for quality has also been given a higher profile since the advent of general management in the NHS: most district health authorities now have a director with a specific responsibility for quality of services and/or customer relations. Attempts to improve the effectiveness of monitoring should focus on the refinement of these and other developments, rather than radical innovations.

MONITORING: TOOLS OF THE TRADE

The test of the effectiveness of current systems for assessing quality is not confined to whether they give sufficient weight to outcome considerations. Also important are criteria for assessment which allow scores (more or less) and therefore more discrimination between shades of performance than absolutes (yes or no). Another consideration is the level of performance expected. It is not always clear whether the (implicit) standards are based on minimum requirements, informed by professional or planning norms, i.e. what could reasonably be expected given the performance of others, or what is required for an optimal service. This is an important issue for nursing homes where inspectors may sometimes require standards higher than those achieved in the elderly patient wards of NHS trust hospitals. There is no categorical answer about the level on which expectations should be based. What is required is more clarity about the level of assessment.

The most important issue is selectivity. If monitoring is to be more effective and meaningful, attention must be focused on key elements which also give a good indication of the general quality of the institutional care. Otherwise, there is always the danger of assessments becoming a compendium of information requiring a laborious form-filling process.

THE MONITORS

There is a need to quicken the pace of improvement in regulation methods. The problem is not the availability of people to review and check standards. In addition to managers, who have this responsibility, there are already a number of external agencies with an interest in quality of care. Professional associations are involved when approving training posts, and the Health Advisory Service has been around for more than two decades. Similarly, in the private sector, there are registration and inspection officers to monitor standards, and reviews of standards are also performed by representatives of nursing home associations on applications for membership.

As health authorities are merged, contract monitoring and inspection work may benefit or suffer. In some areas, the larger units are widening the skills and expertise available for professional monitoring and inspections, while others find the number of inspectors cut, with even fewer resources allocated to this important function. As the RCN report 'An Inspector Calls?' pointed out 'It is difficult to understand how in one authority, one full-time and two half-time inspectors can effectively monitor the standards of care in 167 private healthcare establishments over a large county area. If it is possible, then why does it take seven full-time officers to monitor 163 establishments in another similar rural county area? . . . Those authorities undertaking only the statutory minimum inspections do them all by appointment. It is difficult to see how they assure themselves that standards are adequate.' (RCN, 1994, p. 8).

There may be a case for expanding the remit of registration and inspection officers to cover NHS long-stay units for older people, as already practised in some health authorities, but this will add to the pressure for an independent organization to ensure even-handedness. More important is the preparation of these officers for their responsibilities. The job requires knowledge and a different range of skills to those developed within the NHS. Examples include familiarity with the law on registration, an appreciation of the financial viability of small businesses, and the ability to communicate across organizational boundaries. Better preparation, resourcing, supervision, and reviews of performance would do much to improve the effectiveness of registration and inspection officers. There is officially recognized training for officers responsible for the registration and inspection of nursing homes. The Central Council for Education and Training in Social Work (CCETSW) has published the competencies required by social services inspectors (Davis, 1992) but no national vocational qualification yet exists. These competencies are equally appropriate for nurse inspectors.

The introduction of lay assessors and open reporting of nursing home inspections was due in 1995 but has been delayed despite evidence from open reporting of inspection of residential care homes that it does bring pressure to improve standards.

The advice, support and training offered as part of the inspection service have contributed to improvements in quality in many establishments, and it is vital to note that many inspectors are working to raise standards through quality audit methods. For example, Worcester and District Health Authority developed a quality assurance system which has been widely adopted by local nursing homes, and Oxfordshire Health Authority's Nursing Home Monitoring Unit has adapted the Australian 'outcome standards' to produce seven clear objectives, with 34 specific outcome standards, as the basis of nursing home inspection (Commonwealth/State Working Party on Nursing Home Standards, 1987). The Australian objectives are very similar to those in the SSI's 'Homes Are For Living In':

- health care
- social independence
- freedom of choice
- homelike environment
- privacy and dignity
- variety of experience
- safety

ELIMINATING POOR PRACTICE AND ENFORCING HIGHER STANDARDS

Safety is the 'bottom line' in the legal protection of those cared for in private and voluntary organizations: the law allows for the immediate cancellation of registration of a proprietor who places patients at serious risk. Serious risk is usually self-evident, but it is only by concentrating on processes and outputs that less dramatic failures in care standards emerge. Although influence is the main method of trying to achieve higher standards of care, the law provides for a range of enforcement action; offenders who break the law or fail to provide adequate care may be prosecuted under criminal proceedings. Businesses may be restricted or closed using slow and costly civil law procedures.

Enforcement is becoming more common as inspectors become more confident in applying the law, but delays sometimes result in horrifying instances of neglect and cruelty towards older people being allowed to continue. NHS managers are understandably nervous about taking criminals to court or giving evidence at costly tribunal hearings. All too often, NHS lawyers fail to understand the full extent of the authority's powers to regulate and stamp out unsafe and uncaring practice. Local authorities undertake many regulatory activities, but even here there has been some reluctance to enforce the law against residential care home proprietors, particularly since the local authority may have a contract for service with a less than good home.

Achieving basic standards is enforceable through the magistrates court where failure to provide adequate inputs must be factually proved, for example insufficient staff or failure to observe specific fire safety measures or provide adequate facilities. Civil procedures focus on the process of care, the output standards of health care and the patient's or relative's views about their care. Greater emphasis on outputs and outcomes shifts the balance from the interests of the providers towards the welfare of the service users. Evidence must be factual, but regimes of fear or rigid and authoritarian approaches that deny individual rights are not tolerated by Registered Homes Tribunals and can be reasons to cancel registration.

Much is to be gained by closer collaboration between health and local authority inspectors. Perceptions of differences in approach to standard setting and monitoring between the two public services tend to construct an insuperable barrier. This divide seems to be endemic throughout the system: new national guidelines for good practice are presently being produced, and again nursing and residential care are being considered separately!

FINAL COMMENTS

Institutions will remain a significant element in services for older people. Community care, even if effectively implemented, will not eliminate the need for shelter for the very frail, and some of this shelter will be found in nursing-home-type provision in both public and private sectors.

The chapter started from the premise that standards need to improve. In so doing, it assumed that there is no magic solution. The problem is how to generalize what the good are already doing and turn good intentions into practice.

Perhaps one of the obstacles to quicker progress is a pre-occupation with quality of service, rather than quality of life. This chapter has shown that many people are satisfied with ensuring that there are sufficient inputs and the process of care is up to standard. A counterbalance is needed with more inspection, reinforced by effective review, centred on human values and patients' rights. Both provide a reminder that quality of life, from the vantage point of the individual, is the crucial factor in quality of care.

Tools are available to facilitate the necessary changes. The problem of unacceptable standards for older people in institutions is therefore not one of poor systems and information. It is a problem amenable to the sustained application of what is already known, including the use of legal sanctions.

It would be wrong to leave the impression that little progress has been made or that no quality care is provided in institutions within the NHS or independent sector. Very high-quality individual nursing care is achieved in many places, allowing patients to live out their lives in hospital or nursing homes with dignity, rather than being sent to an institution to die. It is heartening to note that in the market economy for care it is not always the most expensive private homes that achieve the best quality: kindness and skilled individual attention have no price.

REFERENCES

Birkett, R. of Bevan Ashford Solicitors (1996) *Registered Homes Tribunals: Index to Decisions, including a Digest of High Court Judgements*, Anne Davis Associates, Birmingham.

Centre for Policy on Ageing (1984) *Home Life. A Code of Practice for Residential Care. Report of a Working Party*, Centre for Policy on Ageing, London. (Updated 1996 as 'A Bettter Home Life.')

Commonwealth/State Working Party on Nursing Home Standards (1987) *Living in a Nursing Home: Outcome Standards for Australian Nursing Homes*, Australian Government Publishing Service, Canberra.

Counsel and Care (1993) *The Right to Take Risks*, Counsel and Care, London.

Counsel and Care (1994) *Under Inspection*, Counsel and Care, London.

Davis, A. (1992) *Central Council for Education and Training in Social Work Paper 24.1: Exploring Competence in Registration, Inspection and Quality Control*, CCETSW, London.

Day, P. and Klein, R. (1987) Quality of institutional care and the elderly: policy issues and options. *BMJ*, **294**, 384.

Department of Health and Social Security (1990) *Community Care in the Next Decade and Beyond: Policy Guidance*, HMSO, London.

Department of Health and Social Security (1991) *Inspecting for Quality: Guidance on Practice for Inspection Units in Social Services Departments and Other Agencies; Principles, Issues and Recommendations*, HMSO, London.

Department of Health Social Services Inspectorate (1989) *Homes are for Living In*, HMSO, London.

Department of Health Social Services Inspectorate (1990) *Guidance on Standards for the Residential Care Needs of Elderly People*, HMSO, London.

Department of Health Social Services Inspectorate (1990) *Guidance on Standards for the Residential Care Needs of People with a Physical Disability*, HMSO, London.

Department of Health Social Services Inspectorate (1992) *Guidance on Standards for the Residential Care Needs of People with Specific Mental Health Needs*, HMSO, London.

Donabedian, A. (1980) *The Definition of Quality and Approaches to its Assessment*, Health Administration Press, Ann Arbor, Michigan, USA.

Laing, W. (1994) *Review of Private Health Care*, Laing and Buisson Publications, London.

National Association of Health Authorities and Trusts (1985) *Registration and Inspection of Nursing Homes*, NAHAT, Birmingham.

National Association of Health Authorities and Trusts (1988) *Registration and Inspection of Nursing Homes: Supplement*, NAHAT, Birmingham.

Royal College of Nursing, in collaboration with the British Geriatric Society and Royal College of Psychiatrists (1987) *Improving the Care of Elderly People in Hospital*, Royal College of Nursing, London.

Royal College of Nursing (1992) *A Scandal Waiting to Happen*, Royal College of Nursing, London.

Royal College of Nursing (1994) *An Inspector Calls?*, Royal College of Nursing, London.

United Kingdom Central Council for Nursing, Midwifery and Health Visiting (1994) *Professional Conduct – Occasional Report on Standards of Nursing in Nursing Homes*, United Kingdom Central Council for Nursing, Midwifery and Health, London.

Audit and quality management systems for long-term care

3

INTRODUCTION

This chapter deals with specific schemes now available for audit, quality assurance and quality management in long-term care of elderly people. Many of the schemes derive from three major consensus reports: *Home Life* (Centre for Policy on Ageing, 1984), *Residential Care – A Positive Choice* (Wagner, 1988) and *High Quality Long-Term Care for Elderly People* (RCP/ BGS, 1992a). The first two are specifically relevant to residential homes and the third refers to long-term care in hospitals and in nursing homes, but, with increasing overlap of all these areas, the guidelines they contain are generally relevant across the sectors. The schemes vary considerably in cost, time required for their implementation, the extent to which they are audits or management schemes, and whether or not they lead to accreditation. Individual homes and hospitals must decide on their requirements and select accordingly.

DEFINITIONS

There is a confusing array of quality activities. We offer the idea of the 'quality toolbox' to clarify the role and relationships of different approaches and resources (Dickinson, 1997). The quality toolbox contains four tools:

- quality standards
- quality schemes
- quality support systems
- quality measures

QUALITY STANDARDS

These are the standards of care that are sought. Some standards may be external, being derived from national reports, clinical guidelines and other similar documents. Other standards may be internal, reflecting more detailed goals for care.

QUALITY SCHEMES

These are the approaches used to achieve the required quality standards. There is a wide range of examples, such as clinical audit, quality circles, total quality management etc. In addition, initiatives such as the government's 'Investors in People' may have a contribution to quality.

QUALITY SUPPORT SYSTEMS

These tools are concerned with the organizational and administrative underpinning of quality schemes. To operate any scheme effectively, staff require resources, records and other information. There also need to be clear links between quality schemes and the wider management of the service. This requires a commitment by management to support the quality scheme appropriately and act on results.

QUALITY MEASURES

These tools are for measuring outcome and case mix. Despite the difficulties of measuring health and quality of life, there is a need to consider the case mix of residents, i.e. how they vary in important respects, when attempting to make comparisons over time or with others, as this has implications for the quality of care. The issue of case mix is discussed in greater detail in a following section.

USING THE QUALITY TOOLS TOGETHER

All four quality tools should be used together to undertake a credible quality activity. Without quality standards, it would be hard to focus activities and move forward. Without a recognized and organized scheme, staff will find it hard to participate effectively. Without quality support systems, progress is not likely to be made, as staff will waste time on inappropriate activities. Without quality measures, comparisons will be difficult to make.

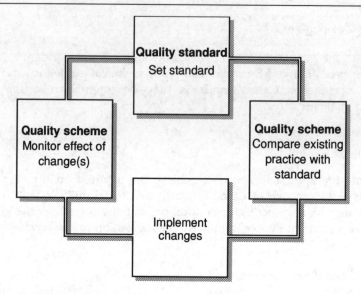

Figure 3.1 The quality cycle.

AN UNDERLYING THEME

Implicit in all quality activities is that efforts are being directed to improving the quality of care. The common theme in all quality activities, whether they be in industry, health care or long-term care, is a cycle of events. In this way people can examine the quality of their work, set objectives for improvement, and re-examine the situation to see whether objectives have been met. Thus, quality activities should not be a 'one-off' event, but should form part of a continuous cycle (Figure 3.1).

THE IMPORTANCE OF CASE MIX

An element of considering the quality of care is making comparisons, but this can be meaningless if differences in residents are not taken into account. There is a greater challenge in providing high-quality care if residents are frailer, more disabled or suffer from dementia. It would be wrong to compare quality of care between a facility with relatively well residents and a facility with very frail residents – a variation known as case mix. In long-term care, the most important indicators of case mix are probably disability and the presence of dementia. The Royal College of Physicians and the British Geriatrics Society have recommended standard scales for the assessment of these two aspects of elderly people's health and these may have some applicability in long-term care (RCP/BGS, 1992b). The abbreviated mental test (Hodkinson, 1972) is a brief way of screening for confusion. The Barthel index (Mahoney and Barthel, 1965) is a simple way of assessing basic activities of daily living, such as walking, transferring, dressing, using the toilet etc. With extremely disabled people, the Barthel index may fail to detect important differences in function and the Clifton procedure for the elderly (Pattie and Gillard, 1976) may be useful.

ACCREDITATION

Important both to the prospective resident and the nursing home itself is recognition that the care it provides meets an authorized standard, or is accredited. Accreditation is especially important in view of the wide choice of homes which is often available, the difficulties a prospective resident or relative will often have in judging the quality of care from one or two short visits, and the absence of any recognized rating system (such as exist for hotels, restaurants and other services). While social service and national health service inspectors regulate the registration of homes, their criteria of satisfactory service vary geographically and do not indicate homes with higher standards than others.

There is one international standard relating to care homes which is recognized by the International Organisation of Standardisation, the European Committee for Standardisation and the British Standards Institution. This is known as ISO9002 (1987) and is accepted also as EN29002 (European) and BS5750 (British) (British Standards Institution, 1987). However, this is a standard for quality support systems, and does not accredit the quality of care. Accreditation to ISO9002 (BS5750) can be sought via agencies approved by the Department of Trade and Industry for this purpose. Other independent agencies, not necessarily with government recognition, which offer accreditation for specific programmes include The IQA Consortium which offers the Inside Quality Assurance accreditation scheme and The British Federation of Care Home Providers which accredits to standards laid down by the association itself. In addition, the King's Fund Organisational Audit is now being piloted in nursing homes (T, Brooks, personal communication).

AVAILABLE QUALITY SCHEMES

Many systems have been produced, some evaluated and a few accredited. The Social Service Inspectorate Scheme (SSI) 'Homes Are For Living In' (SSI, 1989) is specifically intended for registration officers but provides a well-structured system which care staff could benefit from using. Inside Quality Assurance (IQA Consortium, 1992) appears to be unique in deriving its findings from in-depth interviews with the residents. The CARE Scheme (RCP, 1992), and Standards for Care and Practice Audits

(SCAPA) (Worcester District Health Authority, 1989) are primarily clinical audit schemes. Other schemes combine audit with elements of management procedures and staff training, e.g. Quest for Quality (David Pinder plc, 1993), Nursing Home Monitor II (Morton *et al.*, 1991), Evaluating the Quality of Care (National Institute for Social Work, 1994). Arcadia Quality Management (Arcadia Health Care plc, 1994) provides a complete audit and management structure. This list is not exhaustive but these schemes are discussed below and provide a broad cross-section of the genre.

HOMES ARE FOR LIVING IN

This is a system for evaluation of the quality of care and of life experienced in residential homes for elderly people. It was produced by a project team for the SSI in association with a number of social service departments (SSI, 1989). It was intended for the use of inspectors of residential homes (local authority part III homes and independent homes). However, it provides a detailed system which may be used in all forms of long-term care.

The system is built around six basic values, namely privacy, dignity, independence, choice, rights, fulfilment. For each there is an extensive questionnaire with space for written information submitted by the provider, discussion with the staff, residents and relatives, and observations made by the inspector during inspection. For instance, the section on dignity comprises 98 questions covering the physical environment, care practice, staff, staff training and development, procedures, records and documents and meals. The questions are also based on 19 principles as to what should be provided, ways in which residents should be involved and what they should be entitled to receive. Following the questionnaire is a series of suggested criteria for evaluation of the section and space for general evaluation and for conclusions. If this system was used widely by inspecting authorities, it would mark a triumph for registration.

INSIDE QUALITY ASSURANCE (IQA)

This system allows residents to say what they think about their everyday experience and provides a framework for recording and co-ordinating what is said. The package contains an instruction manual, posters to use at discussion meetings, questionnaires and prompt cards for interviews, model information sheets and model agendas (IQA Consortium, 1992). A quality group is established to oversee the whole exercise. This includes 'insiders' (residents and members of the staff including the head of the home), and 'outsiders' (for example a social worker, clergymen, Age Concern member, relatives etc.). The chairperson is an outsider and should be as independent as possible.

The scheme includes confidential interviews with as many as possible of the residents and staff. Interviews with residents are structured around the following seven topics:

- physical care
- choice
- expression of feelings
- the home as somewhere to live
- knowing how things run
- making links
- how the home feels to residents.

For each topic, two main questions are asked, namely 'can you describe (the topic)' and 'how much do you think it needs to be different?'. This avoids the direct and possibly threatening question 'what do you think about the home?' and is more likely to evoke honest criticism which may otherwise be withheld for fear of reprisal. Interviews are carried out by one or two outsiders and are a major commitment for them. Interviews may take up to one hour each (Challiner, 1993) and the interviewer carries the responsibility of reporting back the fears and anxieties in the home. Clearly stamina and tact are required. All this information is then presented to the quality group which formulates the changes that appear necessary. These conclusions are fed back to the residents and staff for their further views and agreement. A plan of action is drawn up by the quality group and implemented by the staff.

The experience of carrying out an IQA programme has been well described by Challiner (1993). She emphasizes staff anxieties about the process and how these were overcome. The whole procedure in a 20-place private residential home took six months to complete. It is clearly a major commitment, providing an almost unique opportunity to determine residents' real experiences and desires about the home that they live in and allowing them to feel involved. An independent accreditation scheme for IQA is available from the IQA Consortium. After IQA has been carried out, a report is submitted by the home and verified by an independent visit. Accreditation may then be awarded for two years.

THE CARE SCHEME

The CARE scheme (RCP, 1992) is a system of clinical audit: the acronym stands for continuous assessment, review and evaluation. The purpose is to improve the quality of life of residents by improving the quality of care. The scheme was produced by the Research Unit of the Royal College of Physicians and is based on their guidelines for long-term care (RCP/ BGS, 1992a). It comprises an A4 booklet containing instruction sheets and clinical audit forms. Once purchased, for a nominal sum, the contents can be copied as required. The instruction sheets give a suggested approach, describe the steps to take and stress the importance of management commitment. There are audit forms for both the facility and individual resident care for each of the nine topics covered by the scheme, along with resident summary forms to summarize the findings of the individual resident audits. The scheme covers nine topics with guidelines for each:

- preserving autonomy
- promoting urinary continence
- promoting faecal continence
- optimizing drug use
- managing falls and accidents
- preventing pressure sores
- equipment and environment
- aids and adaptions
- the medical role in long-term care.

The scheme focuses on empowering staff with the means to examine the quality of their work and establish a system by which to work together in setting and achieving objectives. The scheme elucidates a clear vision and emphasizes the importance of teamwork. Moreover, staff are encouraged to take responsibility for organizing how they use the scheme. A rolling programme of audits is suggested but the exact details are decided locally. Finally, staff are encouraged to set achievable objectives so they can see the fruits of their efforts in trying to improve the quality of care. There is evidence that use of the CARE scheme can lead to tangible improvements in the quality of care. In a recent multi-centre study (Brocklehurst and Dickinson, 1997), the CARE scheme was evaluated in a range of facilities. Every topic was audited over a four-month period and repeat audits were carried out three months later. On average, an audit for 20 residents took about 1½ hours: a mean of approximately 4 min per resident. In most cases (62%), records were made of the audit meeting. The CARE scheme appears to be an acceptable, feasible and effective way of improving the quality of care and is now being revised to take account of experience in its use.

STANDARDS OF CARE AND PRACTICE AUDIT

This audit was devised by inspecting officers of Worcester and District Health Authority (1989) and is intended for nursing homes. It provides individual quantified statements in five settings: general administration, physical needs, psychological needs, social needs and clinical status. Each section then provides a series of statements (e.g. 'staff aim to respond immediately to requests for toilet facilities'). Having read out the statement, the auditor then listens to open discussion among the staff, encouraging them to reach their own conclusions. Each statement should then be finally scored by the auditor once mutual agreement has been reached and the auditor is satisfied that the conclusions of the staff are correct. The scores are entered in a series of boxes with the following headings: correct; requires further attention; no; does not apply. The first two of these carry a percentage score which has been predetermined by the authors of the scheme. On the basis of the total percentage, each subsection is judged as being below satisfactory standards, that standards could be improved or that standards are high. Spaces are provided for the auditor to indicate what should be done, the action agreed and a review date. This system thus provides a numerical assessment of quality, and encourages widespread discussion by staff members leading to guidelines and action for further improvements.

QUEST FOR QUALITY

This system is derived from one developed in the USA by the American Health Care Association in 1983 and used in over 4000 long-term facilities in the USA in the ten years since its inception. The system marketed by David Pinder plc comprises questionnaires for the collection of data on performance indicators in 15 different settings (e.g. activities, administration, dietary services, health and safety, physician services etc) (David Pinder plc, 1993). Each of the questions requires a numerical answer (e.g. the number of complaints about diets from relatives and family). Data are collected monthly, and a mean score and standard deviation are calculated for each performance indicator from the data for the first three months. These serve as a base for comparison with subsequent months' scores. After a further three months, the base is altered on the cumulative scores for that three-month period.

Questionnaires are also provided for review of each service (e.g. 'is there a sufficient number of staff members to manage food service for residents?'; 'are staff recognized for doing a good job?'). Reasons most likely to contribute to identified problems are agreed using these review questionnaires and goals are set in relation to the problems. These include the time for achieving a solution, goals for the person responsible and the date for re-evaluation.

The programme is supervised by a quality assurance committee of at least six members of staff and residents including at least one outsider. This committee allocates tasks, reviews the findings and recommendations, and offers support. In larger homes, a series of quality action teams is also set up. These collect information, monitor the quality indicators, identify good and bad practice and report recommendations to the quality assurance committee. A quality assurance co-ordinator acts as a facilitator for both the quality assurance committee and quality assurance teams to promote good communication, provide advice and support, and act as an executive officer in setting up and carrying out the programme. A manual, training, a helpline, and an accreditation scheme are available.

NURSING HOME MONITOR II

This quality audit (Morton *et al.*, 1991) is based on Senior Monitor (Goldstone and Maselino-Okai, 1986), which was devised and tested in nursing homes in Harrogate. It provides numerical scores that can be used to identify problems. The audit is based on questions which are put to patients (either all those in a home or a random sample), to staff or checked from the records. Examples are 'do you feel that any particular person here on the staff cares for you?' (to patient) and 'are unusual bowel and bladder problems noted?' (to nurse and from records). There are 161 questions under three general subjects: home management, patient welfare and nursing care. Each question is supplemented by a brief clarification note for the nurse or resident. Answers may be 'yes' (scores 1), 'yes, partially' (scores ½), 'not applicable' or 'no'. For each question, a score is allocated for each patient and on completion the total score for each patient is calculated, the number of non-applicable questions subtracted and the score expressed as a percentage based on the number of applicable questions. By aggregating the percentage scores for each patient, an overall percentage figure is obtained for each of the three general subjects, home management, patient welfare and nursing care. The package includes instructions for a steering group, for auditors (two outsiders are recommended) and for a preliminary seminar for staff. Experience has shown that two auditors are able to audit a 50% sample of a 24-bed home in four days. The results are reviewed by the project co-ordinator and relevant staff, and should then lead to remedial action and appropriate strategies for staff training. The package also provides questionnaires for a profile of the home and for the calculation of patient dependency and workload index.

EVALUATING THE QUALITY OF CARE: A SELF-ASSESSMENT MANUAL

This system was created by a working group of inspectors and home managers in some North Tyneside homes (National Institute for Social Work, 1994) from feedback to inspection teams as they worked on a care staff project. The object was to produce a common basis of standards and indicators by which homes might be assessed using common measures and evidence. This should allow home managers to provide their own evidence that they have met the standards and so to allow the inspection process to 'become more focused and objective'. The system may therefore have several uses:

- as a management monitoring and evaluation instrument;
- for joint identification by those inspected and by the inspectors of areas for development and improvement;
- as an independent development tool;
- as a staff development and training tool.

There are four main sections: quality of environment, staff, care, and management and organization, involving a total of 200 quality indicators. Each question allows one of three answers which are provided; e.g. for appearance of the garden the answers provided are 'the garden is neglected' (score 0–1), 'casual or irregular attempts are made to keep the garden tidy and attractive' (score 2–3), or 'the garden is regularly maintained and always tidy and attractive' (score 4–5). For all four sections (maximum score 1000), the grading may be as follows:

- unacceptable: 0–200
- borderline: 201–400
- adequate: 401–600
- good quality: 601–800
- high quality: 801–1000

The home should carry out its own audit at least annually and prior to full inspection. Action plans can then follow. In each of the four sections, a pro forma is provided for noting changes and improvements indicated, and actions to be taken (the tasks, the people to be involved, how, when and where, and the dates for review).

ARCADIA QUALITY MANAGEMENT (AQM)

This programme combines audit with a detailed management system. Both audit and the management system cover separately all departments of a nursing home: nursing, catering, housekeeping, laundry, maintenance, administration, management, staff, finance. The system is presented in a series in nine looseleaf volumes allowing forms to be photocopied and individual pages updated (Arcadia Health Care plc, 1994).

The audit consists of three elements: standard statements, monthly quality assurance review and quarterly audit. The standard statements are formulated in terms of objective, structure, process and outcome. For example:

- objective: medicine is administered in accordance with an agreed policy;
- structure: a standard drug chart;
- process: a registered general nurse will sign the drug chart each time medicine is administered;
- outcome: to ensure that residents receive correct medication at an appropriate time and in correct dosage.

There are eight standards for nursing care, each of them having between one and five process statements, and similar numbers for all other departments. The monthly quality assurance review is carried out by the manager, head nurse and head of the department being audited. It includes questions to individual employees ('in a positive and non-threatening manner'), providing a series of yes/no answers and allowing discussion. There are 17 questions for nursing. The quarterly audit is carried out by the head of the home or a group operations manager, if the home is one of a group, together with senior staff of the home. It includes a numerical auditing system providing a total percentage score for each department. There are 13 questions for nursing (e.g. 'medication is administered in accordance with agreed policy – view ten medicine charts').

The management system provides philosophy statements on choice, rights, fulfilment, privacy and dignity, and models for all procedures carried out in a nursing home. These include admission, discharge, death, staff induction and training, confidentiality, general practitioners, health and safety, lifting and handling, fire, etc. Amongst other things, the personnel manual provides for interviewing, job descriptions, rules and disciplinary procedures, training, planning and organization for all staff. AQM states its objective as maintaining compliance with statutory requirements for registration and with professional codes of practice, meeting the expectations of residents, encouraging good relations between residents, relatives, staff and management, providing good communication throughout the home, and minimizing weaknesses and maximizing strengths in the whole organization. Accreditation can be obtained for certification to BS5750 through implementation of AQM.

CONCLUSION

In this chapter, we have examined practical approaches for improving the quality of long-term care. The concept of the quality toolbox was used to clarify the differing contributions and roles of quality standards, quality schemes, quality support systems and quality measures. This led to brief discussion of the importance of considering case mix when looking at comparisons and the quality of care. After a short look at the role of BS5750, we went on to look in detail at eight quality schemes:

- Homes Are For Living In: based on six basic values, with a questionnaire completed by the statutory inspector.
- Inside Quality Assurance: involving interviews with residents, a quality group and an action plan. An accreditation scheme available. This scheme is thought to be effective.
- The CARE Scheme: a clinical audit scheme with a focus on the health aspects of long-term care. It is cheap to purchase and effective in use.

- Standards of Care and Practice Audit (SCAPA): an audit scheme based on staff discussion which produces a numerical score.
- Quest for Quality: a questionnaire of 15 aspects of care all requiring objective answers. Supervision involves a quality assurance committee, quality co-ordinator and quality team. Numerical and statistical results are generated. A manual, training, a helpline and accreditation are available.
- Nursing Home Monitor II: an audit scheme covering home management, patient welfare and nursing care. It is a lengthy process carried out by outside auditors.
- Evaluating the Quality of Care: a mixed inspection and quality development tool with 200 quality indicators.
- Arcadia Quality Management: a combined audit scheme and quality management system covering nine aspects of nursing homes from finance to nursing. Monthly quality reviews and quarterly audits by senior staff cover all aspects of management. The system can be used for BS5750 accreditation.

The days when the quality of long-term care can be ignored are well and truly over. All long-term care facilities should implement a recognized quality scheme and ensure that this activity becomes an integral part of care.

REFERENCES

Arcadia Health Care plc (1994) *Aracdia Quality Management*, Arcadia Health Care plc, Reigate Heath, Surrey, UK.

British Standards Institution (1987) *British Standard Quality Systems: BS5750 Part II*, British Standards Institution, London.

Brocklehurst, J.C. and Dickinson, E.J. (1997) Improving the quality of long-term care of older people. Lessons from the CARE scheme. *Quality Health Care*, in press.

Centre for Policy on Ageing (1984) *Home Life. A Code of Practice for Residential Care*, Centre for Policy on Ageing, London. (Updated 1996 as 'A Better Home Life'.)

Challiner, Y. (1993) Experience of a quality assurance programme in a private rest home. *J. Br. Soc. Gerontol.*, **3**, 5–6, 14.

David Pinder plc (1993) *Quest for Quality*, David J Pinder plc, Milton Keynes, UK.

Department of Health Social Services Inspectorate (1989) *Homes Are For Living In*, HMSO, London.

Dickinson, E.J. (1997) The quality movement, in *Quality Care for Elderly People* (eds P.P. Mayer, E.J. Dickinson and S. Sandler), Chapman & Hall (in press).

Goldstone, L.A. and Maselino-Okai, C.V. (1986) *Senior Monitor. An Index of the Quality of Care for Senior Citizens on Hospital Wards*, Newcastle upon Tyne Polytechnic Products Ltd, Newcastle upon Tyne.

Hodkinson, H.M. (1972) Evaluation of a mental test score for assessment of mental impairment in the elderly. *Age Ageing*, **1**, 233–8.

IQA Consortium (1992) *Inside Quality Assurance*, IQA Consortium, Newport Pagnel, Buckinghamshire, UK.

Mahoney, F.L. and Barthel, D.W. (1965) Functional evaluation: the Barthel index. *Maryland State Med. J.*, **14**, 61–65.

Morton, J., Goldstone, L.A., Turner, A., Harrison, S. and Morgan, R. (1991) *Nursing Home Monitor* II, 2nd edn, Gale Centre Publications, Loughton, Essex, UK.

National Institute for Social Work (1994) *Evaluating the Quality of Care: a Self-Assessment Manual*, National Institute for Social Work, London.

Pattie, A.H. and Gillard, C.J. (1976) The Clifton Assessment Schedule: Further validation of a psychogeriatric assessment schedule. *Br. J. Psychiatr.*, **129**, 68–72.

Royal College of Physicians of London (1992) *The CARE Scheme: Clinical Audit of Long term Care of Elderly People*, Royal College of Physicians, London.

Royal College of Physicians and the British Geriatrics Society (1992a) *High Quality Long-term Care for Elderly People. Guidelines and audit measures*, Royal College of Physicians, London.

Royal College of Physicians and British Geriatrics Society (1992b) *Standardised Assessment Scales for Elderly People*, Royal College of Physicians, London.

Wagner, G. (1988) *Residential Care – a Positive Choice*, HMSO, London.

Worcester and District Health Authority (1989) *Standards of Care and Practice Audit (SCAPA). Nursing Homes*, 2nd edn, Worcester and District Health Authority, Worcester, UK.

Ethical dilemmas in continuing care

4

It might be thought that the medical and nursing management of older people in continuing care would present few ethical dilemmas. Those working with older residents know that this is not the case, and with an increasing range of caring options becoming more readily available, it seems that ethical issues are likely to become more prominent and the subject of much debate. This chapter discusses some of the dilemmas facing residents, relatives and carers.

TREATMENT VERSUS NON-TREATMENT

Clinicians working in long-term care often have to make decisions relating to treatment or non-treatment of frail patients. It is paramount that the potential benefits of any treatment are carefully weighed against possible adverse outcomes. Such decisions cannot be properly considered unless there is adequate information to make such a decision.

Until recently there has been little guidance on decision-making in this field and many doctors are confused about what is legally and morally required of them. There is no justification in using ethical arguments to ration health care covertly on cost grounds. Likewise, the cost of treatment should not be a factor in judging its appropriateness. If cost is implicated in treatment unavailability, for example being unable to supply state-of-the art pressure-relieving beds for patients who would theoretically benefit, then this should be acknowledged openly and not rationalized from a clinical standpoint. Likewise, age alone should not be used to deny treatment: the key feature should be physiological and not chronological age. Consultants should also be aware that decision-making should encompass an obligation not only to the patient but to his family, carers and society at large (Lantos, 1994), although rationing on the grounds of benefit to society cannot usually be made at the single-physician level.

Ethical problems relating to treatment or non-treatment seldom occur when it is clear that the required or proposed treatment will benefit the patient. However, problems can arise when there is a conflict between the wishes of the doctor and those of the family or other caring individuals. There is often no policy existing to help resolve these problems.

There is no need to discuss the possibility of non-treatment when the proposed treatment is not clinically justified and clearly will not benefit (Williams, 1993). Likewise, there is no difficulty when a competent patient, following a full explanation of the proposed treatment, refuses this treatment, as this refusal is legally valid. To be judged competent, patients must be able to understand a simple explanation of their condition, prognosis and proposed treatment or non-treatment. They must also be able to reason consistently about this information in the context of their personal beliefs. They must be able to act on the basis of this reasoning and communicate this choice and the reasons for it. Finally, they must be able to understand the consequences of the choice they have made. An acceptable level of ability in each of these areas must be present over a period of time for the patient to be judged competent (Doyal and Wilsher, 1993; Re T, 1993). For most patients, it must be presumed that competence exists until proven otherwise, and the reasons for deciding otherwise should be stated in the medical notes. The British Medical Association report 'Assessment of Mental Capacity' is a useful guide to physicians practising in this field and in general medicine (British Medical Association, 1995a).

In the case of a patient judged incompetent, and many elderly people residing in long-term care fall into this category, it is the doctor's duty to make the decision regarding treatment in the best interests of the patient. There is no legal right in England or Wales for a relative to make such a decision on a patient's behalf, although in Scotland there is still legal provision for the appointment of such an attorney. However, good practice dictates that the views of those closest to the patient, including members of the multidisciplinary team caring for the patient, are taken into account when making decisions of this nature. The burden of decision-making should not be placed on the relatives as this often leads to feelings of guilt and may place them under undue duress.

Doyal and Wilsher (1994) have attempted to delineate states in which it would be justifiable not to treat incompetent patients. Scenarios such as those outlined are subject to widely differing interpretations by many physicians but do attempt to encompass the conditions with which practising clinicians are familiar.

The House of Lords Committee on Medical Ethics (1994) has supported the proposal of the Law Commission for the establishment of local judicial forums to consider such issues in the future. It is intended that these would have the power to authorize commencement, withholding or withdrawal of treatment in the best interests of an incompetent patient. The importance of medical and ethical advice to such forums has been noted.

DECISIONS BASED ON QUALITY OF LIFE

Even healthcare professionals acting in their patient's best interests cannot help but make judgements based on 'quality of life', especially when considering whether or not to treat a certain condition. Quality of life is an all-encapsulating term which attempts to describe a uniquely personal perception reflecting feelings about one's personal, physical and spiritual well-being; it is therefore inherently difficult to assess.

Most members of the caring professions are not trained in assessing quality of life, and its uniquely personal attributes compound the difficulties in making such an assessment. Scales using material possessions or social standing are largely irrelevant to those in long-term care. Likewise, attempts to measure quality of life by patient satisfaction with life or state of health are often inappropriate. Well-validated scales of functional ability (e.g. the Barthel index of activities of daily living, see Mahoney and Barthel, 1965) may be used, but once again these do not reflect the global nature of the concept. Thus many attempts at objective measurement have been developed and most fail to address the true nature of that which they seek to measure (for a review, see Gill and Feinstein, 1994). As with any such score, the veracity of using a population-based method for any individual is somewhat suspect. A subjective holistic assessment of morale and motivation may be the best approximation of quality of life status that can be achieved for nursing home patients.

The situation becomes more difficult when patients are severely demented, are unable to care for themselves in any way, and are immobile and incontinent – the so-called pre-death state (Isaacs *et al.*, 1971). Clinicians should once again seek the advice of relatives and those staff caring for the patient in an attempt to gather information to enable them to make a decision based truly on the best interests of the patient.

Decisions surrounding treatment and non-treatment issues may bring medical and para-medical staff into conflict. It is often easier for the physician to take a detached viewpoint, whereas those directly involved in day-to-day patient care are often unable to do this. However, geriatricians must be sensitive to the opinions and feelings of other members of the team when considering such issues surrounding patient care. Time must be taken to discuss areas of contention and come to a mutually agreed solution or plan of action wherever possible. A sound ethical basis of decision-making should be central to all such discussions.

NUTRITION AND HYDRATION

There is no legal distinction between withholding and withdrawing treatment, and both are equally lawful in the appropriate setting. Often clinicians are concerned about starting a treatment (e.g. nasogastric feeding in severe stroke) because of the consequences of having to withdraw it at a later stage. This concern was upheld by the House of Lords Committee on Medical Ethics (1994). However, this is often a very emotive decision; nutritional problems in those nearing the end of their lives often cause severe stresses in the patient–carer relationship and there tends to be a reluctance amongst many caring staff to cease attempts at feeding (Norberg et al., 1980).

Studies such as those by Cassem (1980) and Watts and Cassell (1984) support the view that withdrawal of feeding and hydration may be justified in certain cases. It is important to draw a distinction between those chronically sick, often demented patients who come to refuse food and fluids as part of the natural history of their illness and those who are unable to feed either because of an acute illness or because of sudden neurological damage. Those patients who refuse food and fluids whilst acutely unwell will clearly benefit from artificial hydration or nutrition and this should be provided in such cases.

Where patients are unconscious following a severe stroke or other neurological insult, it has been argued that artificial feeding is a medical treatment much as any other. This view and the lawfulness of withdrawal was supported in the courts (Airedale NHS Trust v. Bland [1993]). However, the likely benefit to the patient from this should be calculated. The Lords Committee on Medical Ethics was unable to come to a definite decision on this matter and felt that 'the progressive development and ultimate acceptance of the notion that some treatment is inappropriate should make it unnecessary to consider the withdrawal of nutrition and hydration, except in circumstances where its administration is in itself evidently burdensome to the patient'. Clearly, the administration of food and fluids to an unconscious patient is not burdensome as the patient is unaware. However, since the 1993 judgment, the same declaratory juris-diction has been invoked in several other cases involving persistent vegetative state (Frenchay NHS Trust v. S [1994]; Swindon and Marlborough NHS Trust v. S [1994]).

For those demented patients who deteriorate in their ability to feed themselves and eventually have to be fed by syringe, sometimes refusing even this method of nutrition, the case is somewhat different. In this situation, it can be argued that force feeding or the administration of artifi-cial methods of nutrition or hydration are burdensome to the patient, i.e. the siting and re-siting of an intravenous cannula or insertion of a nasogastric tube, and are of no medical or other benefit to the patient. There would in this case be an argument for stopping feeding on grounds that the proposed intervention did more harm than good. However, withdrawal of hydration and feeding often produces strong emotional reactions in staff whose prime aim is to treat the patient. Often to do nothing is viewed as neglectful, the provision of fluid and nutrition being essential symbols of care and compassion. There is potential for conflict between those responsible for the day-to-day care of the patient and the person clinically responsible for that patient. On the other side of the coin, it has been argued that provision of artificial feeding actually distances the carer from the patient, with most attention then being given to the mechanism of feeding rather than personal needs (Fox, 1987).

CARDIOPULMONARY RESUSCITATION

The role of cardiopulmonary resuscitation (CPR) in the long-stay setting is very limited because patients in NHS continuing care are the most dependent group of older people (Pattie and Heaton, 1990). Most, if not all, would not be candidates for CPR in the event of a cardiac arrest and the patients are so frail that such an intervention would be futile for any individual and therefore not clinically or morally justifiable. Furthermore, the geographical and staffing situation of NHS long-stay institutions are not conducive to effective provision of such a facility. It may be decided therefore that the difficulties in initiating and performing CPR in such an environment make formal provision impractical. However, there are good arguments that patients, if suitable for CPR, should be able to expect similar treatment to any person suffering a cardiac arrest in the street.

Traditionally it has been felt unnecessary to discuss the decision not to resuscitate with either other members of the healthcare team or with the patient or relatives. It was also felt that there was no need for written, formal policies as patients in the UK trusted their doctors to make decisions in their best interest (Bayliss, 1982). There has been much published literature suggesting that all patients should have their resuscitation status discussed with them and that they should be able to choose whether or not to be resuscitated (Liddle *et al.*, 1994). It has also been shown that patients, when correctly informed of the rates of survival following a CPR attempt, are often more likely to decline CPR (Murphy *et al.*, 1994). It must be remembered that CPR is a treatment like any other and therefore discussion is clearly not warranted if it is clinically inappropriate to offer it. Decisions relating to individual incompetent patients should be made using the same ethical guidelines as for other treatment and non-treatment decisions.

ADVANCE CARE DIRECTIVES

An advance care directive (ACD), sometimes known as 'living will', is a mechanism whereby competent people can make decisions about their healthcare should they become incompetent due to life-threatening illness. ACDs have been promoted in the UK by such organizations as the Terrence Higgins Trust and the Voluntary Euthanasia Society, mainly as a vehicle to refuse life-prolonging measures for a patient who has become incompetent. In 1995, the BMA issued a policy statement stating that ACDs are probably legally binding under case law and issuing guidelines for their use (BMA, 1995b). They have also suggested that persons with ACDs review their decisions with their physician at regular intervals and perhaps carry a card indicating the existence of such a document. The operation of such directives can potentially place the doctor in some difficulty.

Presently, following a ruling from the High Court (Re C, 1993), ACDs are subject to the following provisions: that the patient was competent when the ACD was made, that the person anticipated the circumstances and intended the ACD to apply when they arose, and finally that there were no undue influences acting upon the person when the ACD was drawn up. ACDs specifying treatment demands are not legally binding and are unlikely ever to become so. Likewise, those which appoint a third party to make healthcare decisions on the patient's behalf are not legally binding in England and Wales although the status of such healthcare proxies is recognized in some states of the USA and provision for the appointment of an attorney of the person still exists under Scottish law. In the USA, some states have legally stated hierarchies of healthcare surrogates from within a patient's family (Menikoff et al., 1992). Further legislation in this area is likely following the Law Commission report 'Mental Incapacity' (1995) endorsing the principle of ACDs.

However, the medical profession has treated the subject of ACDs with some caution and is not keen to see legislation on the subject. The profession also confirms the rights of doctors to override these documents on clinical grounds or if their personal beliefs do not agree with the terms of the ACD (although they should communicate this to the patient prior to likely enactment of the ACD).

Despite initial concern that signing such a document would be an acceptance of impending death, it has been shown that execution of ACDs by patients with terminal illnesses was not associated with any significant positive or negative effect on well-being or self-reported health status (Schneiderman et al., 1992). The use of such documents also has the beneficial effect of encouraging frank discussion between doctor and patient regarding their disease and prognosis and treatment. Other recognized advantages are that nurses and other carers arguing for limitation of treatment, which seems unnecessary, have some ethical back-up to their argument, and people in possession of these documents feel they have more autonomy in healthcare decision-making and may relieve their next of kin from the burden of decision-making on their behalf. However, some see the widespread adoption of ACDs as tacit acceptance of euthanasia, or foresee services for frail older people deteriorating as a response to the use of directives. There has also been much discussion about the changing of personal values with the onset of progressive illness, e.g. dementia, the point at which the patient intended an ACD to be acted upon, and the continued validity of an ACD.

In conclusion, the increasing adoption of ACDs can only serve to stimulate open and frank discussion between doctors and patients about their condition. Their use contributes to patient autonomy and reduces the paternalism of the medical profession, however benevolently this is portrayed. Those people entering long-term care who are mentally competent should be given the opportunity to discuss their healthcare wishes and to make an ACD if they feel this is appropriate.

EUTHANASIA

This subject is a very emotive topic with debate hotly contested from both extremes of opinion. The term euthanasia was originally used to describe a good death, but has since been adopted as a term for mercy killing. Euthanasia in this sense has also been split into passive death, i.e. death caused by omission of a potentially beneficial treatment, and active death, i.e. that caused by a definitive treatment act. Atkinson (1983) argues that morally there is no difference between these types of killing. Hastening death by withdrawing a treatment without medical benefit is not euthanasia. Similarly, the administration of a drug with the primary aim of achieving relief of symptoms, which may, as a by-product, hasten death ('double-effect'), cannot be included in this definition.

Doctors faced with looking after extremely dependent patients are faced with the task of deciding whether to carry on with life-sustaining treatments. When it is decided that it is no longer ethical to continue with such treatments, at what stage does it become morally or ethically justifiable to hasten death by the administration of drugs? The Institute of Medical Ethics has presented a justification for active euthanasia or assisted death (1990). The working party felt that such action was justified if the necessity for the relief of pain or other distressing symptoms caused by a terminal illness outweighed the benefit of any further life-prolonging treatment. There were some caveats to this justification: firstly, the proximity to death was felt to be very important, and secondly, it was felt imperative that all members of the healthcare team should be unable to propose any therapeutic method of achieving symptom relief prior to a decision being taken to assist in the death of the patient. In a 1994 survey, 60% of general practitioners and consultants had been asked by competent patients to hasten their deaths (Ward and Tate, 1994). Given the right of competent patients to decline treatment, most doctors in this survey complied with the wishes of their patients. Surprisingly, 32% of doctors in this survey reported that they had been involved in cases of active euthanasia.

The House of Lords Committee on Medical Ethics (1994) has not supported the arguments in favour of voluntary euthanasia, finding it impossible to set secure limits upon such practice. It was felt that to do so would lead inevitably to an erosion of the law in favour of mercy killing. In the Netherlands where active euthanasia, although technically illegal, is practised, there have been several reports of euthanasia being administered without the request of the patient, perhaps illustrating the concerns of the House of Lords Committee (Pijnenborg et al., 1993).

Many caring physicians, certainly in the UK, would consider that there is no role for euthanasia in the context of long-term care for older people. Adequate symptom control is usually possible using the therapeutic techniques of palliative care with which physicians with responsibilities for continuing care should be familiar; if not, they should be able to draw upon specialist advice when needed.

PHYSICIAN-ASSISTED SUICIDE

Fear of growing old and of dying in an age of technological medicine has led to an increasing interest in voluntary and physician-assisted suicide. Physician-assisted suicide (PAS) is different from voluntary euthanasia in that the physician only supplies the means for suicide and is not necessarily present at the death. Suicide is carried out at the patient's own volition and at a time which is convenient to them. To many commentators, this difference is marginal and the same arguments against euthanasia have been used against PAS, often lumping the two practices together as physician-assisted death (Miller et al., 1994).

Many geriatricians have been involved in the debate on physician-assisted suicide via their interest in palliative medicine. Much of the argument against the adoption of these practices comes from this quarter. There is, however, much evidence that palliative support to people dying in a non-hospice setting is poor for many reasons (Callahan, 1993). Singling out those who are dying as the only persons warranting palliative or symptom-relieving care is somewhat iniquitous, particularly in the environment of long-term care. Frail older people who require institutional care may be excluded from provision of formal palliative care, and, if it is available, this care may only be provided to such patients in a fragmented fashion.

Physicians involved in long-term care are likely to be faced with issues of PAS in the coming years as the attitudes of older people change. The era of benign paternalism in medical practice is passing and is being replaced by an environment of increasing patient autonomy surrounding medical decisions. There is evidence from the USA that American attitudes to PAS are shifting towards acceptance (Blendon et al., 1992). Seidlitz et al. (1995) found that elderly people with risk factors for suicide are more likely to express lenient attitudes towards planned or physician-assisted suicide. Also, the attitudes of practising physicians are changing in the USA and many other countries (Shapiro *et al.*, 1994; Ward and Tate, 1994).

The American Geriatrics Society has continued to prohibit both PAS and voluntary active euthanasia in its position statements on the subject (AGS, 1995). The House of Lords Select Committee on Medical Ethics supports continuing prohibition in the UK and sees no reason to distinguish the act of a member of the medical profession from that of any another person with respect to assisted suicide. However, the committee did recommend the creation of a new offence of 'mercy killing' under UK law, such that the mandatory life sentence associated with murder might be avoided in such cases.

At the time of writing, laws permitting the practice of euthanasia and PAS have been passed in Oregon, USA, and the Northern Territories, Australia. Contrary to widely held belief, the practice is still illegal in the Netherlands, but criminal charges are waived if the physician adheres to guidelines concerning correct practice.

Data from Dutch nursing homes suggest that few requests for PAS are made, and that only one in ten of such requests are met (Van der Wal *et al.*, 1994). The desire to exert some measure of control over one's death is not a selfish one, or indicative of serious psychiatric disturbance. Such a request should be explored further and the underlying motives taken into account. Such requests are likely to be rare in the long-term care setting. To make such a request, a patient must be competent and be able to communicate this; thus, many residents in long-term care in the NHS would be automatically excluded. The request must be free from undue influences. The disease from which the patient is suffering must be incurable and unbearable. Finally, all options for other care must have been exhausted or refused. For the incompetent patient, most intervention for palliation of terminal or severe suffering is done in the 'best interests' of the patient and the 'double-effect' principle would be relevant here.

In conclusion, there is little demand at present for PAS within the long-term care setting. Once again, expertise in and access to good palliative care is the overriding requirement to provide a quality service to frail older residents.

RESEARCH IN CONTINUING CARE

Much of the published literature on research in the nursing home comes from the USA, where much geriatric practice occurs within this setting. It is increasingly accepted that research on older patients is becoming ever more relevant to medical practice as much of the morbidity and mortality in the population as a whole is concentrated in late life. Those trials which include older people often include only the fittest members of the population, and this practice often limits extrapolation of the derived data to a general older group. Potential benefits from such research include the improvement of general knowledge about a particular condition, or improving treatment, management or diagnosis within a defined population.

There are, however, special problems associated with research in a group of institutionalized individuals. They are amongst the most vulnerable of their age group and may be subject to coercion, lack the necessary attention span, or lack the mental capacity to give consent to take part in such research. Such people may also consent to research studies as a 'quid pro quo' – 'you have helped me, therefore I will help you' or in order to meet people and pass the time of day. There is also little privacy in many nursing homes and decisions may thus be widely known amongst residents; this may serve to increase the pressure on others considering whether or not to participate.

Clearly, any proposed research must be approved by the appropriate research ethics committee for the institution. The research in question must be methodologically sound and be worth doing. There must be sufficient expertise to carry the study through to completion and the subject under investigation must clearly justify the use of the nursing home population. Such a population must either be necessary for or add something to the study, rather than being a convenient source of patients or subjects. It must also be remembered that the potential subjects are a wide and varied group, many with significant functional impairment. Such people should neither be exploited as subjects for research nor yet prevented from having equal access to participation. Excluding patients with hearing or sight problems when the trial protocol does not call for this leads to bias within the study. With this in mind, it is useful to produce items such as consent forms in large print or to use additional material which might be needed in a different format, perhaps on video or in the form of a case study. There is good evidence that the comprehension of older people, who are often cognitively impaired, can be improved by the method in which the information is presented (Tymchuk and Ouslander, 1990). In addition to adaptation of methods, obtaining consent from older people takes longer and often requires more resources. Many older people are reluctant to sign a consent form although happy to take part in a study (Hoffman, 1983). Some require further discussion with relatives prior to any decision being made. Therefore, in addition to dealing with the patient alone, the researcher may become a family counsellor.

As previously mentioned, in England and Wales there is no provision for a relative or carer to act as surrogate decision maker for an incompetent patient. At present, there is no option but to exclude such patients from studies in this setting. Studies into dementia present their own particular problems. All trials of treatment can only be conducted in those with mild disease who are able to give informed consent. The results of such studies clearly have limited value when extrapolated to the entire population of those with dementia. There is still a need for research into the standards and tests for capacity to give informed consent, particularly for those sufferers who might display fluctuating decision-making capacity.

As in any study setting, the premises of good clinical practice in research must be adhered to. However, a beneficial finding or the discovery of a potentially treatable abnormality in any particular patient raises questions about the confidentiality of research data. There are good arguments for the disclosure of such findings so that the individual might benefit, but such issues should be clear to the relevant ethical committee at the time of approval and should be considered prior to commencement of the study.

Given the problems outlined above, it is perhaps not surprising that the Royal College of Physicians (1990) has recommended that it might be appropriate to conduct research which uses indirect measures of data collection. Much of this is likely to be in the form of clinical audit rather than a randomized clinical trial of an intervention.

In summary then, the proposed study should be methodologically sound and aim to answer an important question. Long-stay residents should be selected because of the particular problems involved in their care or because of a particular diagnosis, not because they are a convenient population to study. Patients with sensory or mobility impairment should not be excluded automatically because of these. The process of consent and the forms themselves should be adapted to the target population where necessary, as should the presentation of relevant information.

CONCLUSION

The ethical dilemmas which present themselves in long-term care are likely to become more, rather than less, frequent in the coming years. Increasing patient expectation of treatment, along with advancing technological intervention, is likely to contribute to this. There will undoubtedly be legislation on surrogate decision makers for healthcare for incompetent patients and a reinforcement of acceptability of advance care directives within the next few years. The UK is unlikely to go down the road of Oregon or the Northern Territories in legislating for physician-assisted suicide or euthanasia. However, none of the above is likely to change the requirement for a holistic, palliative approach to good quality long-term care, whether this takes place within the NHS or the private sector.

REFERENCES

Airedale NHS Trust v. *Bland* [1993] AC 789.

American Geriatrics Society (1995) Position statement on physician assisted suicide and voluntary active euthanasia. *J. Am. Geriatr. Soc.*, **43**, 579–80.

Atkinson, G. (1983) Killing and letting die: hidden value assumptions. *Soc. Sci. Med.*, **17**, 1915–25.

Bayliss, R.I.S. (1982) Thou shalt not strive officiously. *BMJ*, **285**, 1373–5.

Blendon, R.J., Szalay, U.S. and Knox, P.A. (1992) Should physicians aid their patients in dying? The public perspective. *JAMA*, **267**, 2658–62.

British Medical Association (1995a) *Assessment of Mental Capacity. Guidance for Doctors and Lawyers*, British Medical Association, London.

British Medical Association (1995b) *Advance Statements About Medical Treatment*, BMJ Publishing, London.

Callahan, D. (1993) *The Troubled Dream of Life: Living with Mortality*. Simon and Schuster, New York.

Cassem, N. (1980) When illness is judged irreversible: imperative and elective treatments. *Man Med.*, **5**, 154.

Doyal, L. and Wilsher, D. (1993) Cardiopulmonary nonresuscitation: proposals for formal guidelines. *BMJ*, **306**, 1593–6.

Doyal L. and Wilsher, D. (1994) Withholding and withdrawing life sustaining treatment from elderly people: towards formal guidelines. *BMJ*, **308**, 1689–92.

Fox, R.A. (1987) Palliative care and aggressive therapy, in *Medical Ethics and Elderly People* (ed R.J. Elford), Churchill Livingstone, Edinburgh.

Frenchay NHS Trust v. *S* [1994] 1 WLR 601.

Gill, T.M. and Feinstein, A.R. (1994) A critical appraisal of the quality of quality of life measurements. *JAMA*, **272**, 619–26.

Hoffman, P., Marron, K.R., Fillit, H. and Libow, L.S. (1983) Obtaining informed consent in a teaching nursing home. *J. Am. Geriatr. Soc.*, **31**, 565–9.

House of Lords Select Committee on Medical Ethics (1994) *Report of the House of Lords Select Committee on Medical Ethics*, volume 1, HMSO, London.

Institute of Medical Ethics Working Party on the Ethics of Prolonging Life and Assisting Death (1990) Assisted death. *Lancet*, **336**, 610–13.

Isaacs, B., Gunn, J., McKeckan, A. *et al.* (1971) The concept of pre-death. *Lancet* **i**, 1115–19.

Lantos, J.D. (1994) Futility assessments and the doctor patient relationship. *J. Am. Geriatr. Soc.*, **42**, 868–70.

Law Commission (1995) *Mental Incapacity. Item 9 of the Fourth Programme of Law Reform: Mentally Incapacitated Adults*. Law Com No 231. HMSO, London.

Liddle, J., Gilleard, C. and Neil, A. (1994) The views of elderly patients and their relatives on cardiopulmonary resuscitation. *J. R. Coll. Physicians Lond.*, **28**, 228–9.

Mahoney, F.I. and Barthel, D.W. (1965) Functional evaluation: the Barthel index. *MD State Med. J.*, **14**, 61–5.

Menikoff, J.A., Sachs, G.A. and Seigler, M. (1992) Beyond advance directives – health care surrogate laws. *N. Engl. J. Med.*, **327**, 1165–9.

Miller, F.G., Quill, T.E., Brody, H. *et al.* (1994) Regulating physician assisted death. *N. Engl. J. Med.*, **331**, 119–23.

Murphy, D.J., Burrows, D., Sandilli, S. *et al.* (1994) The influence of the probability of survival on patients' preferences regarding cardiopulmonary resuscitation. *N. Engl. J. Med.*, **330**, 545–9.

Norberg, A., Norberg, B., Gippert, H. and Bexell, G. (1980) Ethical conflicts in long term care of the aged: nutritional problems and the patient–care worker relationship. *BMJ*, **280**, 377–8.

Pettie, A.H. and Heaton, J. (1990) *A Comparative Study of Dependency and Provision of Care for the Elderly in the State and Private Sectors in York Health District*, York Regional Health Authority, York.

Pijnenborg, L., van der Maas, P.J., van Delden, J.J.M. and Looman, C.W.N. (1993) Life-terminating acts without explicit request of patient. *Lancet*, **341**, 1196–9.

Re C 1993 News report *BMJ* 1993; **307**, 1023.

Re T (Adult : Refusal of treatment) 1993 Fam 95, 115.

Royal College of Physicians (1990) *Research Involving Patients*, Royal College of Physicians, London.

Schapiro, R.S., Derse, A.R., Gottlieb, M., Schneidermayer, D. and Olson, M. (1994) Willingness to perform euthanasia: a survey of physician attitudes. *Arch. Intern. Med.*, **154**, 575–84.

Schneiderman, L.J., Kronick, R., Kaplan, R.M. *et al.* (1992) Effects of offering ADs on medical treatments and costs. *Ann. Intern. Med.*, **117**, 599–606.

Seidlitz, L., Duberstein, P.R., Cox, C.C. and Conwell, Y. (1995) Attitudes of older people toward suicide and assisted suicide: an analysis of Gallup poll findings. *J. Am. Geriatr. Soc.*, **43**, 993–8.

Swindon and Marlborough NHS Trust v S, *The Guardian* 10 December 1994.

van der Wal, G., Muller, M.T., Christ, L.M., Ribbe, M.W. and van Eijk, J.Th.M. (1994) Voluntary active euthanasia and physician assisted suicide in Dutch nursing homes: requests and administration. *J. Am. Geriatr. Soc.*, **42**, 620–3.

Tymchuk, A.J. and Ouslander, J.G. (1990) Optimising the informed consent process with elderly people. *Educ. Gerontol.* **16**, 245–7.

Ward, B.J. and Tate, P.A. (1994) Attitudes among NHS doctors to requests for euthanasia. *BMJ*, **308**, 1332–4.

Watts, D.T. and Cassel, C.K. (1984) Extraordinary nutritional support: a case study and ethical analysis. *J. Am. Geriatr. Soc.*, **32**, 237–42.

Williams, F. (1993) Medical futility in context. *Br. J. Hosp. Med.*, **50**, 50–3.

Role of the purchasers in continuing care 5

BACKGROUND

Long-term care has been part of the health services provided in this country for many years, originating in the Poor Law infirmaries in the 18th and 19th centuries. In hospital terms, these were the poor relations when compared with the voluntary hospitals, where the bulk of the acute medicine and surgery and all the teaching took place. Considerable efforts were made to keep such long-term patients out of the voluntary hospitals in earlier centuries. Long-term care hospitals were developed in the late 1940s by the new specialty of geriatric medicine.

THE PURCHASERS OF LONG-TERM CARE

Efforts to improve the efficiency of the health and social services over the past 10 years have led to the emergence of the concept of an 'internal market' for both health and social services. The reason for this change was a belief that the health and social services, by having the total budget for the health or social services in their area and managing those services, would be unlikely to take criticism seriously. It was felt that any problems with the service would reflect on the budget holders themselves as much as on the people providing the service. The overseeing role, originally performed by the Department of Health, was transferred to the health authorities and social services departments. They are known as the purchasers or commissioners of health and social care. The departments and health authorities are also required to consider all providers of services, whether privately run or voluntary organizations.

In social services, the government even went so far as to stipulate that the great majority of services in some areas, especially community care, should not be provided directly by the departments. For health services, the private and voluntary alternatives are tiny in comparison to the large

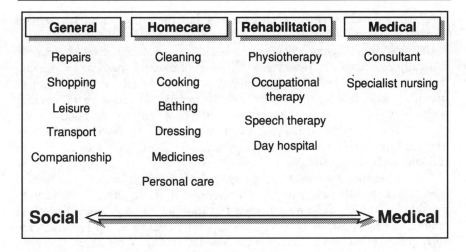

General	Homecare	Rehabilitation	Medical
Repairs	Cleaning	Physiotherapy	Consultant
Shopping	Cooking	Occupational therapy	Specialist nursing
Leisure	Bathing	Speech therapy	
Transport	Dressing	Day hospital	
Companionship	Medicines		
	Personal care		

Social ⟵⟶ Medical

Figure 5.1   Range of long-term care services.

NHS hospitals and community providers. Because of this, the only adjust-ment was to ensure that NHS trusts paid similar amounts for their capital developments as private organizations. They were then expected to be able to compete for price and quality.

Part of the problem of defining who should provide long-term care revolves around the wide range of services involved. Figure 5.1 outlines some of these. Over the past five years or so, social services departments have moved away from providing general services, leaving voluntary or private organizations to provide most of those labelled 'general'. There has also been a move for social services departments to take over personal tasks, such as bathing, overseeing medicines and cutting toenails. Previously, these were the province of nurses. Some social services depart-ments now offer some rehabilitation facilities in day centres.

DEFINITION OF THE NEED FOR HEALTH CARE

There is no satisfactory definition of health care that separates it from social care, although the difference is easily discernible in many fields. There are a number of grey areas, and long-term care for dependent people is one of these. It is certain that long-term health care for groups of older people may be very poor. Where performed properly, it requires considerable skill in the management of their skin, bladder and bowels, and assistance with mobility, cleanliness and feeding. The government has avoided defining what it means by a health need; it has left this to local planning groups and legal precedent. On 1 October 1992, the then Minister for State for Health, Dr Mawhinney, said 'it must be a matter of collaborative judgement in each case whether the health or social element of need is paramount'.

Defining the difference between a health and a social need is certainly difficult. For instance, relatives with no professional medical or nursing training and often with minimal assistance from health or other services provide most long-term care for elderly people. The degree of tending required is of an intensity that only a devoted relative or relatives can provide for an individual. For groups of such people, only the relatively high staffing levels found in health service facilities appear to be able to contend with such difficulties.

There therefore appears to be no agreed objective definition of a person who has a health need for long-term care. It is therefore necessary to provide a working definition. It seems to me that an older person needing long-term care must, of necessity, be dependent upon others for their care and quite severely so. Isaacs and Neville (1976), with their 'interval' approach, described the best way of defining dependency. A need for assistance at short notice at any time is defined as 'critical interval need'. Even this degree of dependency does not automatically suggest that an older person requires the assistance of long-term health services. Such individuals are quite common in the community. Figure 5.2 shows the prevalence of such older people by age and sex in a study of over 650 people aged 70 and over in a small market town in South Wales (Vetter *et al.*, 1986). Forty per cent of women over the age of 85 fall into this

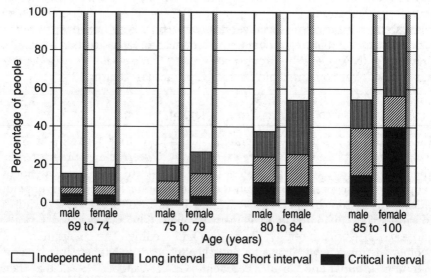

Figure 5.2 Interval dependency by age and sex.

category. It is obvious that the need for long-term health care needs to be further defined.

PRINCIPLES OF PURCHASING

A number of different sources have suggested principles for purchasers. In England, the Health of the Nation report (DoH, 1991) emphasized the need for purchasers to plan health care. It recognized that the UK health service is predominantly concerned with illness, not health, and spends the great majority of its time trying to satisfy the immediate demand of patients for treatment. It stressed the importance of influences outside the health service upon health, such as poverty and poor housing, and the importance of working with organizations trying to tackle these.

In 1984, Maxwell also suggested a series of principles that should underlie a service:

- access to services
- relevance to the needs of the whole community
- effectiveness of individual patients
- equity
- social acceptability
- efficiency and economy.

THE PROCESS OF PURCHASING

Purchasing health care within the health services divides naturally into a number of processes. These are assessment of the needs of the population served, development of a service specification and production of a full specification, which may be thought of as a tender. Providers then negotiate with the purchaser regarding a price for the tender and a contract is agreed. Once the contract is under way, it is monitored and feedback from the monitoring process is used to develop new service specification data.

ASSESSMENT OF NEED BY THE COMMUNITY

Epidemiologists would, for preference, start with data about the degree of disability and hence dependency present in the locality. They would include data about the known responses of families and friends to this dependency. They would try to take into account the degree to which relatives in a particular area, whether inner city or village, can cope with a given degree of dependency. A further factor would be the extent to which relatives should reasonably be expected to contend with such difficulties.

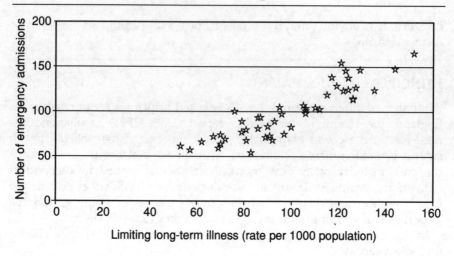

Figure 5.3 Emergency admissions by long-term illness rates in Cardiff electoral wards, 1991.

Few such data are locally available. The best that can be done in most districts is an estimate, using national data, such as the OPCS surveys of disability in Great Britain (Martin *et al.*, 1988) or the 1991 census data on limiting long-standing disability. These indicate differences between areas and may be a useful indication of the need for long-term care in one small area compared with another. Figure 5.3 shows that for small areas, in this case the 26 electoral wards in Cardiff, the data for long-standing disability standardized by age and sex are related to emergency hospitalization rates. There appears to be a degree of consistency between two very different measures of 'need' in these small areas.

WHAT IS THERE TO PURCHASE?

A rapid expansion of private residential and nursing homes occurred during the 1980s. There was a doubling of the number of places taken up over the period, especially in the private sector. If the effect of ageing of the population is taken into account, the increase is less marked. Nevertheless, almost one-third more elderly people were in long-term care establishments than would have been if the rates for different age groups had remained unchanged from 1981 (Laing, 1991). As the demand for private residential care increased due to its increasing availability, the costs of such care began to soar.

The other alternative is long-term care wards in hospitals, which still tend to have very poor facilities, often in modified 'Nightingale' wards partitioned poorly into four- and six-bed units. They are particularly unsuitable for long-term care as they lack privacy. They also tend to be noisy, for a group that specially appreciates quietness. They were originally designed for young war-wounded men in the 19th century who did not expect much from life and that is what they are good for.

PRAGMATIC PURCHASING OF LONG-STAY HEALTH CARE

The principles to be applied for purchasing care in any specialty or sector of a specialty have been described above. I intend to use the Maxwell criteria to assess the facilities available for long-term care.

ACCESS TO SERVICES

Older people may have some problems with obtaining services available to assist them at home for a number of reasons. The most immediate of these is that many older people do not know of the existence of some services. The older the person is, the more likely this is (Figure 5.4) (Salvage *et al.*, 1988).

Many people were unaware of the existence of many services that have for years formed the mainstream of facilities provided for elderly people. Especially worrying in this regard was the use of day centres and sheltered housing, where the impetus to take up these services often rests with older people themselves. Some basic services were known to virtually all the people questioned and their function appeared to be well

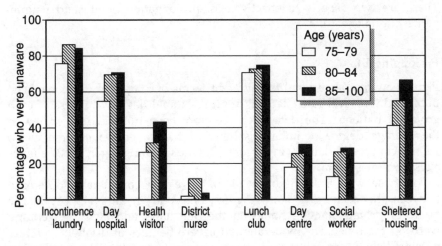

Figure 5.4 Awareness of the availability of various community services in those over 75 years old.

understood. General practitioners, chiropodists, home helps and 'meals on wheels' were well known, as were their functions.

RELEVANCE TO THE NEEDS OF THE WHOLE COMMUNITY

General acceptability

It seems self-evident that the long-term workhouse-based hospital ward must disappear as quickly as possible. No purchaser of services who had ever visited one would choose it if there were any other options. Health authorities will be looking for cost-effective alternatives and the simplest approach for most will be to use voluntary and private sector nursing homes or extra-care sheltered housing.

Acceptability to family and other carers

Some studies have shown that carers feel that their elderly relatives are being well cared for once admitted to residential care, whilst others seem to suffer considerable guilt. The lives of carers in some studies have often been changed immeasurably for the better as a result of the older person being admitted to institutional care. One factor in this must be the lack of support available at present to carers of dependent older people. What support is available has had a tendency to be stereotyped and limited both in quality and quantity.

EFFECTIVENESS FOR INDIVIDUAL PATIENTS

There are two aspects to effectiveness: prolongation of life and maintenance of quality of life.

Prolonging life

Figures on annual survival for different forms of long-term care have been published. Survival rates depend upon the initial degree of illness of each group of patients. The data have therefore been published according to the average degree of initial disability of the patients, measured as an ADL (activities of daily living) score (Donaldson and Jagger, 1983). Figure 5.5 shows these data.

For those with little disability (0–2), there is a considerable difference between the chances of surviving for one year in an NHS psychiatric home or private nursing home on the one hand and an NHS geriatric ward on the other. For moderate and severe degrees of disability, private nursing homes come out best. It may be expected that the NHS acute sector would do badly as many older people have acute illnesses that

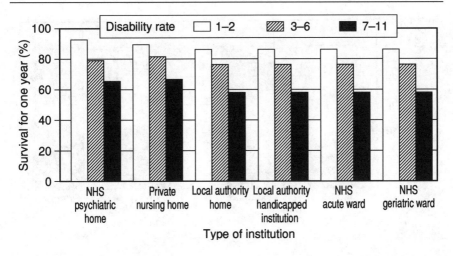

Figure 5.5 Survival for one year in various types of long-stay accommodation, by disability rate.

are not well reflected by an ADL score. In addition there may be differences, even within the ADL score groupings, as they were defined quite broadly, for those in one form of residence compared with others. Nevertheless, a purchaser taking the evidence at face value would need to be persuaded that it was not the poor environment in the geriatric hospital, with problems of cross-infection from chest complaints, or the generally depressing atmosphere of the place, which led older people to take to their beds.

Mortality rates have been measured in alternatives to long-stay hospitals although sadly some studies have been small and did not constitute a randomized trial (Gibbins *et al.*, 1982; Challis *et al.*, 1991). The study set up in Darlington concerned 101 patients given supported home care instead of long-term hospital care (Challis, 1991). Figure 5.6 shows the outcome, in terms of the placement of the patients at 6 and 12 months. It can be seen that there is a dramatic difference in the numbers who remain at home in the project group (home care) compared with controls (hospital care) at both 6 and 12 months. There is also a dramatic difference in favour of those in hospital in terms of a lower death rate at 6 months, although this difference is reduced at one year. The researchers explain this by making the point that a much higher proportion of the project group was receiving care for terminal illness than the control group. The major difficulty with this, apart from invalidating the information on deaths, is that it suggests that the two groups may have been different in other ways.

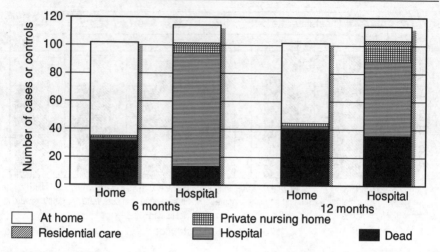

Figure 5.6   Comparing long-term hospital care (controls) with home care in terms of outcome.

Maintaining the quality of life

Quality of life was also measured in the Darlington study (Challis *et al.*, 1991). The high early mortality rate meant that only 42 cases were available at 6 months for proxy measures of quality of life. There was considerable advantage to the patients in terms of their subjective well-being, especially their morale, if those in the project (home care) group were compared with those in the control (hospital care) group. The overall CAPE scores, a measure of physical disability, were not different (Pattie and Gilleard, 1979). Social activity levels were greater for the project group. There is no doubt that some long-term hospital facilities effectively discourage social activities for patients, often due to the physical layout of the ward. The description by the carers of the hospital care given in this study suggests that the control hospital was not an exception.

EQUITY

Older people with the same problems that require long-term care will be treated differently in different places in the UK. Those who are judged to have a 'need for health care' will be given free care without an external test of their physical or financial status. Those who are not so judged will be cared for in private or voluntary nursing homes. They may be given social services support at home, and both their physical needs and financial needs will be externally assessed by social services before they are able to receive these services. The definition of a 'need for health care' is agreed between local health authorities and social services departments. Recent advice from central government has underlined the importance of local agreements. It has hinted that the need for 'continuing and specialist medical or nursing supervision' brought about by the 'nature and complexity of their health care needs' should be the central point at issue. The decision should depend on a multidisciplinary assessment of their needs (DoH, 1994).

However, objective physical measures of physical disability show a considerable overlap between patients living in the various settings available for long-term care. Work by the Health Care Research Unit in Newcastle has shown the disability characteristics of people in local authority residential homes, geriatric wards, acute wards and private nursing homes (Atkinson et al., 1986). Although there were differences in the scores for those treated in different places, there was considerable overlap. The authors stated that 'it is obvious from our comparisons of elderly people in residential and hospital care that the same needs are being met in a variety of different settings'.

The inevitable differences between areas in the definitions of 'the need for health care' will mean that some older people will be disadvantaged compared with others. The odd thing is that some observers believe this to be a new phenomenon (Warden, 1995).

SOCIAL ACCEPTABILITY

A group of 75-year-old people were asked under what circumstances they would consider going into some form of institutional care (Salvage et al., 1988). One-third could think of a situation where they might consider it. A quarter of the people asked said they would consider it if they were too ill to manage at home. Slightly fewer than that said they would prefer to go into a home rather than living on their own. Half of the people claimed that they would not think of entering a residential home even if they were incontinent and unable to get out of bed. Virtually all the people questioned said that they had somebody who would be available to help them and that this person or persons would look after them, allowing them to remain at home.

One of the main reasons for older people wishing to be treated at home is the poor image that they and many other people have of hospitals and nursing homes. The older people suggested that geriatric units, in particular, lead to a loss of dignity and self-respect. Indeed, whilst many older people accept the need for hospital care for specific ailments, they are much less happy to be seen as part of geriatric care, especially long-stay geriatric care. They clearly feel labelled and wish to avoid this by being admitted, if they have to be admitted, to general medical or surgical wards in hospital.

The study showed that people who had been into general acute hospital care were happier about their admission than those who had entered a geriatric ward. Two-thirds of those who had been treated in geriatric units were unhappy with their experience compared with less than a quarter who had been cared for in a general medical ward. The main advantage of general medical care mentioned was the company. The most common and linked disadvantage of geriatric care was the presence of other disabled or disturbed older people. This was one of the elements in the general distaste of older people for care in hospital.

Studies about private and council-run residential homes have suggested that, although there were some differences, older people did not like either form of institutionalized care because of a loss of independence (Sinclair, 1990).

EFFICIENCY AND ECONOMY

The costs of different types of long-term care have been studied by a number of researchers. Donaldson and Bond (1995) have looked at the costs of NHS-based nursing homes and compared them with the costs of long-term hospital wards. The results show that the costs are very similar.

The costs of the home-based long-term care and the hospital-based care for the Darlington study, mentioned above, are shown in Figure 5.7. The group treated at home had an average agency cost (cost to statutory services) much below that of the hospital-treated group. Fascinatingly, and this may be the most important finding of this study, the social

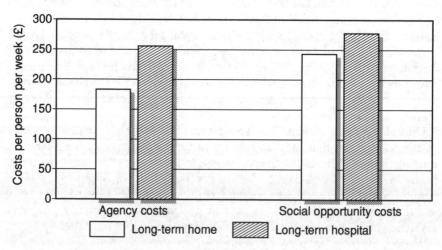

Figure 5.7   Costs of long-term hospital and home care.

opportunity costs (costs to relatives and friends) were also lower for the home-managed group.

CONCLUSIONS

As a purchaser of long-term care for older people following the guidelines above, I would suggest the following procedure.

1. An assessment system would be used to identify the small proportion of older people who require a high level of medical attention and are most suitably cared for in a health-oriented facility. The assessment would have two tiers, with a screening test applied by nurses and a multidisciplinary team of professionals to assess those who passed the screening assessment. People thought to have acute remediable problems would receive suitable help. The final say must depend on the opinion of a skilled clinician.
2. People thought to require such a high degree of care would receive it under existing NHS arrangements, in a small NHS nursing home, modelled on existing units. If they preferred, they could choose research-based extended home care.
3. Health authorities unable to afford their own facilities could contract to use a small number of local private or voluntary nursing homes. These would specialize in the care of very dependent patients and have a proven track record at doing so. The health authority would pay for the patients' care. The nursing homes in question would have to accept, as part of the contract, supervision from a local geriatrician.
4. Less dependent people would come under the assessment and case management system set up under the NHS & Community Care Act (1990) and organized by the social services department and would be subject to a measure of financial means.

REFERENCES

Atkinson, D.A., Bond, J. and Gregson, B.A. (1986) The dependency characteristics of older people in long-term institutional care, in *Dependency and Interdependency in Old Age* (eds C. Phillipson, M. Bernard and P. Strang), Croom Helm, London.

Challis, D., Darton, R., Johnson, L. *et al.* (1991) An evaluation of an alternative to long-stay hospital care for frail elderly patients: 1. The model of care. *Age Ageing*, **20**, 236–44.

Department of Health (1991) *Health of the Nation*, HMSO, London.

Department of Health (1994) *NHS responsibilities for meeting long term health care needs. HSG (94)*, Department of Health, Leeds.

Donaldson, C. and Bond, J. (1991) Cost of continuing care facilities in the evaluation of experimental National Health Service nursing homes. *Age Ageing*, **20**, 160–8.

Donaldson, L.J. and Jagger, G. (1983) Survival and functional capacity: three year follow-up of an elderly population in hospitals and homes. *J. Epidemiol. Community Health*, **37**, 176–9.

Gibbins, F.J., Lee, M., Davison, P.R. *et al.* (1982) Augmented home nursing as an alternative to hospital care for chronic elderly invalids. *BMJ*, **284**, 330–3.

Isaacs, B. and Neville, Y. (1976) The needs of old people – the 'interval' as a method of measurement *Br. J. Preventive Soc. Med.*, **30**, 79–85.

Laing, W. (1991) *Empowering the elderly: direct consumer funding of care services*. IEA Health and Welfare Unit, Institute of Economic Affairs, London.

Martin, J., Meltzer, H. and Elliot, D. (1988) *The prevalence of disability among adults. OPCS surveys of disability in Great Britain. Report 1*, HMSO, London.

Maxwell, R. (1984) Quality assessment in health. *BMJ*, **288**, 1470–2.

Pattie, A.M. and Gilleard, C.J. (1979) *Manual of the Clifton Assessment Procedures for the Elderly*, Hodder and Stoughton, Sevenoaks, UK.

Salvage, A.V., Jones, D.A. and Vetter, N.J. (1988) Awareness of and satisfaction with community services in a random sample of over 75s. *Health Trends*, **20**, 88–92.

Salvage, A.V., Vetter, N.J. and Jones, D.A. (1988) Attitudes to hospital care among a community sample of people aged 75 and older. *Age Ageing*, **17**, 270–4.

Sinclair, I. (1990) Residential care, in *The Kaleidoscope of Care* (eds I. Sinclair, R. Parker, D. Leat and J. Williams), HMSO, London.

Vetter, N.J., Jones, D.A. and Victor, C.R. (1986). A health visitor affects the problems others do not reach. *Lancet*, **ii**, 30–2.

Warden, J. (1995) BMA criticises guidance on long term care. *BMJ*, **310**, 550–1.

The ageing population: the mixed economy in long-term care

6

INTRODUCTION

The last 20 years have witnessed a transformation in the way that long-term care is provided in the UK. Twenty years ago, the old welfare state model was alive and well. Most people needing long-term care received it in local authority part III accommodation, or in long-stay hospitals. There was a strong voluntary sector, acting as an adjunct to local authority social services departments, but the private sector was small and catered almost exclusively for privately paying individuals. Now, in contrast, it is the private sector which dominates supply, and although privately paying individuals remain an important segment of the market, accounting for some 20% of private care home residents, the great majority of private providers' customers are funded by the state. How this transformation started is described briefly below. It owes something to the pro-market ideology of successive Conservative governments which have been in place since 1979. However, it probably owes more to the state of the British economy and the strains that would have been placed on the public purse if the state – via local authorities or the NHS – had sought to fund the massive capital investment necessary to expand the supply of long-term care services to cater for the rapidly growing population of very old people.

In this sense, therefore, the ageing population was the trigger for the transformation of long-term care delivery from the mid-1970s to the mid-1990s, from the old welfare state model to a mixed economy in which the state pays and private, voluntary and public sector providers compete as suppliers. Moreover, the demographic factor will continue to underpin the mixed economy of long-term care as the very old population continues to increase (according to latest official population projections) until the middle of the 21st century. This conclusion on the effect of demography seems likely to hold regardless of the political persuasion of the government. In July 1995, the Labour Party published a review of health policy (Labour Party, 1995). Although the review was principally about health care, and long-term care was limited to a couple of pages at the end of the document, the contents clearly signalled that, under Labour, there will be no roll-back of the frontiers of the private sector of long-term care. A Labour government may well halt the current decline in local authorities' own in-house provision of part III residential homes. However, in the present political climate, it seems that the option of substantially increased investment in public sector-owned care facilities is a non-starter.

In the last few years, the focus of the debate on long-term care has tended to shift away from delivery and towards funding. There has been much talk of a 'demographic time-bomb' and concern about how the country can afford to pay for long-term care, whether privately or out of state funds, in the future. My own view, explained in more detail below, is that there is no impending funding 'crisis', and no reason to believe that long-term care will not be as affordable in the future as it is now. Nevertheless, there is no doubt that the issue of who should pay for long-term care has risen rapidly up the political agenda. Partly, this is to do with the community care reforms, implemented in April 1993, which have raised the profile of long-term care at the same time as creating higher expectations. However, the underlying reason for heightened media coverage and political debate has been the steady withdrawal of the NHS from its role as a purchaser of continuing care for people with long-term nursing needs, a process which has been going on for at least 20 years. NHS withdrawal from long-term care has a number of implications, clinical and otherwise. Viewed from a wholly political perspective, however, the essence of the 'problem' is that middle-class property owners' expectations are being disappointed. Instead of being offered an NHS place at no charge, those who need care in a residential setting have to undergo a means test prior to entering a private or voluntary care home and may have to spend down their property and other assets before they qualify for state funding. As a result, there may be nothing left for family members to inherit. To date, the government's response when faced with this argument is that long-term social care has always been means tested since the inception of the welfare state, under the 1948 National Assistance Act. This is, of course, true. However, it is also the case that the definition of what qualifies as health care, to be provided without charge by the NHS, has become much narrower. The point is best illustrated by reference to statistics. In 1970, an estimated 24% of people entering long-term care in the UK received that care without charge in an NHS long-stay hospital. By the mid-1990s, the proportion had decreased to 10% (Laing, 1994).

Middle-class property owners and prospective inheritors are justified, therefore, in saying that the financial goal posts have shifted during their lifetimes. Where the goal posts should finally be placed will continue to be a matter of active public debate. The government has set in train a process by which individual health authorities will define local eligibility criteria for receiving long-term care paid for by the NHS (Department of Health, 1995). Meanwhile, two enquiries into the funding of long-term care started in 1995, one by the House of Commons Health Committee and the other by the Joseph Rowntree Foundation. It is not within the remit of this chapter to rehearse the arguments for and against different approaches to long-term care funding, from social insurance to private insurance to simple refinement of the existing, largely means-tested balance of state and personal funding. Whatever funding changes are brought in, it seems likely that long-term care will continue to be supplied on a mixed economy model, with the dominant position occupied by private sector providers.

HISTORICAL BACKGROUND: EMERGENCE OF THE CARE HOME INDUSTRY

The first 30 years of the welfare state, up to the mid-1970s, witnessed a broad expansion of state-financed residential and non-residential care services for elderly people, almost exclusively provided in public sector facilities. Public sector capital was available to create local authority old peoples' homes (typically newly built with 40–50 places), and these so-called 'part III' homes became virtually synonymous with residential accommodation offering personal care. At this time, most nursing care for people with higher levels of dependency was also provided in the public sector in NHS geriatric and mental illness hospitals. These were, and still are, typically 19th century buildings with open 'Nightingale' wards. With the development of a professional consensus on the merits of community care, old geriatric hospitals were already on the decline by the early 1970s and were losing some of their clientele to part III homes. Official statistics are less clear about trends in mental illness hospitals, but it is believed that the number of NHS beds occupied by older severely mentally ill people, typically people suffering from severe dementia, actually rose in the 1970s and 1980s in line with demographic change, against a background of declining numbers within mental illness hospitals as a whole. On balance, therefore, combined NHS geriatric and psychogeriatric provision showed only a gradual decline in those years.

Alongside the expanding local authority sector in the early 1970s there was a voluntary sector, largely financed by local authorities, and a private sector catering mainly for people with their own means. The private sector experienced periodic difficulties, for example in the mid-1970s when BUPA changed its rules to prevent such a large proportion of its benefits being spent on supporting older subscribers in long-stay nursing homes.

The private sector could at that time be characterized almost exclusively as a cottage industry. There was little corporate activity and proprietors often experienced great difficulty in getting loan finance. It was even common for a vendor of a home to offer a private mortgage to the purchaser.

Despite the expansion of local authority services in the 1950s, 1960s and 1970s, there was mounting pressure on resources as a consequence of demographic change. Access to local authority part III accommodation for older people was rationed and 'bed blocking' became a major problem for NHS hospital wards unable to discharge older patients to alternative care.

The stresses in the system became overwhelming when, following the UK monetary crisis in 1976, capital for the expansion of part III accommodation ceased to be available. In the years that followed, voluntary organizations also found their income from cash-strapped local authorities rapidly dwindling. In 1974, local authorities paid for about 60% of voluntary sector residential home places in England. By 1983, it had dropped to 34%. Voluntary organizations started to look for an alternative source of money and found it in the social security system. Responding to pressure orchestrated and articulated by voluntary organizations, local social security offices started to pay supplementary benefits to people unable to afford their own fees and for whom local authorities were unwilling to foot the bill. Initially there was no national policy governing what were known as board and lodging allowances, but the practice became so widespread that policy was formalized in 1983 when, in effect, the government set up a voucher system for public funding of private and voluntary care homes. The rules that were introduced allowed people with less than £3000 in capital and who qualified on income grounds to apply as of right for supplementary benefits to pay for admission to a residential or nursing home of their choice, provided it was a private or voluntary home. The benefits were not available to pay for local authority residential homes, nor, of course, could they be claimed to pay for NHS long-stay hospitals, since the NHS cannot charge for in-patient care of NHS patients. No assessment of need for residential or nursing care was required. In its essentials, this new source of public funding remained in place until April 1993, although the initially generous local income support limits were subsequently replaced by much lower national limits, annually reviewed, while the £3000 capital limit was subsequently raised to £16 000 in April 1996.

Although voluntary organizations led the campaign for the new source of public funding, the principal beneficiaries in a business sense have been private providers of care homes. There is no doubt that the availability of supplementary benefits (renamed income support with the 1988 social security changes) fuelled the rapid expansion of private residential care, followed a few years later by an even more rapid expansion of private nursing care (Figure 6.1).

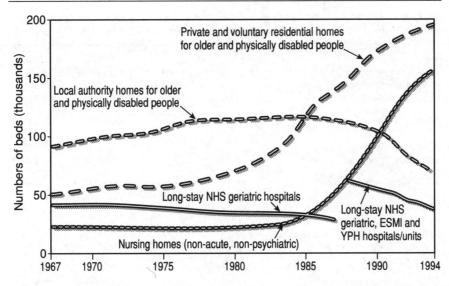

Figure 6.1 Number of nursing and residential care places for older, chronically ill and physically disabled people by sector: England and Wales, 1967–1994. The discontinuity occurs at the time of change to Korner aggregates. After 1988, separate figures for acute/rehabilitation geriatric beds and long-stay geriatric beds are no longer available. Long-stay beds have therefore been estimated since 1988 on the assumption that acute/rehabilitation geriatric beds in England have remained constant and all the decline in beds in England in the speciality of geriatrics overall is attributable to loss of long-stay beds. ESMI, elderly severely mentally ill; YPH, young physically handicapped.

RECENT TRENDS AND MARKET SIZE

MARKET SIZE – CARE IN RESIDENTIAL SETTINGS

Over 30 years of uninterrupted growth in overall UK capacity for long-stay care of elderly and physically handicapped people came to a halt in the year to April 1994, the first year of the community care reforms. At April 1994, there were an estimated 556 300 places across all sectors (556 900 in April 1993), and the value of the market had changed little compared with the previous year at an estimated £8.0 billion, of which the private sector accounted for £4.6 billion (Table 6.1).

Within the static total across all sectors, however, private nursing home capacity continued to expand in the year up to April 1994, and into 1995. There has also been continued capacity growth in the private residential sector, although at a much slower pace. Public sector capacity, in both local authority part III accommodation and NHS long-stay hospitals, has continued to decline (Table 6.2).

Table 6.1   Expenditure on nursing and residential care of elderly, chronically ill and physically disabled people, and the number of places at April 1994, UK

	Places	£ million
Private nursing homes	178 800	2762
Private residential homes[a]	167 500	1820
Total private supply	346 300	4582
Voluntary nursing homes	16 000	253
Voluntary residential homes[a]	50 700	591
Total voluntary supply	66 700	844
NHS long-stay geriatric	34 700	866
NHS mentally ill older people	20 100	502
NHS younger physically disabled	2 100	52
Local authority older people and younger physically handicapped	86 400	1196
Total public supply	143 300	2616
Total care in residential settings	556 300	8042
Plus non-residential care		3685
Grand total (Residential and Non-residential)		11 727

[a]Excludes 'small homes' of less than four beds, estimated at some 5000 beds for the elderly and physically handicapped client group at April 1994.
Source: *Care of Elderly Market Survey 1995*, Laing & Buisson.

MARKET SIZE – CARE IN NON-RESIDENTIAL SETTINGS

Information on the scale and growth of the non-residential care market is less readily available than for the care home market. The size of the state-funded sector can be estimated from government statistical sources (Table 6.3), although figures for recent years have to be extrapolated as there is a long delay before expenditure figures emerge into the public domain.

Information on personally financed and privately provided services is poor. Private market size cannot at present be estimated from the supply side because it is so highly fragmented. No survey has yet been carried out which satisfactorily separates out the domiciliary care element of nursing and employment agencies' revenue from the remainder of their business. Nor is there any continuing statistical series that enables private market size to be estimated from the expenditure side. In the absence of any such statistical series, private market size is estimated in Table 6.3 from data on expenditure on care services given in the OPCS report on the financial circumstances of disabled people (Martin and White, 1988).

Table 6.2 Nursing, residential and long-stay hospital care of elderly, chronically ill and physically disabled people, places by sector, UK, 1970–1994

	Residential home places[a]			Nursing home places[b] private/voluntary			Long-stay geriatric places NHS	Long-stay psycho-geriatric places NHS	Long-stay young physically disabled places NHS	Total places
	Local authority	Private	Voluntary	private/voluntary						
1 April										
1970	108 700	23 700	40 100	20 300			52 000	23 000	2 500	270 300
1975	128 300	25 800	41 000	24 000			49 000			
1980	134 500	37 400	42 600	26 900			46 100			
1981	135 600	40 200	44 500	26 900			46 400			
1982	136 200	46 900	44 400	27 200			46 300			
1983	136 500	54 700	45 300	29 000			46 900			
1984	137 200	67 100	45 900	32 500			46 500			
1985	137 100	85 300	45 100	38 000			46 300			
1986	136 900	99 500	46 600	47 900			45 600			
					Private	Voluntary				
1987	135 500	114 600	42 200		52 000	8 300	43 000[c]	29 300	2 500	465 800
1988	133 500	127 900	43 000		68 700	9 600	51 400[c]	28 200	2 500	492 100
1989	129 800	143 200	39 900		88 600	10 400	49 500[d]	27 000	2 500	521 000
1990	125 600	155 600	40 000		112 600	10 500	47 200[d]	24 500	2 400	539 100
1991	117 400	161 200	41 900		135 200	12 100	44 400[d]	23 500	2 300	547 000
1992	105 200	162 400	46 900		152 800	13 700	40 200[d]	22 300	2 200	556 900
1993	95 000	165 400	51 000		168 200	15 000	37 800[d]	20 100	2 100	556 300
1994	86 400	167 500	50 700		178 800	16 000	34 700[d]			

[a] Includes residential places in dual registration homes; excludes 'small homes' of less than four beds, estimated at some 5000 for the elderly and physically handicapped client group at April 1994.
[b] Includes nursing places in dual registration homes.
[c] The increase in 1988 is an artefact caused by re-classification of hospital types when Korner aggregates were introduced.
[d] NHS long-stay geriatric beds estimated since 1988 on the assumption that acute/rehabilitation geriatric beds in England have remained constant and all the decline in beds in the speciality of geriatrics overall is attributable to loss of long-stay beds.
Source: *Care of Elderly People Market Survey 1995*, Laing & Buisson.

Table 6.3 Expenditure on non-residential care of elderly and physically disabled peoples, UK estimates April 1994

	< 65 £ million	65 + £ million	all ages £ million
NHS expenditure on non-residential care (community health)			
district nursing	292	878	1170
day care	35	115	150
chiropody	13	117	130
Total NHS expenditure on non-residential care	340	1110	1450
Local authority expenditure on non-residential care[a]			
home care	90	810	900
day care (local authority and other provision)	95	180	275
other local authority domiciliary care	70	200	270
meals on wheels	–	90	90
aids and applications	30	40	70
Total gross local authority expenditure on non-residential care	285	1320	1605
Personal expenditure on private non-residential care[b]			
aids and applications	70	90	160
home care	90	380	470
Total public and personal expenditure on non-residential care	785	2900	3685
[Informal care]	[7000]	[34000]	[41000]

[a]Gross of user charges.
[b]Excluding user charges for local authority services.
[c]Calculated following a method originally used by the Family Policy Studies Centre (1989), valuing each hour of informal care at £7.00 per hour (based on local authority pay rates).
Source: *Review of Private Healthcare 1995*, Laing & Buisson.

The estimate, however, is subject to considerable error because the survey work took place in 1985 and projections for more recent years must adjust both for inflation and for volume growth of services resulting from an ageing population.

Until the community care reforms implemented in April 1993, the non-residential care market for for-profit providers was effectively limited to the estimated £470 million of personal expenditure on home care in 1994. The much larger state-funded non-residential care budgets were almost entirely spent in-house on directly provided services. This is now changing rapidly, with local authority contracting of non-residential care

Table 6.4 Volumes of local authority-funded community care services directly provided and contracted out during a survey week, England 1992–1994.

			Under contract using		
	All sectors	Direct	Voluntary sector	Private sector	NHS
Number of home care contact hours in week					
September 1992	1 687 000	1 647 800	6 800	32 300	–
September 1993	1 780 800	1 694 300	16 100	70 400	–
October 1994	2 214 400	1 787 500	62 200	364 700	–
Number of day care attendances in week[a]					
September 1992	146 800	121 100	25 300	500	–
September 1993	159 800	125 500	33 700	500	–
October 1994	174 400	131 400	41 400	1 500	–
Number of clients served meals in week					
September 1992	275 700	156 000	106 500	11 300	2000
September 1993	286 900	155 100	118 100	11 100	2600
October 1994	300 400	152 100	130 000	16 100	2200

[a]A person attending more than once during the week is counted on each occasion.
Source: Community Care Statistics 1994. Department of Health Statistical Bulletin, May 1995.

growing fast from a very small baseline (Table 6.4). Among the various non-residential services, home care is the largest expenditure category and the area in which contracting activity is the greatest. By October 1994, 16.5% of all local authority-funded home care hours were contracted out to for-profit home care providers and a further 2.8% to not-for-profit organizations. This implies that local authorities across the UK were contracting out home care to the value of over £150 million per annum at the time of the survey. It is also of interest that for-profit provision is concentrated at the more intensive end of the home care spectrum, delivering 7.9 hours of care per household per week compared with an average of 4.8 hours for voluntary sector providers and 3.7 hours for direct local authority provision. The delivery of day care is changing less quickly, and voluntary sector providers dominate what contracted day care services there are.

For the future, the local authority-funded home care market clearly has much more potential for growth for for-profit home care operators than their traditional privately funded market. It is likely that those for-profit home care operators who succeed in this new state-funded market will see the profile of their businesses rapidly changing from virtually 100%

privately funded, as it was before the community care reforms, to predominantly state-funded.

The NHS community care market, on the other hand, looks unlikely to open up to for-profit providers for the foreseeable future. Although community health services, including district nursing, are now included in general practitioner fundholder budgets, fundholders are specifically restricted to purchasing community health services from NHS providers only. Independent sector providers will not, therefore, be able to pay an active role in this market until the government changes the ground rules.

THE AGEING POPULATION

The principal driving force behind the growth of long-term care provision in the past has been the ageing population. A less important, but nonetheless significant, factor has been the funding system. As noted above, the emergence of open-ended income support funding greatly stimulated demand. The extent to which this new demand was additional to demographic pressure is illustrated in Figure 6.2. This shows that, after adjusting for the effect of the ageing population, there were 27% more long-term care places per unit population by the beginning of the 1990s than there had been before income support started to come on stream at the end of the 1970s. This statistic can, of course, be interpreted in different ways. On the one hand, it could be seen as evidence of income

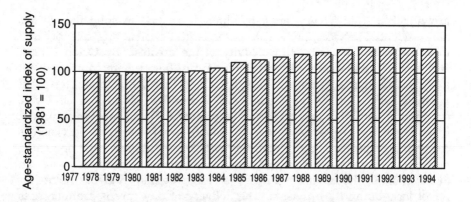

Figure 6.2　Age-adjusted index of supply of private, voluntary, local authority and NHS long-stay places for older people: England, 1977–1994. The index is the ratio of observed to expected places, the latter being the number that would have been observed in a given year if age-specific rates of occupation of residential homes (grossed up to places of all types for long-term care of older people) are applied to the population in that year. Source: *Care of Elderly People Market Survey 1995*, Laing & Buisson).

support allowing more people to go inappropriately into care homes. On the other hand, it could be seen as evidence that public sector provision was too tightly constrained before, and that income support offered much needed funding for pent-up demand which had previously led to chronic bed-blocking in the NHS.

Whichever interpretation is closer to the truth, it seems from Figure 6.2 that one of the effects of the community care reforms in April 1993, which replaced open-ended income support funding for care homes with cash-limited local authority funding, has been to halt growth in long-term care provision across all sectors combined. In fact, the index of age-adjusted demand was pushed down by two percentage points in 1994 compared with 1992. It may be assumed that this reduction in age-adjusted demand was brought about by the introduction of local authority assessments prior to care home entry under the new system, and thus represents avoidance of inappropriate placements.

However, this interruption to the growth trend in long-term care provision can only be temporary. Underlying demand for care services will continue to expand throughout the remainder of the 1990s and beyond as the number and proportion of very old people in the community grows (Figure 6.3). However successful local authorities are in diverting care home placements to home care, demand for the former can hardly fail to grow because rates of disability and dependence escalate so rapidly with increasing old age. The latest figures (1994) indicate that 1% of the 65–74-year-old population lives in some form of institutional setting, whether a local authority old people's home, an NHS hospital or a

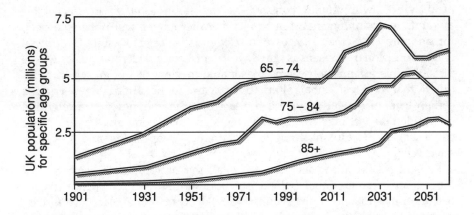

Figure 6.3 UK population 1901–2061 (projected) for specific age groups. (Sources: 1901–1986 census data; 1991–2061 *National Population Projections*, Office of Population Censuses and Surveys, Series PP2 No. 18, HMSO).

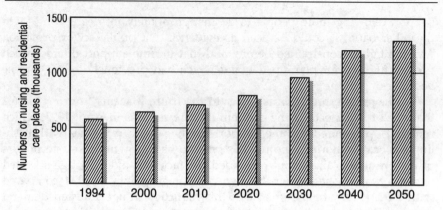

Figure 6.4   Projected numbers of places for nursing and residential care of older chronically ill and physically disabled people: UK, 1994–2050 (all sectors). Numbers are calculated by applying age-specific rates of supply to official population projections. Age-specific rates of supply are derived by applying the age distribution of care home and long-stay hospital residents to the number of beds in all sectors. The age distribution of care homes is estimated by combining the age distribution of care home residents (from Department of Health Residential Accommodation Statistics) and the age distribution of nursing home residents (from Communal Establishments report of the 1991 census).

private or voluntary residential or nursing home. For people aged 85 and over, the proportion is estimated to reach 26%.

The projections in Figure 6.4 illustrate potential demographic-led growth in care home places to the year 2050. They assume that age-specific rates of provision will remain constant at the same level as in 1994. This amounts to assuming that non-residential alternatives will not make deep inroads into the demand for care in residential settings. Despite the official and professional consensus in favour of non-residential care where possible, this assumption seems reasonable in view of the growing recognition that non-residential alternatives cease to be affordable beyond a certain level of dependency, and the fact that the volume of care provided in residential settings in Britain remains low compared with other countries, in the Organization for Economic Co-operation and Development (OECD).

Looking as far ahead as the year 2050, the projections indicate that, if other things remain equal (which is a bold assumption for such a distant projection), a total of approaching 1 300 000 care home places would be required to serve the needs of the UK population at that time. It is clearly not possible to estimate how much private, voluntary and public sector provision there will be then, although, taking a shorter time horizon, the assumption of private sector operators is that they will provide all the additional net demand for care facilities until at least the end of this decade.

At first sight, the projection of 1 300 000 long-term care beds may look quite horrifying, and may even be adduced as evidence of an impending funding 'crisis' by those who support the demographic time-bomb hypothesis. However, a closer look at projected funding requirements in relation to the economy as a whole does not reveal such a pessimistic picture. In a recent book commissioned by Age Concern England (Laing, 1994), I calculated that 1.5% of gross domestic product was being spent on care services for elderly people in 1992, and that this may rise to a peak of 3.5% by 2050, using the same method of projection (constant age-specific utilization) as outlined above. At present, the state pays for some 70% of long-term care costs, but on present means-testing rules, this proportion will presumably decline in the future as succeeding cohorts of people with higher rates of owner occupation reach old age. In summary, provided medical science does not succeed in greatly prolonging the life expectancy of dependent people, and provided relatives do not opt out of informal care in large numbers, there is no reason to believe that funding this level of demand would place intolerable strains on either the tax payer or the economy as a whole.

WHERE IS THE MIXED ECONOMY TAKING US?

Most professionals involved in the long-term care of older people are aware of the rapid expansion of the private care home sector over the last 20 years. However, there is perhaps less awareness of changes in the make-up of the private sector itself. Twenty years ago, the private sector consisted almost entirely of owner managers. Groups of care homes scarcely existed, aside from some local clusters of a handful of homes under the same ownership. By 1994, however, major for-profit providers of care homes – defined as groups of three or more care homes – operated 30% of all private sector nursing home places. These groups, including 16 stock exchange quoted companies and 11 companies with more than 1000 beds each, have concentrated their activities principally on the nursing home sector. Ownership of residential homes by major providers with three or more homes each is much less extensive, accounting for just 6% of private residential home beds in 1994.

There is no doubt that major providers will increase their penetration of the care home market in the next few years, and this has major implications for the style and quality of long-term care provision. Major providers are expanding both by acquisition and development of entirely new care homes. One way in which major providers differ markedly from 'mom and pop' or 'cottage industry' operators is that their homes are significantly larger, with an average of 51 beds per nursing home in 1994 compared with 36 for the nursing home sector as a whole. Most new developments have about 60 beds and some are as large as 120 or 150 beds. Investment in larger homes is driven primarily by economies of scale, and some professionals have expressed concern about the possible recreation of institution-like environments in such larger establishments. The counter-argument to this is that everything depends on the design of the interior and the nature of the care and it is certainly true that new purpose-built care homes are totally unlike older NHS institutions in their design. They are usually split into separate units, with a number of lounge areas, and rooms are predominantly or entirely single, often with their own *en suite* toilet facilities. Additional communal facilities such as an activity room or hydrotherapy pool can also be included in larger care home designs, which would not be viable in smaller establishments. There can be little doubt, therefore, that major provider investment is having the effect of raising the quality of the physical environment of care homes. Certainly, the privacy and amenities that they afford is greatly superior to that which was in the past, and is still, typically available in NHS long-stay hospitals. There is also a strong case that new, purpose-built, 60-bed care homes developed by major providers are preferred by many if not most customers to the alternative of smaller, converted care homes.

Of course, it is always possible to provide a still better physical environment, at a price. Most corporate operators now build single rooms of at least 12 m^2, in order to ensure compliance with inspection standards for the foreseeable future. But there are care home models which are yet more generous. Anchor Housing Association, for example, builds to a 20 m^2 per room specification in its 'housing with care' developments. Other private and voluntary providers have experimented with 'close care' or 'assisted living' models, in which more generous specifications are linked with features such as own front doors and kitchenettes in order to maximize opportunities for independent living. Most major providers are not at present developing facilities of this type, generally because they do not perceive a market for them.

Physical environment is one aspect of quality, but the quality of care itself is of more fundamental importance. How does the private sector in general – and corporate providers in particular – compare with voluntary and public sector providers? The answer is that we simply do not know. Certainly, there is huge variability in all sectors, but such indicators of quality as have been used in comparative studies of private, voluntary and public sector provision are inadequate. What can be said, however, is that many private and voluntary providers, as well as their representative organizations, are very much alive to the issue of how best to promote quality. There are now about half a dozen well-established quality assurance packages available, most of them backed up by external verification and accreditation. They range from the clinically oriented CARE package developed by the Royal College of Physicians, through care-oriented Inside Quality Assurance, to multi-sector quality assurance systems such as Investors in People and BS5750–ISO9000. Although it is true that quality assurance and monitoring is in its infancy, and there is not yet any wholly satisfactory definition of what 'quality' of long-term care is, at least it can be said that larger operators in the private and voluntary sectors are at the leading edge in exploring mechanisms for achieving quality goals.

The reservation is that care that is specifically medical does not form part of quality assurance packages and there is a danger that the continuing process of privatization of supply may lead to a loss of medical expertise in dealing with the needs of the frail older population of care homes. The danger becomes greater the more the NHS withdraws from long-term care and the more dependent the recipients of care in private and voluntary homes become. There is certainly a challenge here for NHS consultants in those specialities dealing with older and physically disabled people to devise strategies whereby, if long-term care patients are no longer located in NHS beds, appropriate medical monitoring and management can be delivered to the care homes where they are located.

It should also be recognized that many private care home operators, particularly the larger major providers, are keen to build up their own expertise and capability to manage patients in need of more active treatment and rehabilitation than is normally provided at present in nursing homes. Already, specialist private and voluntary nursing homes cater for significant numbers of difficult-to-place patients with challenging behaviour, under contract to the NHS. Other specialist services could well be developed outside NHS hospitals. Post-stroke rehabilitation, for example, is an activity that may in the future be contracted out by NHS purchasers to appropriately qualified private sector providers. With the whole future of NHS district general hospitals now open to question, and the possibility of emergency treatment being increasingly concentrated in 'super-hospitals' serving much larger catchment populations, the concept of contracting out this and other forms of 'sub-acute' care to remodelled nursing homes may be an attractive one. It has already been widely adopted in the USA as a cost-effective alternative to acute hospital treatment. If a similar shift takes place in the UK, the private nursing home sector will enter into yet another stage of development and diversification which will bring ever closer contractual and professional ties with the core of the NHS.

REFERENCES

Department of Health (1995) *NHS Responsibilities for Meeting Continuing Health Care Needs. HSG (95)8*, Department of Health, London.

Labour Party (1995) *Renewing the NHS: Labour's Agenda for a Healthier Britain*, The Labour Party, London.

Laing, W. (1994) *Financing Long Term Care: the Crucial Debate* Age Concern England, London.

Laing & Buisson (1995) *Care of Elderly People Market Survey 1995*, Laing & Buisson, London.

Martin, J. and White, A. (1988) *The financial circumstances of disabled adults living in private households*, OPCS surveys of disability in Great Britain, Report 2. HMSO, London.

PART TWO
General and specific
aspects of care

The chapters in this section help to set the scene in continuing care. Structure and process are considered but many authors concentrate on outcome; i.e. those activities which can help older people enjoy life and look forward with optimism to the future.

Patients' and residents' rights

7

SETTING THE SCENE

An older resident in a home tells how she came to be there. Admitted to hospital following a fall, she was judged after a two-week stay not to be in need of further treatment. It was equally clear that she could not return to her own flat where she had lived alone, so she agreed to move to the nursing home to complete her recovery. She was visited there by her daughter who brought her some of her personal belongings, but after several visits she began to question why she needed so many clothes. The daughter prevaricated; eventually she confessed that she had terminated the lease on her mother's flat. 'So that's how I'm here,' the story concludes. Such a client, it is clear, has exercised little choice or self-determination over decisions which profoundly affect the rest of her life.

Meanwhile, in one of a diminishing number of long-stay NHS geriatric units, another woman in her eighties lives in fear. She has 'learning difficulties'; a few years ago she was termed 'mentally handicapped'; when originally admitted, she was said merely to be 'simple'. She has heard that the unit will close sometime soon but she does not know where she will be moved to; there was talk a couple of years ago of a new home soon to be built, but those plans seem to have been cancelled. The uncertainty, she feels, might be her own fault. She is getting forgetful these days and sometimes confuses staff with distantly remembered family members. Her relatives don't visit any more; is that because they don't want to see her now, or are they dead? Her new resting place might of course be better than the ward she shares with eight other patients. There are screens but the hard-pressed staff sometimes appear not to have the time or energy to pull them into place when she is transferred to the commode from the bed to which her worsening arthritis often confines her. It would be nice, she thinks to herself, to go out sometimes – shopping, or to a park, or just to a real street where someone might push her up and down in a wheelchair. What, by any standard, is the quality of life of such a patient?

Out in what that hospital's staff would probably call 'the community', a man recalls two world wars, the first in which his father died, and the second in which he served himself. Society seems to pay little regard to the sacrifices he and others of his generation made, and his situation now shows scant sign of the freedom he thought he fought to save. The stroke he suffered a year ago effectively ended his capacity to live alone, confirming the vulnerability his daughter had been warning him about since his wife died some years previously. It's true, his housekeeping and cooking had been rudimentary towards the end, but the flat had been a place he could really call his own. He still doubts whether moving into the so-called spare room in his daughter's house was wise. Sharing a living room with noisy grandchildren and knowing that his son-in-law resents his inability to eat tidily invades his peace of mind. Having to be bathed by his daughter doesn't seem right. He's alive and safe and looked after, but is this enough?

It is surely clear to any observer that the rights of these elderly people – to choice, to dignity in front of others, to privacy when they want it, to a fulfilling lifestyle – are not being achieved in practice. The concept of rights is a slippery one. To assert that someone has a right is very far from saying that they actually possess what they have a right to. Indeed, rights are most often claimed when they are threatened. It is wholly appropriate that we should be concerned for the rights of older people; our concern should be all the more acute when we see so many older people deprived of the benefits that possession of those rights would bring them.

DIFFERING VIEWS ON RIGHTS

There have been many attempts to set out the rights of older people in relation to the health and social services. One of Age Concern's best-selling, and regularly revised, publications rejoices in the straightforward title 'Your Rights'; its contents tabulate the entitlements of pensioners to a variety of social security and related benefits (West, 1995). The word 'rights' occurs very frequently in both the titles and text of publications written over the last decade (Harris and Hyland, 1979; Norman, 1980; Counsel and Care, 1993b). This is clearly an issue which has lately, and quite appropriately, preoccupied practitioners in the caring professions.

Two documents from Age Concern, both published in 1992 on the eve of community care implementation, set out statements of principles for the delivery of help in the home for older people, and the provision of day care services (Age Concern England, 1992a, b). The second of these summarizes the Age Concern basic principles for working with older people who need care: 'the right to a life which retains respect for him or her as an individual, and which retains independence, safeguards privacy, offers genuine and informed choices, encourages the forming and continuation of friendships, gives the chance to develop new skills and knowledge, and meets his/her social, cultural and individual needs'.

At more or less the same time, the Department of Health's Social Services Inspectorate published a handbook addressed to managers and others on developing quality standards for home support services (Social Services Inspectorate, 1993a). This detailed a different set of fundamental values. In summary, these were: autonomy and independence of decision-making; choice of lifestyle; respect for intrinsic worth, dignity and individuality; participation and integration in society; knowledge; fulfilment of personal aspirations and abilities; privacy; and equality of opportunity.

There is a similar profusion of statements of rights and values in relation to the residential field. Home Life, an enormously influential code of practice produced by a working party funded by the Department of Health in the wake of the Registered Homes Act in 1984, set the tone for a decade of writing about the quality of care in residential establishments (Centre for Policy on Ageing, 1984). Its opening chapter listed the rights of residents as fulfilment, dignity, autonomy, individuality, esteem, quality of experience, emotional needs, and risk and choice.

It is difficult now to understand how radical and thoroughgoing was this statement and how influential Home Life was in contributing to rising standards of care over the years which followed its publication. If it is to be faulted, it is for the failure consistently to relate the framework of rights it so boldly set out to its equally trenchant and detailed recommendations. The call for the phasing out of multi-occupied bedrooms, for example – quite a controversial demand at the time, which, however, has still not been achieved in full – was not set in the context of the initial value statement and therefore lacked the authority it merited. This weakness was not altogether corrected in 'A Better Home Life' published 12 years later (Centre for Policy on Ageing, 1996).

The Wagner Committee Report, an independent review of residential care commissioned by the Secretary of State for Health and Social Services, is open to the same criticism (National Institute for Social Work, 1988). Its recommendations concerned with 'the rights of the individual' repeat Home Life's call for single rooms along with detailed suggestions for trial periods, complaints procedures and the handling of financial affairs. These are sensible and worthy, but again they lack any underpinning framework of principles.

BASIC VALUES FROM THE DEPARTMENT OF HEALTH

This omission of a framework of principles was splendidly rectified by publication of Homes Are For Living In (Social Services Inspectorate, 1989). HAFLI, as it has come to be known, tabulates six fundamental principles, key values or basic rights: privacy, dignity, independence, rights of citizenship, choice and fulfilment. These should form the basis of an establishment's approach to the planning of its task, to the organization of its environment and to its relations with its clients.

Subsequent work within the Social Services Inspectorate relating to care in establishments has built on this approach to very good effect (Social Services Inspectorate, 1992a, b, 1993b). Although originally designed for local inspections of homes, the HAFLI rights make a logical basis for considering the quality of service provision and the quality of the lives of older people from various perspectives. Material has also been devised to make the framework one which is accessible to practitioners at all levels.

For example, on the basis of Homes Are For Living In, it is possible to develop a series of questions which can be asked by an inspector to assess the extent to which any one of the rights is given practical weight and value in a home's regime. In considering privacy, an inspector (or a manager, relative, service purchaser or prospective resident) may appropriately ask whether residents have private storage space for personal possessions or whether staff knock on the doors of residents' rooms and wait for a reply before entering. To assess the respect for dignity, one may ask whether all residents are dressed appropriately and have a choice in the name by which they are addressed by staff and introduced to visitors.

Similarly, Standards for the Residential Care of Elderly People with Mental Disorders includes practical suggestions for implementing each of the rights (Social Services Inspectorate, 1993b). For independence, for example, it proposes 'Encourage as much decision-making as possible'; for choice, it suggests 'Show users food, clothing and other objects to aid choosing'. Far from being merely an abstract statement of general principles, the Homes Are For Living In table of rights has become an operational device and a tool of highly practical use in aiming for high-quality care.

INCONSISTENCY IN STANDARD SETTING

It is regrettable that the HAFLI statement of rights has not become more generally accepted as the start of the process of standard setting for services for older people. A document setting standards for registration for domiciliary care produced in 1993, for example, reverts to Home Life's longer list of rights, and then fails to use them as anything other than an introductory statement (Joint Advisory Group, 1993). This much needed initiative therefore presents workers in the home care field with a starting point for setting quality standards which is structurally different from that used in residential care, although the issues are recognized to be very similar.

Even within the output of the Social Services Inspectorate, various tabulations of principles or values proliferate, many of them differing only marginally, but sometimes confusingly for hard-pressed practitioners, from those of HAFLI. The good practice statement in Developing Quality Standards for Home Support Services, for example, claims to 'synthesise common elements from a number of sources'; it then complicates the picture by covering much the same ground as HAFLI but under eight rather than six headings (Social Services Inspectorate, 1993a). The list starts with 'autonomy and independence'. If this is intended to imply that these qualities are distinguishable from each other, the difference is not explained. For fieldworkers with limited time, and perhaps limited energy for conceptualization, such complexity and lack of consistency is at best annoying, at worst seriously discouraging.

Other approaches to quality assurance use terminology similar to some of the HAFLI values but set them into different contexts even when the purposes appear to be almost exactly those for which the HAFLI framework was devised. The Research Unit of the Royal College of Physicians working with the British Geriatrics Society, for example, produced a series of guidelines and audit measures for long-term care for older people in 1992 (Royal College of Physicians, 1992a, b). The section on preserving autonomy is very close in spirit to the HAFLI work on independence. Other sections on continence, drug use, falls and accidents, pressure sores, the environment, equipment and aids, and the medical role in long-term care, although containing much useful material and practical advice, lack the sort of theoretical framework that enables a practitioner to review the totality of an establishment's regime and its impact on its residents. Perhaps this reflects the almost exclusively medical composition of the group concerned with the drawing up of the initial documentation, a bias happily corrected in subsequent work.

In another part of the forest of experts seeking to lay down systems for inspecting and assessing the quality of care in homes for older people, the National Association of Health Authorities and Trusts, the body which has responsibility for defining standards for the registration and inspection of nursing homes, has adopted a somewhat different system. NAHAT groups its questions defining 'the relationship between staff and the patient' under the broad headings of 'dignity; social needs; spiritual needs; social aspects of physical needs – food, sleep; recreational and diversional activities' (NAHA, 1988). Many of the questions in this list cover very similar territory to that subsequently surveyed in Homes Are For Living In. The groupings, however, are quite different, and the approach is focused much more on staff responsibilities than on patients' rights.

Practitioners engaged in work with older people are therefore faced with an array of advice on the principles that should form the basis of their practice. Although almost all of the formal statements of quality mention the rights of service users, their authors have come from a variety of directions and give differing emphases. Sometimes these derive from differences in professional backgrounds, sometimes from less definable, even arbitrary, factors. Under a welfare economy increasingly operating on free-enterprise principles, such richness and diversity is perhaps inevitable, and doubtless welcome to some, but it would be useful if the experts and advisors could now work more diligently than they seem to have done in the past towards some greater degree of consensus. The HAFLI framework probably provides the best starting point, as its definitions are widely accepted and used in welfare practice. It would be a pity if those coming from predominantly nursing and medical backgrounds were to continue to ignore HAFLI because of its origins in social work.

PRIVACY

Of all of the rights that older people should have, privacy is the one most easily defined: 'to be left alone, undisturbed and free from intrusion and public attention'. Privacy is immediately under threat for people who enter an institution. Research on residential care and nursing homes carried out in 1991 produced evidence of widespread sharing of rooms, residents having to use commodes in front of others often without even the protection of a screen or curtain, bathrooms and lavatories without locks (or having only locks without keys), limited private storage facilities, and restrictions on the use of even relatively private space (Counsel and Care, 1991).

Entering any sort of residential community involves some sacrifice of privacy, which makes the maintenance of what remains all the more important. Hospitals, with a history of large – even mixed – wards, a pattern of work based on expectations of relatively short stays, a tradition within which therapeutic demands take precedence over all other considerations, and rather rigid hierarchies and role definition, tend to score poorly for privacy. Nursing homes, with nurses perhaps carrying some of the culture of hospitals into supposedly more homelike environments, are sometimes not much better. Residential homes, and even sheltered housing schemes where the residents' ownership of their part of the facility is generally accepted and indeed enshrined in tenancy agreements, also often needlessly offend.

Privacy is by no means guaranteed for older people who remain in private houses, as disability brings the need to depend on others, sometimes for quite intimate functions. An older person who has to leave the front door unlocked to let in a home help or who has to be bathed by a stranger, perhaps of the opposite sex, necessarily has their privacy invaded. Caring services need to do all they can to compensate for this loss.

Privacy, however, is an ambiguous quality. It might indeed be said to be best preserved by total isolation, so privacy is best in moderation. The degree of privacy which is welcomed before it degenerates into oppressive loneliness is very much an individual matter. People living in their own homes are often left alone for long periods, and for some the effect is understandably depressing. Their privacy is assured, but at what price for their general quality of life? (Chester and Smith, 1995.) Some homes, drawing perhaps on the model of life in hotels, leave their residents relatively unattended, who, if they have few other visitors, may even feel unbefriended by staff. In contrast, others advertise their 'homeliness' although this can develop into annoying and constant intrusion. One man, for example, complained that he and his wife who had dementia were made to feel snobbish if they left the communal lounge to listen to music in their own bedsitting room.

DIGNITY

Dignity overlaps heavily with privacy, and perhaps too with independence. Recognition of one's intrinsic value, uniqueness and personal needs, and being treated with respect in all contacts are major features of dignity. An often quoted example is the freedom of residents to choose their own preferred style of address by staff, although, even in otherwise sensitive regimes, it is too often assumed that residents will never change their minds or do not want to vary the name by which they are known between different individuals. For older people from ethnic minorities, the maintenance of dignity demands that staff should be knowledgeable about and sympathetic to their specific cultural needs.

Carers, care staff and organizations providing care can do much to undermine, or alternatively to reinforce, the dignity of those they care for (Twigg, 1992). One valuable indicator is the extent to which a service user's previous life history and behaviour have been studied and taken into account. The partner of an Alzheimer's patient who had cared for his wife for seven years before she entered a home remarked on his surprise that the home's staff asked him nothing about her; this was an insensitive snub to a committed carer, but it was also evidence that the home paid little regard to elements of a new resident's background which may have been vital to her dignity. When a Jewish resident in a home died on the Day of Atonement, staff found themselves without any information on what steps they should take to respect the demands of his religion.

Older people with mental disorders may of course undermine their own dignity by, for example, failing to dress or present themselves appropriately, or in situations where they have lost control of aspects of their behaviour or their bodily functions. Here, it is the responsibility of staff or carers to help to restore damaged or forfeited dignity, perhaps through careful research into earlier lifestyles and sensitive persuasion to modify a way of behaving or a style of dress. The HAFLI definition of dignity neatly encapsulates this process: 'a recognition of the intrinsic value of people regardless of circumstances by respecting their uniqueness and their personal needs'.

INDEPENDENCE

It will immediately be apparent that to preserve dignity in such circumstances may involve some restriction on independence, a good illustration of the way in which rights are never absolute and frequently conflict with each other, so that balances have often to be struck. Independence is a quality much valued by older people, and the right they most often identify as threatened by ageing and its consequences. It is the failure of institutions – homes of all sorts and more particularly hospitals – to allow their patients and clients to retain reasonable degrees of independence which often makes them so hated and feared.

Many older people who are experiencing grave privation through disability cling to what they perceive as central to their independence, which often means trying to stay in their own homes. Even if their disabilities make them heavily dependent in other ways, their perception that power over their own lives would be fatally compromised by living in any sort of establishment is often a true one. People who move into the homes of friends or relatives, thinking such a setting will avoid the limitations of an institution, may find the sense of being on someone else's territory even more oppressive on a domestic scale. There are many sad stories of older people living with a loving daughter who find their presence hurtfully resented by the son-in-law or grandchildren.

There is much that residential and nursing homes can do to empower their residents, or at least to resist the disempowering effects of institutions and institutionalization. The facility to get up and go to bed at times that residents select for themselves, to entertain visitors whenever they wish, or to go out without having to tell anyone demand flexibility, generosity and perhaps courage on the part of the staff responsible. It needs also to be clear in the home's contract with its residents, and clear too to relatives, purchasers of services and the wider community, that the home does not accept total responsibility for those who live there since they retain at least a degree of accountability for their own actions.

This sort of independence should include the capacity to incur risks.

Risk-taking is an inevitable part of a full lifestyle, and homes cannot and should not attempt to provide a risk-free environment. HAFLI thus defines independence as 'opportunities to think and act without reference to another person including a willingness to incur a degree of calculated risk'.

Institutions, it needs to be remembered, have the capacity to institutionalize not only their residents but also their staff. Rules and regulations can proliferate, often ironically to no-one's benefit. Once set, the norms of an institution may be difficult to shift, even if many of those involved appear to want change. One home advertised that its residents were allowed, indeed encouraged, to entertain visitors at any time; all of the staff were aware of this arrangement and sincerely tried to make it a reality. However, a notice in the porch of the building stated the limited visiting hours that had once been in force. Staff who passed the notice frequently either failed to observe it or imagined that its non-operational status was somehow clear, but the visitors, who were the people most seriously affected by the out-of-date regulation, may well have taken it literally.

It requires constant and perceptive vigilance to strip institutions of their institutionalism. Generally, the larger and more contained they are, the greater the dangers. If homes and hospitals can remain permeable to the attitudes of the community outside, there is less chance that they will develop into worlds of their own. Relatives, visiting practitioners, students, entertainers, even tradespeople, have an important role in questioning practices which seem at odds with normality. Those within the system, however well-intentioned, can quickly lose this critical capacity.

RIGHTS OF CITIZENSHIP

It is easily assumed by agencies in the wider community that all of the needs of older people living in hospitals or homes are met within the institutions themselves. This of course is not true, and special efforts need to be made to ensure that patients and residents preserve as far as possible all entitlements associated with citizenship. Voting in elections, the use of public libraries, and access to mainstream health services are rights that may easily be lost to people living in establishments, partly because they may lack the boldness to demand them, and partly because the organizations responsible for supervising services easily overlook the less visible potential consumers. Older people from ethnic minority groups may find themselves particularly disadvantaged (Norman, 1985). Chiropody, dentistry, audiology and eye care are often, ironically, less readily available in homes than to older people living in their own homes. General practitioners' services may be restricted to the one doctor willing to visit that home, offering little chance to exercise the right to select a general practitioner that the health service theoretically offers.

Again, it should not be assumed that people who go on living in their own homes necessarily retain all of their civil rights. Mobility and access to information are critical constituents in the capacity to claim one's rights, and older people are often in a weak position in these areas. Those living with or intensively helped by a carer may have their options communicated through someone who thinks they know what the older person would want but is effectively filtering out the right to self-determination. Relatives and carers are not necessarily good advocates since they have agendas of their own, and on occasions their interests may diverge sharply from those of the person they care for, a point that the 1995 Carers (Recognition and Services) Act explicitly recognized.

CHOICE

In devising the arrangements for community care, the right to which legislators and planners most often referred was choice, i.e. the opportunity to select independently from a range of options. Providing a wider choice of services was seen as a central objective of the reforms. Choice, it was claimed, would flow from the creation of the mixed economy of welfare which was progressively to replace what was perceived as the near-monopoly supplier status of the NHS and local authorities. Social services departments, appointed as lead agencies in the provision of community care, were obliged to spend a high proportion of their available resources in purchasing services from independent sector providers, with the expectation that a greater diversity of provision would result. Indeed, one of the six key objectives of community care identified by the Department of Health was the promotion of 'a flourishing independent sector', so as to 'increase the available range of options and widen consumer choice' (Department of Health, 1989).

The market, however, proved an inadequate mechanism for ensuring that the consumer was in control, not least because the consumers' demands had to be both communicated through and rationed by care managers (Baldock and Ungerson, 1995). Indeed, in one important respect, the narrowing of choice had been built into the objectives of the re-organization. During the 1980s, places in residential care and nursing homes were funded, for those fulfilling the necessary financial criteria, through the social security system without any test of social need. The rather worthy argument then applied was that it was the task of an income maintenance agency to maintain income not determine how it was spent! The result, however, was what came to be known as the perverse incentive in favour of places in residential accommodation over the much more difficult-to-fund packages of domiciliary services.

The exposing of this anomaly by the Audit Commission and Sir Roy Griffiths formed the basis of the subsequent government action (Audit Commission, 1986; Griffiths, 1988). However, during the course of implementation of the legislation, concerns began to be expressed that some people who might previously have opted to go into a home would in future be denied this resource. The critical fear was that the necessarily local focus of local authorities and their strictly controlled financial resources would make it difficult for them to offer clients places outside their areas or of the required type and quality. The guidance on choice which swiftly followed by no means answered the anxiety that service options for older people had in some respects definitely narrowed. (Department of Health, 1992).

Of course, for many older people, effective choice is constrained not only by limits to what is provided but also by the nature of their own disabilities. A client with severe arthritis may no longer be able to engage in activities that demand dexterity or mobility. A disabled person in their own home may be dependent on a carer to help them get up and wash, which could limit the hours at which such tasks are accomplished to within the carer's tightly constrained schedule. Several research studies have demonstrated that high proportions of older people who have entered residential care or nursing homes experienced the decision as having been taken by someone else, they themselves having exercised little or no choice over either the move itself or over the selection of the home (Counsel and Care, 1992).

FULFILMENT

Privacy, dignity, independence, rights of citizenship and choice – if these are all constrained what chance is their of achieving fulfilment, the sixth of the rights listed in Homes Are For Living In? Fulfilment is the most idiosyncratic of the rights. While it is reasonable for each of the other rights to devise general questions which establish the extent to which that right is preserved or eroded, this process only makes sense for fulfilment if the questions are individualized to the situation of each client. A lifestyle consists of a patchwork of hobbies, activities, likes and dislikes, aspirations, memories and so on, and true fulfilment allows for the full expression of each of these. Carers and caring agencies thus need to study the particular elements which would contribute to a sense of fulfilment for individual clients. There is no way in which fulfilment, defined in HAFLI as 'the realisation of personal aspirations and abilities in all aspects of daily life', is amenable to generalization; its essence lies in personalized detail.

This apparently obvious truth is nevertheless one missed by many institutions. A degree of communal provision is perhaps an inevitable element to life in any home or hospital, but the extent to which individuals are still sometimes robbed of their individuality is frightening and reprehensible. Within living memory, many long-stay units provided only communal clothing for their patients; some, it is reported, even failed to individualize dentures and hearing aids (Robb, 1967). But too many homes still provide very few opportunities for activities for their residents, and the sight of a sitting room offering nothing but a circle of chairs and a flickering television set to its bored occupants is not uncommon. Some homes provide only very limited menu choices at mealtimes, no opportunity for new residents to furnish their own rooms, limited access to paramedical and community health services, and low paid and undermotivated staff who can provide residents with little more than a custodial and basic care service.

This is greatly to be regretted. For many elderly people living alone or with a carer in an inadequately resourced setting, life in a home of good quality could offer splendid new opportunites, providing precisely the positive choice of which Lady Wagner and her colleagues dreamed (National Institute for Social Work, 1988). Many older people at home are lonely, but a residential home potentially provides plenty of company. The effects of the loss that often accompanies ageing can be substantially alleviated by the companionship of fellow residents; supportive interaction between residents is indeed a much neglected resource. The imminence of death may be easier to face in an environment where counselling and sensitive discussion are easily available. Imaginative and resourceful homes provide many opportunities for participation in group activities including exercise, games, outings, crafts and cultural events (Counsel and Care, 1993a). There are many examples of homes which have successfully modified their regimes to accommodate minority tastes. One home in a coal-mining area, for example, provides breakfast early each morning for a small group of residents who are ex-miners and who like to rise in line with life-long habit at 4.00 a.m.

Responding as sensitively and flexibly as that to the needs of individual clients requires well-developed listening and assessment skills in carers and caring staff. One elderly woman entering a home was very depressed, not an unusual state following the trauma of a move, the loss of home and possessions, and the sudden shift of relationships. Staff talked with her and found eventually that she was particularly missing the garden she had known and loved. Acting swiftly, they went to the house in which she had lived, and, only hours before its sale was negotiated, dug up a selection of plants and replanted them outside her new bedroom window. A link between the old and new chapters of her life was thus firmly forged, and the right to have a past and to have it recognized and respected immediately reinforced.

To help clients with dementia communicate requires even more highly developed skills, including the willingness to explore unconventional ways of stimulating the senses of those with damaged brain functioning (Chapman *et al.*, 1994). An elderly man with Alzheimer's disease in a home was regularly visiting the room of a female resident in the middle of each night, frightening and annoying her. Nocturnal wandering by such clients is not uncommon, but to understand the objective of obviously anti-social behaviour requires thoughtful analysis, and certainly not an immediate jumping to conclusions. In many homes, restraint – mechanical or chemical – would be the immediate resort. In this case, careful observation revealed that the only purpose of the strange nightly journey was to look at the lady's clock; providing the man with a clock of his own so that he could tell the time from the comfort of his bed immediately resolved the problem. Enhancing his independence incidentally preserved his fellow resident's dignity.

SECURITY

Useful as the HAFLI rights are in reviewing the quality of life of an older person or the quality of the environment provided to care for them, they seem to ignore one crucial factor – the vulnerability of older people to danger. When carers and care staff talk about their task, this is the quality in their clients or patients to which they most often refer, and the need to provide protection is often perceived as overriding all other considerations. Bedrooms and lavatory doors which lack locks clearly threaten privacy, but, it is argued, a confused older person might lock themselves in and what then? In contrast, doors of living areas are often firmly secured, denying their occupants the independence to wander at will, a precaution justified by the perils – real or imagined – that they would face if they escaped to the world outside. Many regimes offer no activities involving risk or unpredictability, but it is argued that, given the frailty and vulnerability of older people, safety must come first.

Such caution is not to be dismissed out of hand. In asking to be admitted to a home or to enter any sort of arrangement for care, an older person is acknowledging honestly their need for something beyond what they could entirely provide for themselves. Recent research has demonstrated that a predominant factor in the psychology of entering a home is fear: fear of living alone, fear of street and neighbourhood crime, fear of falling, fear of being ill, fear of loneliness, fear even of being harmed by a carer (Department of Health, 1994). For such clients, a residential care or nursing home is indeed a refuge, almost, to resurrect an old and now somewhat devalued word, an asylum.

It is clear that we need to identify a seventh right to encapsulate this aspiration. It might be called security, the right to an environment and support structure which provides comfort, readily available assistance when required, and reasonable protection from danger. Clients seeking security are entering into a contract which involves a degree of caring surveillance. This is not the routine use of sedating drugs, imprisonment in restraining chairs or beds, or the imposition of a regime totally devoid of risk, but the willingness of staff or carers to come swiftly when assistance is needed, advice and help with personal safety, even if necessary a modest degree of restraint in perilous situations in which a client might not exercise wise judgements of their own. Establishments need clear policies on these matters and the subject needs to be covered in the individual care plan of each resident (Counsel and Care, 1993b).

Ensuring that sort of positive security may involve some trade-off of other rights such as independence and privacy, but such are the balances to be struck. Carers and the staff of establishments providing care need to be ready to help their residents decide their personal priorities by giving individual weightings to the rights they value. Hospitals generally have a poor record in preserving or restoring the rights of their patients, which is why they usually form unsuitable environments for long-term care. Experience of the lack of autonomy that patients experience in hospital gives many potential candidates for care in a home an expectation of similar deprivation.

ASSESSMENT

When the new arrangements for community care were introduced in 1993, it was recognized that accurate assessment of clients would be central to the appropriate provision of services. Assessment had previously too often consisted of fitting an older person into a pre-existing pattern of services. The new system was to turn this arrangement on its head by giving priority to identifying the needs of clients and then devising services which met those needs. This did not prove an easy task (Social Services Inspectorate, 1993c).

Practitioners lack a framework for structuring the needs they encounter other than by the remedies they know about. Thus, the essentially stigmatizing process of requiring the clients to rehearse their need for help continues. They may be accorded a more dignified status than mere providers of information, but a comprehensive setting out of their needs remains the ultimate objective (Smale and Tuson, 1993). A more radical analysis of aims and roles is required for the end users of services to achieve anything like the dignity and power enjoyed by consumers in more conventional commercial environments, which is the alleged aim.

If those undertaking assessment would use the rights of older people instead of their needs as the starting point, a true revolution in service provision could begin to take place. The questions to a potential consumer become not 'what do you need?' or 'what services do you need?', but 'are the rights you should be enjoying protected or eroded by your way of life?' and 'what can we do to enhance, or at least preserve, your rights?'. Such a formulation would transform assessment from a gatekeeping to an empowering process.

REGISTRATION AND INSPECTION

Inspection and regulatory systems should, and often do, adopt an approach to homes based on a list of the rights that residents should enjoy. The framework of rights outlined in Homes Are For Living In was devised to give those inspecting residential care homes a system from which to derive standards to assess the care provided in the establishments they visit. Over recent years, many other systems of internal audit of care procedures and quality assurance have been devised, for example by the King's Fund (King's Fund Organizational Audit, 1996). However, a major criticism of some of these systems is that they are often not grounded in the sort of theoretical framework that a stronger reference to the rights of residents would provide.

Regrettably, despite strong pressures from within the industry, the government has resisted the creation of a comprehensive system of inspection for domiciliary care services, leaving clients in their own homes in some ways more vulnerable to poor standards of care than those in institutions. It should certainly not be assumed that, because independence is nominally assured for a client remaining at home, their other rights are sufficiently attended to. Dependence on informal or professional carers can lead to major invasions of privacy and dignity. Living alone in an environment characterized by a diminishing social circle, few opportunities for new experiences and little access to external stimulation, can result in a lifestyle very far from any concept of fulfilment.

AGEISM

Older people, it needs to be frankly stated, face massive discrimination in our society. Practices of the sort which would be socially quite unacceptable, and probably also illegal, in the fields of gender and ethnicity, are accepted without criticism in advertising, personnel and the media in praise of youth and in disparagement of old age.

Attitudes towards older people in service delivery systems often echo these prejudices. Why is it, for example, that homes with 50, 100, or more places are still being built to accommodate older people, many of whom have or will develop dementia? Research evidence clearly indicates that mentally frail clients suffer worse confusion in such inevitably institutional environments, and such large units have long been discarded for other groups with clearly similar needs such as adults with learning difficulties

(Chapman *et al.*, 1994). How can it be justified that expenditure per week on a child in public residential care is over twice the sum allowed for nursing homes fees for an older person needing constant care? Why are the promoters of otherwise laudable schemes to involve consumers in service planning so often satisfied with participation by younger physically disabled people, leaving older customers unrepresented? (Hoyes *et al.*, 1994). It is difficult not to draw the conclusion that the traditions of the Poor Law and the workhouse are by no means erased from contemporary policies (Walker, 1995).

INDIVIDUAL PLANNING

How then should an older person who feels their situation to be vulnerable plan a future? For all except those requiring specific short-term medical treatment, the sort of care that used to be provided by the NHS and which was free at the point of delivery has now almost disappeared, with the result that any sort of care is likely to have to be paid for. Only those without significant income and with very low levels of capital can expect any subsidy towards care costs. Fees in residential care and nursing homes, even at minimum levels, are likely to run down the resources of all but the richest clients.

The case for expanding community care used to include the expectation that caring for clients in their own homes would be cheaper than the cost of residential places. The equation, it is now generally agreed, is considerably more complex, and for highly dependent people, assembling a comprehensive package of domiciliary care services can be extremely costly. 'Packages of care', a convenient professional term, conceals the intricacies of the arrangements needed to achieve satisfactory co-ordination of services, particularly when – as is often the case – many agencies, accountable to different hierarchies of management, are involved. The complicated structure of the social security benefits system and the diverse patterns of charging for or subsidizing services make the arithmetic even more difficult to summarise.

Where cost considerations can be ignored, clients' preferences between long-stay hospitals, residential homes and their own homes almost invariably favour the domiciliary option. Of course the choice is wider and still widening, including sheltered and very sheltered housing, schemes with varied forms of tenancy, leasing or freehold ownership, residential care, nursing or dual-registered homes, and a wide variety of home caring arrangements including differing patterns of partnership between informal, voluntary, private and statutory services. The addition of respite care, providing relief to carers and a change of regime or location for the older person in need, creates further permutations.

Although this diversity is designed theoretically to provide varying forms of care for varied levels of dependency, many older people who enter the system remain with approximately the initially chosen pattern of care until they die. It is a tribute to the flexibility of many homes that they ignore the over-fine distinctions drawn between their respective functions and in the process protect clients who become more disabled from a succession of disruptive moves. Similarly, some carers cope admirably with apparently impossible burdens of care, and some older people insist on sustaining their independence with amazing extremes of fortitude.

Long-stay hospital provision has been largely discredited as a way of caring for older people. This derives largely from the failure of nursing and medical regimes within highly structured and institutionalized settings to address the needs of patients in terms which recognized their wider rights as people. Some of the stigma of the institution attaches still to other forms of residential care, although many units now provide a style of life for their residents which responds to their desire for continued autonomy, and many residents, even some who entered care reluctantly, report life in a home to be dignified and fulfilling. Care at home, although widely considered by practitioners and potential service users alike as the naturally preferred option, has more drawbacks than are sometimes acknowledged: isolation, low levels of stimulation, poor access to facilities and high risk among them.

Inadequate advice on what is available, uncertainties over resources, misinformation about services, ancient prejudices, critical media coverage, or the inaccurately reported experiences of others may add to the confusion of an older person in need of help. Theoretically, the mixed economy of welfare has widened the choice available, but it is not yet clear whether older people are always able to make wise and informed choices between the diverse services which should be available to them.

REFERENCES

Age Concern England (1992a) *Home Help and Care: Rights, Charging and Reality*, Age Concern England, London.

Age Concern England (1992b) *Standards in Day Care Services*, Age Concern England, London.

Audit Commission (1986) *Making a Reality of Community Care*, HMSO, London.

Baldock, J. and Ungerson, C. (1995) *Becoming Consumers of Community Care: Households within the Mixed Economy of Welfare*, Joseph Rowntree Foundation/Community Care, London.

Centre for Policy on Ageing (1984) *Home Life: A Code of Practice for Residential Care*, HMSO, London.

Centre for Policy on Ageing (1996) *A Better Home Life: A Code of Good Practice for Residential and Nursing Home Care*, Centre for Policy on Ageing, London.

Chapman, A. Jaques, A. and Marshall, M. (1994) *Dementia Care*, Age Concern England, London.

Chester, R. and Smith, J. (1995) *Older People's Sadness*, Counsel and Care, London.

Counsel and Care (1991) *Not Such Private Places*, Counsel and Care, London.

Counsel and Care (1992) *From Home to a Home*, Counsel and Care, London.

Counsel and Care (1993a) *Not Only Bingo*, Counsel and Care, London.

Counsel and Care (1993b) *The Right to Take Risks*, Counsel and Care, London.

Department of Health (1989) *Caring for People: Community Care in the Next Decade and Beyond*, HMSO, London.

Department of Health (1992) *Local Authority Circular, LAC (92)27*, Department of Health, London.

Department of Health (1994) *The F Factor*, HMSO, London.

Griffiths, Sir R. (1988) *Community Care: Agenda for Action*, HMSO, London.

Harris, D. and Hyland, J. (eds) (1979) *Rights in Residence*, Residential Care Association, London.

Hoyes, L., Lart, R., Means, R. and Taylor, M. (1994) *Community Care in Transition*, Joseph Rowntree Foundation/Community Care, London.

Joint Advisory Group of Domiciliary Care Agencies (1993) *Standards for Registration for Domiciliary Care*, Joint Advisory Group, London.

King's Fund Organizational Audit (1996) *Nursing Homes: Organizational Standards and Criteria*, King's Fund, London.

National Association of Health Authorities (1988) *The Registration and Inspection of Nursing Homes (Supplement)*, National Association of Health Authorities and Trusts, Birmingham.

National Institute for Social Work (1988) *Residential Care: A Positive Choice (The Wagner Committee Report)*, HMSO, London.

Norman, A. (1980) *Rights and Risks*, National Corporation for the Care of Old People, London.

Norman, A. (1985) *Triple Jeopardy: Growing Old in a Second Homeland*, Centre for Policy on Ageing, London.

Robb, B. (1967) *Sans Everything*, Nelson, London.

Royal College of Physicians and British Geriatrics Society (1992a) *High Quality Long-Term Care for Elderly People*, The Royal College of Physicians of London, London.

Royal College of Physicians (1992b) *The CARE Scheme (Continuous Assessment Review and Evaluation)*, Royal College of Physicians of London, London.

Smale, G. and Tuson, E. (1993) *Empowerment, Assessment, Care Management and the Skilled Worker*, National Institute for Social Work/HMSO, London.

Social Services Inspectorate (1989) *Homes Are For Living In*, HMSO, London.

Social Services Inspectorate (1992a) *Update of Homes Are For Living In*, HMSO, London.

Social Services Inspectorate (1992b) *Caring for Quality in Day Services*, HMSO, London.

Social Services Inspectorate (1993a) *Developing Quality Standards for Home Support Services*, HMSO, London.

Social Services Inspectorate (1993b) *Standards for the Residential Care of Elderly People with Mental Disorders*, HMSO, London.

Social Services Inspectorate (1993c) *Inspection of Assessment and Care Management Arrangements in Social Services Departments*, HMSO, London.

Twigg, J. (ed) (1992) *Carers: Research and Practice*, HMSO, London.

West, S. (1995) *Your Rights*, Age Concern England, London.

Walker, A. (1995) *Half a Century of Promises*, Counsel and Care, London.

Quality of life: assessment and improvement

8

INTRODUCTION

Those providing long-term care would no doubt agree that the aim is to give the patients or residents the best possible quality of life. However, just as there will be universal agreement as to this general goal, there will be a thousand and more views on just what this means and how it should be achieved. In this chapter I shall attempt to answer four questions: why measure quality of life, how can it be defined, how can it be measured, and how can such measures be applied to the evaluation of long-term care?

THE NEED FOR MEASUREMENT

It is an unfortunate paradox that the more successful we are in raising standards, the more difficult it becomes to demonstrate that what we are doing is effective. If our standards of care are so appalling that we fail to feed people adequately, then we can measure any improvement in terms of basic physiological parameters. We can, for example, use mortality rates just as we might when examining the treatment of a potentially fatal illness. However, if we assume that we are already meeting the patients' basic bodily needs so that, for example, they are not dying of starvation, measuring outcome solely in terms of mortality is unlikely to be appropriate. We know that there is more to good care than this but how do we define and measure this?

In measuring the outcome of acute care, we can judge our success in terms of measures such as the average length of stay or the number of patients treated. The better our care, the shorter the stay or the more patients receiving treatment. Quite the opposite trend will be true of long-term care. The better our care, the longer will people live, and the lower the numbers receiving care in that particular ward or home. In the care of long-stay patients, our outcome measures must be much more wide-ranging and are necessarily a little more difficult to construct.

We cannot use these difficulties as an excuse for not assessing the efficacy of long-term care. There is no universally held concept of what constitutes 'high-quality care' or what steps should be taken to achieve this. It is no good simply assuming that other people will agree with us in what we think is an effective method for improving care. Even if most of our contemporaries do share some such view, later generations may show us all to be wrong. The history of care in general, and medicine in particular, is littered with outmoded treatments that were once thought to be effective.

The scientific progress that has achieved so much in acute care depends at its core on evaluating different treatments and altering our management accordingly. This is important both to see that the treatment works and to see that it does no harm. In the case of long-term care, the side-effects of a change in pattern of care are unlikely to be serious, at least in terms of mortality, although even here there may be exceptions. However, it is just as important that we ensure that we do no harm in other respects such as emotional well-being.

Perhaps even more importantly, the needs of long-term patients have always to be met from the finite resources available. If we are successfully to argue that resources should be devoted to some new form of care, or just to more of an existing type of care, we must justify the effort and expense. The cool breeze of evaluation grows ever stronger and it is no longer enough for an 'expert' to say 'We need more money for . . .' for resources to be made available. It is necessary to show what the outcome is and how effective a particular method is in achieving this.

It is widely recognized that the measurement of efficacy is a considerable problem in health care. This is true for many different types of care but none more so than that which concerns us here. Perhaps because of this, the parameters that have been used to evaluate care depend at least as much on how easy they are to measure as on their relevance to outcome.

Indeed, health care as a whole has not very often been described in terms of outcome at all. More often it has been described in terms of the input of resources and the process of care. This is more easily understood if we draw a comparison with the evaluation of a manufacturing business. Let us suppose that, instead of providing long-term care, we were running a factory making teapots. In this case we have a clear aim in mind, namely to maximize our profit. This we can do by selling as many teapots as possible at as high a price as we can. We need to balance the price against sales but at least we know that if we are successful, the bottom line, net profit, will increase. Contrast this with long-term care. We are often in possession of only a vague idea what we are producing. I would suggest that a good quality of life might be one way of describing this. However, this is difficult to measure so we look for other ways of measuring what we do. We may look at the number of staff we employ, the cost of the food or some other measure of input. This describes our service but no more so than would detailing the amount of clay or electricity we use in making our teapots each year.

We may look then at the number of times we bath people or the time we spend talking to patients. These tell us about the process of care, but again, this is only like counting the number of teapots we decorate each year or how many enquiries we get from customers. It does not indicate directly any effect on outcome. If we are making lots of teapots and then simply storing them in a big warehouse, we will not be making much profit.

The answer in the end must be to measure outcome, although not simply in terms of the number of patients treated, as this is not the right measure for long-term care. We must decide on a definition of what it is that we are really trying to do and measure this.

THE AIM OF LONG-TERM CARE

The ultimate aim of nearly all care for older people is quality rather than quantity of life. In practice there is rarely any conflict between these two goals, although when this does arise it is quite usual for people to assert that it is quality that is the more important. Thus, if we are to evaluate the efficacy of our interventions, we must look for improved quality of life as one, if not the most important, yardstick.

As is all too often the case, the thing that seems to be most important as a measure of outcome is also that which it is most difficult to define, let alone measure. However, this should not deter us because how we approach these issues can reveal much of what we hold at the centre of our philosophy of care. To try to duck the issue, for example to measure only the process of care rather than its outcome, can be a particularly dangerous failing. We may have a set of procedures, a pattern of care which in its individual elements is excellent but which, as a whole, quite fails to achieve its overall aim.

WHAT IS QUALITY OF LIFE?

Asserting the importance of quality of life as an outcome measure rather begs the question, 'What is it?'. We all have some notion of what it is but might find it hard to put this into words. The sort of words that are used to define quality of life include independence, privacy, choice, dignity and freedom of action. A life which is short of all or any of these is not seen to be very good. In evaluating the quality of life of those receiving medical care, we also need to include things such as freedom from pain and disability.

Just as we may find it easier to measure inputs and processes rather than outcome, so many of the attempts to define quality of life include parameters that are thought to be related to quality of life rather than being direct measures of this construct. Adams (1969) defined quality of life as the degree of satisfaction or dissatisfaction felt by individuals about various aspects of their lives. Such a subjective element is surely crucial to any definition of quality of life. Likewise, Ziller (1974) saw self-esteem as central, and Andreas (1974) related quality of life to the extent to which pleasure and satisfaction characterized peoples' lives.

Havighurst (1963) took a slightly broader view, including both inner factors concerning the individual's subjective view of life and external factors such as the nature and extent of behaviours such as social contact and other activities. We do know, however, that mood and activity are by no means simply related. Low levels of activity do not, for example, necessarily imply depressed mood (Simpson *et al.*, 1981).

The measure of subjective experience is always difficult, and quality of life is no exception. There are problems of response bias, where there is a tendency to use only certain points on a rating scale, typically the mid-point or the extremes. Likewise, there may be demand characteristics whereby the subjects tell the interviewer what they think the interviewer wants to hear. Responses to questions aimed at assessing a presumably fairly stable construct such as quality of life may be influenced by short-term variables such as mood state.

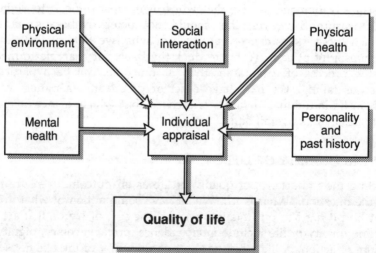

Figure 8.1   Factors that influence quality of life: a causal model.

In addition to all of these problems, there may be cross-cultural, including socio-economic, differences in how individuals view quality of life. A question which works well for retired North Americans may mean something quite different to older British men and women.

None of these, however, are reasons for abandoning any attempt to measure quality of life. Rather, they suggest ways in which we must be fastidious in both developing and applying measures. This is of course true of all measurement, be it psychological or physiological.

Despite all these difficulties, we can identify a number of factors that influence quality of life. These are each important and can be represented in a causal model as shown in Figure 8.1. This model includes several known determinants of life satisfaction, such as physical health, and allows for the influence of personal and mental health factors on individual appraisal. The assumption being made here is that quality of life depends ultimately on how individuals perceive their own lives. Thus it can only ever be this perception, and the factors influencing this, that we can hope to measure.

MEASURES OF QUALITY OF LIFE

It will come as no great surprise to find that there have been many and varied attempts to measure this elusive concept. Some have been designed to measure the concept itself; others, perhaps the majority, have focused on those parameters that are thought, or known, to be related to it.

HEALTH MEASURES

It is well known that one of the best predictors of well-being in later life is health status. It is at least as important, for example, as money in predicting how people feel. Thus many workers have chosen to look at measures of health in order to measure quality of life. This is particularly relevant to the care of long-stay patients who, almost by definition, have suffered some major deterioration in their physical or mental health.

MORTALITY AND SURVIVAL

At the high reliability end of the measurement spectrum must surely be the binary measure 'dead or alive'. It has, despite its obvious inelegance, many virtues to recommend it. In particular, the data are generally easy to collect and there is little or no disagreement about which is the desired outcome value.

On the negative side, it is not always clear whether length of life is necessarily compatible with quality. This is particularly the case in the evaluation of treatments such as those for cancer (Clark and Fallowfield,

1986). On the other hand, there is some evidence that psychometric variables, particularly those relating to cognitive function, are related to time until death in older people (Botwinick *et al.*, 1978). Similarly, it is well-recognized that the early mortality following admission to institutional care may be very high. This is in part, of course, because those who have to be so admitted are among the frailest of those in the population. However, effects of the institution can also be demonstrated following such a move. The topic of relocation and its effects on mortality in older people has been the subject of considerable study, often using survival data as the most important measure. Early studies seemed to show almost universal bad effects from relocation and led some to conclude that this should be avoided whenever possible. Later studies have, however, shed more light on this phenomenon, and a more balanced view would seem to be appropriate (Nirenberg, 1983). It seems that relocation may have either good or bad effects. This depends on such things as whether the individual makes the move out of personal choice, and on the benefits of the receiving environment. Having to move to a deprived environment without preparation can be very bad. Good preparation and, just as important, attention to improving the environment, can have positive benefits including increased survival.

PERCEIVED HEALTH

As with quality of life, one's own perception of one's health is at least as important in determining well-being as objectively defined medical status. Several studies have shown, for example, that such perception of one's own health is a significant predictor of life satisfaction (Palmore and Luikart, 1972; Spreitzer and Snyder, 1974), the measurement of which I will consider in more detail later. Furthermore, it appears that self-assessed health is especially important in settings where there is less choice and individual autonomy (Wolk and Telleen, 1976). It seems therefore reasonable to suppose that good health, or more accurately, thinking you are in good health, is an important determinant of quality of life.

Several scales have been developed to measure general health status, although in some cases this has been for quite different purposes. Both the Cornell Medical Index (Brodman *et al.*, 1951) and the General Health Questionnaire (Goldberg, 1978) are concerned with perceived health as an initial measure of personal well-being. One aim has been to screen people for psychiatric morbidity. In so far as this tends to pick up psychological distress as well as frank mental illness, such measures may seem to have relevance to measuring quality of life. This is probably a fair assumption, but the higher prevalence of physical dysfunction in older people, or indeed any in long-stay care, can rather invalidate the usual norms and cut-offs. Thus, for example, the first factor on the General Health Questionnaire relates to somatic complaints. In a general population of younger people living at home this may be a good way of screening for distress. In older and frailer groups it may simply reflect concurrent illness.

Whilst chronic physical illness is related to risk of depression (Murphy, 1982), not even the majority of those with such illness are depressed. Just because you have some physical symptoms does not mean that you have a poor quality of life. Nonetheless, it is true to say that assessing physical health is a very important dimension in evaluating any care programme and has been included in such studies (Kane and Kane, 1981). Improving someone's overall physical health is likely to be perceived as increasing their quality of life.

Of course, such health assessments are not necessarily self-ratings. For example, whereas the Guttman Health Scale (Rosow and Breslau, 1966) assesses health in relation to day-to-day functional activities by means of a self-administered questionnaire, the Stockton Geriatric Rating Scale (Meer and Baker, 1966) relies on ratings made by others such as nurses. The latter has been modified and combined with some simple measures of cognitive function to provide a general picture of dependency (Pattie and Gilleard, 1979). These Clifton Assessment Procedures for the Elderly (CAPE) have been validated on a wide range of older people. The results show both differences between groups in various settings, for example at home, in residential care or in hospital, and considerable overlap between them. Again, however, it seems reasonable to suppose that a lower level of dependence allows more autonomy, and that achieving this should be part of improving quality of life.

The items on the Stockton Geriatric Rating Scale and its derivative relate to basic tasks such as bathing, dressing and eating, to the presence of disturbed behaviour such as wandering or withdrawal, and to cognitive difficulties – for example, those affecting communication. As such, they give rather a coarse measure of overall function that is better suited to the description of groups of people than to the evaluation of individual ability. Moreover, the factors on the shortened scale seem to be different from those of the original (Twining and Allen, 1981).

For individuals, the use of a more detailed assessment of the activities of daily living and mental state is much more likely to be appropriate. This is included in many sets of procedures such as OARS (Duke University Center for the Study of Ageing and Human Development, 1978), CAMDEX (Roth et al., 1988) and others (Lawton, 1971). In all of these procedures, there is an attempt not simply to assess an individual's basic physical abilities but also their application to the ordinary everyday activities that enable each of us to function independently. These include physical activities such as walking, bathing and dressing, together with other skills such as cooking, handling money and using public transport. It can been seen that, in respect of quality of life, these abilities are permissive, i.e. they define the limits of independence. Of course, the individual's ability to make choices, which is central to most ideas of a high quality of life, depends not simply on physical capacity but also on the availability of prosthetic aids and the person's ability to use these. Thus, someone who is physically unable to walk may, given the correct aids and environment, be able to get around very well with minimal help. Someone with less of a physical limitation may have poorer functional ability because of mental or environmental factors. If you need someone there to prompt you to make a cup of tea, you may be just as dependent as someone who needs physical help to do this.

How the measurement is carried out can make quite a lot of difference to the results. Occupational therapists take great care to match the surroundings to the individual's personal circumstances. It is no good expecting frail older people to perform at their best with a gas cooker when they have always used an electric one. Home assessment has much to commend it, and by 'home' we may mean the nursing home, residential home or hospital ward.

MENTAL HEALTH

Besides physical capacities and environment, the individual's mental state is a very important determinant of their activities and their own perception of their quality of life. It has already been noted that how we feel about our own health can be used as a screening tool for mental health problems. The two most common mental health difficulties for older people are of course depression and dementia. These have both similar and very different implications. Depression is generally the more common, especially in younger old people, for example those aged under 75. It could in many ways be seen as a fairly direct measure of quality of life since we would be unlikely to say that someone with marked dysphoria has a good quality of life. Even if all the other variables are positive, their depressed mood will be reflected in their seeing things differently. In marked depression, they may seek to end their life because they feel it is no longer worth living.

There are several ways that depression can be identified, ranging from an extensive structured assessment of mental state such as the Geriatric Mental Status Schedule (Copeland et al., 1976), through specially designed screening scales (Yesavage et al., 1983) and severity ratings (Hamilton, 1960), to checklists aimed at assessing mood which may or may not be a part of formal depressive illness (Beck et al., 1961; Zung, 1965). There has even been an attempt to measure happiness formally (Kozma and Stones, 1980). Given that we are concerned here with general well-being, and not just with mental illness, the latter would seem to offer more use as a means of measuring whether we are achieving a good quality of life for our clients. Put simply, if we offer people a better quality of life, we would expect them on the whole to feel happier.

Of course, the most common reason for this not happening is the other major mental illness of late life, namely dementia. Again, there are very many ways of assessing the severity of cognitive impairment, varying from a lengthy research tool such as CAMDEX (Roth *et al.*, 1988) to brief questionnaires examining mainly orientation and memory. For a brief, but slightly wider ranging, assessment there are procedures such as CAPE (Pattie and Gilleard, 1979) and the Mini Mental Status Test (Folstein *et al.*, 1975).

The real problem with dementia is of course that it affects the individual's appraisal of their situation, which is of course crucial to that person's understanding of their quality of life. Not only does this make it difficult to use self-report measures, it can produce all kinds of discrepancies between what that person thinks of their life and the way that others view things. Thus people suffering from dementia may be distraught even when well cared for in their own home because they no longer recognize it as such. Conversely, someone who, before developing dementia, was fiercely independent and solitary may show a 'personality change' and appear quite contented sitting doing nothing on a crowded, run-down hospital ward. It can be very hard to know how we are to define what that individual sees as a good quality of life in such cases.

Not surprisingly we tend to come to some sort of compromise and to apply those standards which, dementia notwithstanding, we think lead to a better quality of life. However, we need to be flexible and to recognize that not only is each dementia sufferer an individual but that their needs can and most likely will change over time. We need to be sensitive to each individual's right to choose, even if that means that they do not join in the wonderful activity which we have so carefully designed to improve their quality of life. Even the inarticulate need to be allowed to vote with their feet.

ENGAGEMENT

Although it may seem obvious that someone can be happy without doing things, it is by no means always perceived to be so. Studies of frail older people and others, such as persons suffering from a mental handicap, have shown that, in institutions, there is very little going on. This is seen as a bad thing, and, on the whole, such a generalization seems reasonable. Most of us find our lives more satisfying if we are doing things. Certainly, depressed people tend to do less than people who are not depressed.

As far as institutions for frail older people are concerned, the lack of activity should not surprise us. When people are in their own homes, the greater proportion of their time is taken up by sleeping and 'obligated time', that is cooking, cleaning, bathing and so on. When one takes away the need to do these latter tasks, doing nothing and sleeping are what tend to remain.

If inactivity is bad, then activity must be good. Following such logic seems to have left some workers determined to demonstrate that frail older people can do things if given the opportunity to do so. There have been careful attempts to measure the extent to which people do things, including talking to other people, and such measures are generally referred to as measurements of 'engagement'.

However, much of this work originates from studies of those with a mental handicap, and the translation to older people is not always appropriate. Although it may be quite possible to show that, given the opportunity and encouragement, older people in a residential home will do things like polish coins (Jenkins et al., 1977), it is not clear whether they feel better for this. Such a suspicion is confirmed by work showing that engagement and depression are not inversely correlated in such residents (Simpson et al., 1981). Some people are quite happy to spend a lot of time simply sitting and thinking. The lesson here must be that, if we are to use non-verbal activity measures to assess quality of life, we must complement this by measuring such things as covert reminiscence.

LIFE SATISFACTION

There is good reason to believe that how people feel about their past life relates to how they feel now. Although not all old people spend a lot of time reminiscing, many do, and for many of these people it is a pleasurable activity (Coleman, 1986). Certainly, the comparison with how things used to be is a useful way of judging how you feel about life now. The other way of judging things now is how one's own life compares with others of the same age.

Both these comparisons figure strongly in the most well-known measures of life satisfaction in old age. Neugarten et al. (1961) published two approaches to the measurement of perceived quality of life which have been strongly influential in very many subsequent studies. The measures they developed, the Life Satisfaction Indices, consisted of a series of self-ratings and a set of ratings by an interviewer on the basis of a structured interview. Both of these measures were designed to assess five areas of life satisfaction, namely:

- zest for life
- resolution and fortitude
- congruence between desired and achieved goals

- level of self-esteem
- happy, optimistic mood.

The self-assessment questionnaire has been the more widely used, and several authors have suggested amendments. Bigot (1974) reported that a shorter eight-item questionnaire was sufficient, and that this seemed to measure two components: acceptance/contentment and achievement/fulfilment.

It is worth noting here that another study (Wood *et al.*, 1969) has indicated that there may be marked age and gender differences in the validity of Life Satisfaction Indices. These authors correlated the results from the questionnaire with ratings made by trained observers following a lengthy interview. There was a much higher correlation between the two types of measures for those aged over 70 years and for men. The authors were using the ratings to assess the validity of the questionnaires, and these results do pose some interesting questions. Why should it be that interviews disagree more with the self-ratings of women and the younger elderly? It is of course legitimate to argue that the self-ratings may be 'correct' and that all this shows is how useless trained inter-viewers are. However, this does little to help solve the knotty problem of validity.

One other problem with the original measures, for British workers at least, is that they are written in American rather than in English. Luker (1969) made some amendments for use with a British population but concluded that further refinement might be justified. These differences in language may be of more than passing interest. Some studies have suggested, for example, that British samples tend to show higher levels of life satisfaction than do North American ones. However, it is very hard to judge the significance of this when correctly adjusted forms have not been used.

Lohmann (1977) compared the results of using no less than seven different measures of life satisfaction, some being the familiar question-naires, some being measures of morale (e.g. Kutner *et al.*, 1956), and one being a simple global self-rating (How satisfied are you with your life now?). There was at best only a modest correlation between this rating and the other measures. The size of this correlation varied according to the number of items in the questionnaire. This may indicate that, as Neugarten *et al.* and subsequent authors have found, life satisfaction is multi-dimensional, and that to reduce it to a single number is to simplify beyond utility.

Studies originating in Britain (Abrams, 1973; Andrews and Withey, 1974; Hall, 1976) have also started from a large pool of items and identi-fied a smaller number relating more directly to life satisfaction. The most common areas relating to life satisfaction were family, home life, marriage and health. The longer the interval since the last visit to the doctor, the higher the life satisfaction.

Retirement perhaps has less impact on life satisfaction than we might imagine, although obviously the amount of income for those on a pension is a significant factor. Indeed, only about 10% of those who are retired have significant problems in adjusting to this transition (Braithwaite and Gibson, 1987). Similarly, overall, the effects of housing and leisure activities seem to be lower down the priority order in determining how older people feel. Of course, some of these may be cohort effects, i.e. how you feel now depends on when you were born, how you were brought up, and what you have been used to. This could, for example, explain partly the findings in relation to Life Satisfaction Indices and interview ratings to which I referred earlier. The views of the younger old people may, by virtue of their experience, be closer to those of the interviewers. Such a hypothesis does not bode well for the future. It suggests that as we achieve ever higher standards of material well-being, we may become progressively more reluctant to put up with material deprivation in later life. Such a shift, the logical conclusion of ageing and consumerism, could have at least as strong an effect on the demand for resources as any change in the numbers of very elderly people.

THE ENVIRONMENT

Studies of older people in hospital have shown that the greatest causes of dissatisfaction tend to be interpersonal rather than physical aspects of the environment. Thus, Raphael and Mandeville (1979) found that the furniture, ward and sanitary accommodation were rated by elderly patients as being the most satisfactory, while diversional activity, noise and nurses' care gave most cause for complaint or irritation. The one exception to this general rule was that day-space was also rated as a source of dissatisfaction, although even this may reflect problems in terms of the social effects of inadequate day-space. In this study, staff were also asked to give their views on the satisfaction, or otherwise, of aspects of hospital life. Interestingly, there was no correlation between the rank ordering of topics by staff and patients. This does not bode well for staff trying to act as patient advocates.

Certainly the physical environment is important, not only for its direct effect on residents but indirectly via its influence on staff. The direct influence on residents' social interaction has been demonstrated in terms of the arrangement of furniture (Peterson et al., 1977) and the layout of day-space (Harris et al., 1977). The latter study showed that the arrangement of space influenced the interaction of residents in old people's homes and that residents themselves are, as we always knew, a powerful force. In particular, their work demonstrated the vulnerability of mentally frail older people. The prime space, i.e. the day-spaces nearest to day-to-day activity, was dominated by mentally alert residents who effectively segregated themselves from the confused. The latter were confined to day areas away from the mainstream of activity, thus compounding their handicap. However, as we might expect, whatever the design of the home, the attitudes and policies of the staff were of crucial importance.

Indirectly, the environment affects residents by way of its influence on staff behaviour, recruitment and morale. Knapp and Harissis (1981) have shown that the likelihood of there being vacancies among the supervisory staff in a home is related to the size of the home, the amenities it offers, and its contact with the rest of the community. A small home with plenty of amenities and an adequate supply of toilets, and which provides meals-on-wheels for the surrounding community, is less likely to have problems in recruiting senior staff.

Of course, there may need to be a balance struck between the philosophy of 'small is beautiful' and the economies of scale. An Israeli study (Weihl, 1981) showed that the 'functionally independent elderly' tended to be more satisfied if they lived in homes with more than 90 places. To take one example, the author suggests that the greater level of satisfaction with personal friendships found in the larger homes may be because the residents have a larger pool of persons from whom to find a kindred spirit. The difficulties to be found in maintaining good personal relationships in some small group homes tend to confirm that this could be a valid point.

Nonetheless, there are many arguments in favour of smaller units – perhaps not least because of the influence this has on staff behaviour and attitudes. In a small unit, staff will find it much easier to see each person as an individual rather than as an anonymous member of a large group. This may not matter much for the functionally independent, but it is very important for the very frail. They must depend to a much greater extent on others for their preservation of individuality and the opportunity to exercise choice and control.

It should be clear by now that consideration of 'the environment' for long-stay older patients must include both the physical surroundings and the social milieu of both fellow patients and staff. Of these three areas, there is no doubt that it is a lot easier to measure the first rather than the second and third. Very few people are not familiar with how to use a tape measure and a thermometer. Conversely, many would have trouble knowing how to begin measuring social climate or staff policy. It may be this which has led to much greater emphasis being given to the physical aspects of care. Nonetheless, attempts have been made to take a broader approach and these deserve to be more widely applied.

In Britain, the significant expansion in private sector residential and nursing homes has meant that much more attention has been paid to the registration and monitoring of such homes. Detailed guidance has been given as to how local authorities should assess residential homes (Centre for Policy on Ageing, 1996) and how health authorities should assess nursing homes (National Association of Health Authorities, 1985).

The code of practice for residential care, Home Life (Centre for Policy on Ageing, 1984), includes a checklist of 218 items covering five topics: social care, physical features, client groups, staff and registration. The first of these, social care, actually includes a third of all the items in the checklist and more than twice the number covering physical features. This seems a reasonable balance in view of what we already know of the importance of interpersonal interaction to residents' well-being. This checklist is not, of course, a measurement instrument in its own right. It cannot be compared with a tape measure or a thermometer. However, it does provide a most useful guide to checking on an institution, whether this is for the formal purpose of legal registration or for other reasons.

If we are looking to measure the environment of elderly people, one instrument is available which does offer more than a checklist of features. The Multiphasic Environmental Assessment Procedures (MEAP) (Moos and Lemke, 1984a, b) have been developed from studies of older people in institutional care, and they provide both a conceptual framework for the evaluation of these environments (Moos, 1980) and a set of measuring instruments. The scales comprising the instruments cover five topics. The first four are measures of the institutions based on the reports of residents and staff, and the fifth is a set of ratings for use by an outside observer covering the same areas. The four dimensions measured by the scales are physical features, policy and programme factors, resident and staff characteristics, and social climate. There have been many studies on North American groups using these scales, and these studies have demonstrated good discrimination between different homes and allow for the design of appropriate intervention programmes (e.g. Lemke and Moos, 1980; Moos and Igra, 1980; Brennan et al., 1988). Because the scales consist of parallel forms for completion by residents, with help where necessary, and by staff, it is possible to compare and contrast these different views of each setting. In addition, the social climate scale has separate forms for the residents to rate the real (what is this home like now?), the ideal (what would an ideal home be like?) and the expected (what do I think it will be like when I move to this home?). This enables major discrepancies to be identified and allows prospective residents to express their expectations of the intended home.

Social climate is an important area of care. When frail older people ask for advice on choosing a home, it is rarely in terms of judging whether it looks pleasant or is adequately heated. These things they can generally judge fairly quickly for themselves on the basis of a brief visit. What is much more helpful to them is some indication of how warm and friendly is the atmosphere. Because this is usually based on loose subjective impression, this is just the sort of information that professionals are reluctant to impart. Use of this kind of structured measurement could help a great deal.

Similar approaches have been used to look at the problems of those with long-term psychiatric disability (Wing and Brown, 1970). Of course, by no means all of these people are elderly, but the problems of achieving a good quality of life are in many ways similar. Provided ideas are chosen carefully with the client group in mind, they may come from a wide variety of sources.

It is also easy to see how these kinds of techniques can be used to evaluate care and suggest change. Quality of life for residents and patients is the most relevant outcome measure for long-term care. How do we bring about positive change?

IMPLEMENTATION AND EVALUATION

We saw earlier (Figure 8.1) how a number of factors may be seen to influence quality of life. These are not neatly independent in practice, but considering them separately does help us to consider the options in a manageable way. Thus it is also useful to take the same structure and examine some of the ways in which improvement can be brought about.

Before turning in detail to each area, however, it is worth pausing to remind ourselves of some of the general principles of change that are relevant. Psychology can help us not only to understand how clients change but also how to bring about changes in what staff do. First we must remember that change is more noticeable than the status quo. Our nervous systems are built to detect change, be it movement, sound, touch or taste. We rapidly adapt to the world around us and focus our attention on what changes – not what stays the same. This habituation to things which stay the same is very important in helping us to cope with the great complexity of the world. It helps us to keep things manageable and stops us coming to harm. However, in the context of long-term care it can be a mixed blessing. We can rapidly become unaware of problems, inadequacies or even bad practice when we stay a long time in one place. Most of us can remember what impression a large old hospital made the first time we walked through the door. The sights, the noise and the smell may well have moved us greatly, and probably not for the better. We find this kind of experience stressful and may have difficulty sifting the important information from the irrelevant detail. Unfortunately, if we work in that setting, we rapidly adjust to the situation. Even things that should give us cause for concern no longer attract our attention. What really is a grubby wall in need of a coat of paint can fade into the background. However, for those who are coming into that setting for the first time, be they new staff, patients or relatives, the impression will be much closer to that which we first had and then have forgotten. Somehow we have to try and keep that sensitivity alive and turn it to our advantage.

Similarly, many of the abilities and even the clinical condition of patients in long-term care change only slowly. It may be very hard to pick out a threshold which can alert us to someone needing extra help until the change, whether it be positive or negative, is quite pronounced.

Conversely, if we are trying to change some way of doing things then that change will stand out a mile, however minor the thing we seek to change. For example, even rearranging the chairs to facilitate social inter-action may be resisted both by residents and staff. This resistance may arise not because the change is for the worse but just because it is change. We have to think actively about how to bring about change and how to maintain it.

Change is unsettling. Indeed, in the case of the enforced relocation of frail older people, there is some evidence to suggest that it may, if handled badly, be fatal. Change can be threatening, especially if it is seen as being imposed from outside. We all need to feel that we are in control of at least a substantial portion of our lives. If we find that constantly we are out of control we may become increasingly helpless or indeed frankly depressed. People who believe that they make things happen generally feel much better that those who feel that the outside world determines what happens to them. These general principles apply both to staff and to residents or patients. Both are powerful groups who play a crucial role in what happens in long-term care. Those who are not with change are against it, and few innovators can achieve much if there are many who are opposed. Bearing these principles in mind, we can now consider the various factors, some internal, some external, which influence quality of life, and what can be done to improve these.

THE PHYSICAL ENVIRONMENT

From the examples that have already been given, it is clear that the physical environment is both easy to measure and yet difficult to change. Certainly there are plenty of instruments available, and it is at least possible to set standards and to determine whether these are being achieved. We have explicit guidance available both in the form of the kinds of checklists mentioned earlier and in the building notes and regula-tions published by bodies such as the Department of Health (DHSS, 1980).

Of course, whereas such notes tend to ensure that buildings do not fall down or are not otherwise actively dangerous, they do not in themselves ensure a homely environment which supports appropriate individual and social behaviour. Such guidance is rather more complex but can nonetheless be developed (DHSS, 1976). That these matters ought to be considered carefully need hardly be emphasized. Buildings are important and remarkably enduring. Could the Victorian Britons who designed and built so many workhouses and asylums have foreseen just how many older peoples' lives their work would dominate and for how long? However many times you change the wallpaper, and however many sanitary annexes you build on, a ward in a lunatic asylum still looks like a series of large rooms at the end of long corridor. There are some situations where the right agents for meaningful change must be the bulldozer and the pneumatic drill.

In designing and evaluating environments we must ensure that the needs of the particular client group are properly considered. Those with physical frailty may need compact accessible facilities, while those with mental frailty may need plenty of room to wander. It may be impossible to achieve both, and priorities must be decided. If we do not know what we are trying to achieve, we are unlikely to be successful.

PHYSICAL HEALTH

In the case of physical health, there are likewise well-established techniques for measuring outcome. In the case of long-term care, however, it is important to be aware of potentially conflicting priorities. A simple literature search of medical publications yields a very respectable number of studies which explicitly consider the concept of 'quality of life'. However, closer examination reveals that many, indeed possibly the majority, of these papers relate to terminal care, especially the care of those suffering from cancer. At first this may seem a little disappointing, since the issues in the care of older people are very much broader than just the management of terminal care. However, these studies do address one of the recurring questions, namely, how to balance the benefits of applying treatment – for example, the relief of pain or the prolonging of life – against possible adverse effects (such as unpleasant side-effects or pain arising from invasive procedures).

Evaluation of the outcome of physical health care in long-term settings must include the measurement of phenomena such as pressure areas and contractures and whether there is an appropriate balance between quality and quantity of life. Of course, this begs the question: who is to decide? Here, the answer is not simple, and indeed no one person, not even the physician, can decide alone on the best course of action for each and every patient. Nurses, relatives and, most importantly, the patients themselves have a contribution to make. Perhaps the only thing that can be definitely stated is that care which gives good quality of life must include opportunities for these difficult issues to be considered. Nobody involved, including the patient and family, should feel either excluded or left to decide such matters alone.

SOCIAL INTERACTION

Mention has already been made of how important this is in promoting well-being. It is a fairly simple matter to measure what is, or is not, going on in a long-term care setting. This may take the form of simply noting the programme of activity that might give opportunity for interaction, or, in much more detail, using behavioural methods such as event or time sampling. One word of caution here is that low levels of interaction are the norm, and one must not be too ambitious in trying to achieve change. It is very easy to carry out such measurement and produce a report highly critical of staff, managers and even patients. Staff are very often all too well aware of what is lacking. What they need is help to put things right.

The other important points to remember are that the lack of observable activity is, as we have already seen, no indication of individual client dissatisfaction, and that activity should be meaningful – especially if it is designed to promote social interaction.

The remaining influences on quality of life may be broadly described as being more internal rather than external. They relate particularly to psychological processes and, therefore, psychological approaches are of particular relevance (Twining, 1988).

MENTAL HEALTH

Improving the mental health of older people mostly means alleviating depression and minimizing the effects of dementia. Of these two, the more intractable is undoubtedly dementia – although there is good evidence that depression often goes unrecognized in both the physically frail in hospital (Robinson and Price, 1982; Lim and Ebrahim, 1983) and among older people in the community (Murphy, 1982).

Approaches to dementia have tended to concentrate on the development of reality orientation programmes which have become very popular in recent years (Holden and Woods, 1988). There are some question marks regarding the efficacy of this in overcoming the deficits of dementia (Powell-Procter and Miller, 1982), although there may be some gains to be made in the attitudes and behaviour of staff. Much the same could be said of other interventions for the severely confused. Matters such as personalized clothing and the encouragement of personal belongings can be seen as having two major effects. First, they give the patient or resident a sense of identity, familiarity and security, and second, they help the staff to see that person as an individual with an unique history. The resulting change in staff behaviour is likely to be just as important as the rather small and relatively short-term gains in orientation.

One way of helping staff to see people as individuals and to improve their interactions with the patient is to ensure that detailed information is available on each resident or client. A detailed personal history form can be useful for this purpose.

Reminiscence has also been the focus of a good deal of attention and has, like reality orientation, generated much enthusiasm (Coleman, 1986). It is a common, but by no means universal, activity among older people, and can generate both positive and negative emotions. By drawing on the considerable past experiences of older people, it can provide at least a valuable meaningful activity and, under careful guidance, be the means of psychological therapy.

INDIVIDUAL APPRAISAL

The relationship between cognition and emotion has likewise been shown to be of great value in enhancing well-being. There has been what can only be described as an explosion of work in psychological therapy, much of it soundly based on psychological knowledge and experimental evaluation (Woods and Britton, 1985). The techniques have the potential for application not only to frank disorder, notably anxiety and depression, but also for the promotion of positive adjustment to a wide range of life events. No doubt admission to long-term care could be included in this, but, as yet use in this situation remains to be developed.

There is also the need to develop advocacy schemes similar to those being promoted in the care of those suffering from mental handicap. This would enable the interest of frail older people to figure more in the determination of care.

PERSONALITY AND PAST HISTORY

Being rooted in the past, personality and past history may not seem to be amenable to change and therefore not directly relevant to the improvement of quality of life. However, they do have a very significant impact on how individuals adjust to different settings. Thus we should at the very least give these weight in trying to provide the right sort of long-term care for individual older people.

Again, there may be special problems in the case of those suffering from dementia or other acquired brain damage. Such disorders can lead to considerable personality change and, as a result, a form of care which previously would have been rejected outright may now be the most suitable for current needs. We have to remain flexible in our approach, not only to provide for the wide range of individual differences but also to allow for individuals to change over time.

THE ROLE OF MANAGEMENT

Good management is vital to the success of any complex enterprise. In the case of long-term care, this includes monitoring that care and the implementation of change. There are very many ways of achieving this, but most involve some form of generating ideas and providing appropriate feedback to staff. The specific project may have almost any title, including Positive Monitoring (Porterfield, 1987), a Merit Gram Scheme (Reingold *et al.*, 1987), the introduction of residents' committees (Wells and Singer, 1988), or the use of a staff training programme (Open University, 1988).

Ultimately, promoting a good quality of life may be seen by some as best achieved by the introduction of performance-related funding. The studies by Kane *et al.* (1983a, b) have at least tackled some of the methodological issues which must be addressed if this is to be feasible. In particular they make the point that patient outcome depends on patient condition. Thus, any evaluation of care must take into account the initial level of function of those receiving care. Care must be evaluated as better or worse than expected for such clients if we are to avoid automatically rewarding those who provide care only for the least in need.

Whether this or some other approach proves to be possible and effective remains to be seen. For the present, we must seek to consider all those things which may indicate quality of life and to ensure that these are central to our assessment of the outcome of the care that is provided.

CONCLUSIONS

By now it is probably clear to even the most optimistic reader that there is no easy answer to the question 'what is quality of life?', nor is there any single simple way of measuring this (Gill and Feinstein, 1994). We live and work in a world where the benefit of compromise often outweighs that of pursuing the ideal. It is therefore reasonable to put philosophy temporarily to one side and to suggest which of the available approaches seem the most useful.

As there are several dimensions to quality of life, a short combination of measures seems best. Thus it is appropriate to choose:

1. a self-report measure either of mood (e.g. Beck *et al.*, 1961; Yesavage *et al.*, 1983), life satisfaction (Bigot, 1974) or happiness (Kozma and Stones, 1980);
2. a measure of behaviour or activity either from observation (Simpson *et al.*, 1981) or by the completion of an activity timetable showing the pattern of the residents' days each week;
3. a measure of the environment based on a checklist (Centre for Policy on Ageing, 1984) or a rating scale for social climate (Lemke and Moos, 1980).

Obviously it is also possible to use one of the comprehensive packages (Moos and Lemke, 1984a, b; Kane and Kane, 1981) but these are time-consuming and are likely to appeal only where personnel are available to spend quite a lot of time on their completion.

Whatever the situation, it is clear that there is no excuse for not making at least some attempt to address the fundamental question 'How successful are we in providing a good quality of life for those under our care?'

REFERENCES

Abrams, M.A. (1973) Subjective social indications. *Social Trends*, **4**, 35–56.

Adams, D.L. (1969) Analysis of a life-satisfaction index. *J. Gerontol.*, **24**, 470–4.

Andrews, F.M. (1974) Social indicators of perceived life quality. *Social Indicators Res.*, **1**, 279–99.

Andrews, F.M. and Withey, S.B. (1974) Developing measures of perceived life quality: results from several national surveys. *Social Indicators Res.*, **1**, 1–26.

Beck, A.T., Ward, C.H., Mendelson, M. *et al.* (1961) An inventory for measuring depression. *Arch. Gen. Psychiatry*, **4**, 561–7.

Bigot, A. (1974) The relevance of American life satisfaction indices for research on British subjects before and after retirement. *Age Ageing*, **3**, 113–21.

Botwinick, J., West, R. and Storandt, M. (1978) Predicting death from behavioral test performance. *J. Gerontol.*, **33**, 755–62.

Braithwaite, V.A. and Gibson, D.M. (1987) Adjustment to retirement: what we know and what we need to know. *Ageing Society*, **7**, 1–18.

Brennan, P.L., Moos, R. and Lemke, S. (1988) Preferences of older adults for physical and architectural features of group living facilities. *Gerontologist*, **28**, 84–90.

Brodman, K., Erdmann, A.J., Lorge, I. and Wolff, H.G. (1951) The Cornell Medical Index – health questionnaire. *JAMA*, **145**, 152–7.

Centre for Policy on Ageing (1984) *Home Life: A Code of Practice for Residential Care*, Centre for Policy on Ageing, London.

Centre for Policy on Ageing (1996) *A Better Home Life: A Code of Good Practice for Residential and Nursing Home Care*, Centre for Policy on Ageing, London.

Clark, A. and Fallowfield, L.J. (1986) Quality of life measurements in patients with malignant disease: a review. *J. R. Soc. Med.*, **79**, 165–9.

Coleman, P.G. (1986) *Ageing and Reminiscence Processes*, Wiley, Chichester.

Copeland, J.R.M., Kelleher, M.J., Kellett, J.M. and Gourlay, A.J. (1976) A semi-structured clinical interview in the elderly: the geriatric mental status schedule. 1. Development and reliability. *Psychol. Med.*, **6**, 439–49.

DHSS (1976) *A Life Style for the Elderly*, HMSO, London.

DHSS (1980) *Hospital Accommodation for Elderly People, Draft Building Note No. 37*, HMSO, London.

Duke University Center for the Study of Ageing and Human Development (1978) *Multidimensional Functional Assessment: the OARS Methodology, A Manual*, The Center for Ageing, Durham, NC, USA.

Folstein, J., Folstein, S. and McHugh, P. (1975) Mini-mental state. *J. Psychiat. Res.*, **12**, 189–98.

Gill, T.M. and Feinstein, A.R. (1994) A critical appraisal of the quality of quality-of-life measurement. *JAMA*, **272**, 619–26

Goldberg, D. (1978) *Manual of the General Health Questionnaire*, NFER-Nelson, Windsor, UK.

Hall, J. (1976) Subjective measures of quality of life in Britain, 1971–1975: some developments and trends. *Social Trends*, **7**, 47–60.

Hamilton, M. (1960) A rating scale for depression. *J. Neurol. Neurosurg. Psychiatr.*, **23**, 56–62.

Harris, H., Lipman, A. and Slater, R. (1977) Architectural design: the spatial location and interactions of old people. *Gerontology*, **23**, 390–400.

Havighurst, R. J. (1963) Successful ageing, in *Process of Ageing: Social and Psychological Perceptors* (eds R.H. Williams, C. Tibbits and W. Donahue), Atherton Press, New York.

Holden, U.P. and Woods, R.T. (1988) *Reality Orientation: Psychological Approaches to the 'Confused' Elderly*, Churchill Livingstone, Edinburgh.

Jenkins, J., Felce, D., Lunt, B. and Powell, E. (1977) Increasing engagement in activity of residents in old peoples' homes by providing recreational materials. *Behav. Res. Ther.*, **15**, 429–34.

Kane, R.L. and Kane, R.A. (1981) *Assessing the Elderly: a Practical Guide to Measurement*, DC Heath Lexington, MA, USA.

Kane, R.L., Bell, R., Riegler, S. *et al.* (1983a) Assessing the outcomes of nursing-home patients. *J. Gerontol.*, **38**, 385–93.

Kane, R.L., Bell, R., Riegler, S. *et al.* (1983b) Predicting the outcomes of nursing home patients. *Gerontologist*, **23**, 200–6.

Knapp, M. and Harissis, K. (1981) Staff vacancies and turnover in British old peoples' homes. *Gerontologist*, **21**, 76–84.

Kozma, A. and Stones, M.J. (1980) The measurement of happiness: development of the Memorial University of Newfoundland scale of happiness. *J. Gerontol.*, **35**, 906–12.

Kutner, B., Fanshel, D., Togo, A.M. and Donovan, J.D. (1956) *Five Hundred Over Sixty*, Russell Sage Foundation, New York, USA.

Lawton, M.P. (1971) The functional assessment of elderly people. *J. Am. Geriatr. Soc.*, **19**, 465–81.

Lemke, S. and Moos, R. (1980) Assessing the institutional policies of sheltered care settings. *J. Gerontol.*, **35**, 96–107.

Lim, M.L. and Ebrahim, S.B.J. (1983) Depression after stroke: a hospital treatment survey. *Postgrad. Med. J.*, **59**, 489–91.

Lohmann, N. (1977) Correlations of life satisfaction, morale and adjustment measures. *J. Gerontol.*, **32**, 73–5.

Luker, K.A. (1969) Measuring life satisfaction in an elderly population. *J. Adv. Nurs.*, **4**, 503–11.

Meer, B. and Baker, J.A. (1966) The Stockton Geriatric Rating Scale. *J. Gerontol.*, **21**, 392–403.

Moos, R. (1980) Specialized living environments for older people: a conceptual framework. *J. Soc. Issues*, **36**, 75–94.

Moos, R. and Igra, A. (1980) Determinants of the social environments of sheltered care settings. *J. Health Soc. Behav.*, **21**, 88–98.

Moos, R. and Lemke, S. (1984a) *Multiphasic Environmental Assessment Procedure (MEAP): Manual*, Stanford University Medical Center, Palo Alto, CA, USA.

Moos, R. and Lemke, S. (1984b) *MEAP Supplementary Manual: Ideal and Expectation Forms*, Stanford University Medical Center, Palo Alto, CA, USA.

Murphy, E. (1982) Social origins of depression in old age. *Br. J. Psychiatr.*, **141**, 135–42.

National Association of Health Authorities (1985) *A Code of Guidance for the Inspection and Registration of Nursing Homes*, NAHA, London.

Neugarten, B.L., Havighurst, R.J. and Tobin, S.S. (1961) The measurement of life satisfaction. *J. Gerontol.*, **16** 134–43.

Nirenberg, T.D. (1983) Relocation of institutionalized elderly. *J. Consult. Clin. Psychol.*, **51**, 693–701.

Open University (1988) *Working with Mental Health Problems in Old Age*, Open University, Milton Keynes, UK.

Palmore, E. and Luikart, C. (1972) Health and social factors related to life satisfaction. *J. Health Soc. Behav.*, **3**, 68–80.

Pattie, A.H. and Gilleard, C.J. (1979) *The Clifton Assessment Procedures for the Elderly*, Hodder and Stoughton, London.

Peterson, R.G., Knapp, T.J., Rosen, J.D. and Pither, B.F. (1977) The effect of furniture arrangement. *Behav. Ther.*, **8**, 464–7.

Porterfield, J. (1987) *Positive Monitoring*, British Institute of Mental Handicap, Kidderminster, UK.

Powell-Procter, L. and Miller, E. (1982) Reality orientation: a critical appraisal. *Br. J. Psychiatr.*, **140**, 457–63.

Raphael, W. and Mandeville, J. (1979) *Old People in Hospital*, King Edward's Hospital Fund, London.

Reingold, J., Grossman, H.D. and Burros, N. (1987) Merit Gram: a form of recognition in a long-term care setting. *Gerontologist*, **27**, 147–9.

Robinson, R.G. and Price, T.R. (1982) Post-stroke depressive disorders: a follow-up study of 103 patients. *Stroke*, **13**, 635–41.

Rosow, I. and Breslau, N. (1966) A Guttman health scale for the aged. *J. Gerontol.*, **21**, 556–9.

Roth, M., Huppert, F.A. Tym, E. and Mountjoy, C.Q. (1988) *The Cambridge Examination for Mental Disorders in the Elderly*, Cambridge University Press, Cambridge.

Simpson, S., Woods, R.T. and Britton, P.G. (1981) Depression and engagement in a residential home for the elderly. *Behav. Res. Ther.*, **19**, 435–8.

Spreitzer, E. and Snyder, E.E. (1974) Correlates of life satisfaction among the aged. *J. Gerontol.*, **29**, 454–8.

Twining, T.C. (1988) *Helping Older People: a Psychological Approach*, Wiley, Chichester.

Twining, T.C. and Allen, D.G. (1981) Disability factors among residents of old people's homes. *J. Epidemiol. Community Health*, **35**, 205–7.

Weihl, H. (1981) On the relationship between the size of residential institutions and the well-being of residents. *Gerontologist*, **21**, 247–50.

Wells, L.M. and Singer, C. (1988) Quality of life in institutions for the elderly: maximizing well-being. *Gerontologist*, **28**, 266–9.

Wing, J.K. and Brown, G.W. (1970) *Institutionalisation and Schizophrenia*, Cambridge University Press, Cambridge, UK.

Wolk, S. and Telleen, S. (1976) Psychological and social correlates of life satisfaction as a function of residential constraint. *J. Gerontol.*, **31**, 89–98.

Wood, V., Wylie, M. and Sheafer, B. (1969) An analysis of a short self-report measure of life satisfaction: correlation with raters' judgements. *J. Gerontol.*, **24**, 465–9.

Woods, R.T. and Britton P.G. (1985) *Clinical Psychology with the Elderly*, Croom Helm, London.

Yesavage, J.A., Brink, T.L., Rose, T.L. *et al.* (1983) Development and validation of a geriatric depression screening scale: a preliminary report. *J. Psychiatr. Res.*, **17**, 37–49.

Ziller, R.C. (1974) Self–other orientations and quality of life. *Soc. Indicators Res.*, **1**, 301–10.

Zung, W.W.K. (1965) A self rating depression scale. *Arch. Gen. Psychiatr.*, **12**, 63–70.

Community care

9

INTRODUCTION

As far as older people are concerned, 'the primary objective of depart-
mental policies . . . is to enable old people to maintain independent lives
in the community for as long as possible. To achieve this high priority is
being given to the development of domiciliary provision and the encouragement of measures designed to prevent or postpone the need for long
term care in hospital or residential homes' (DHSS, 1978, p. 13). Thus, it is
argued, the care of older people is a responsibility that should be shared
by all and is not one that solely involves statutory services. Community
care is the policy by which, it is hoped, this objective of helping older
people to live independent lives within their homes for as long as possible
can be achieved.

In this chapter, we briefly review the development of community care
policy, describe the current system for the provision of community care,
consider some of the factors that influence the need for community
care by older people, describe the current levels of service provision and
consider the relationship between the formal and informal sectors in the
provision of care to older people in the community. Issues concerned
with institutional provision, the methods of entry into long-term care and
the characteristics of those people in this sector are not covered as they
are considered elsewhere in this book. This chapter deals exclusively with
the situation in the UK. However, it is important to remember that many
of the issues noted in this chapter, such as the relationship between the
formal and informal sectors, may also be observed throughout Europe
and indeed further afield. Policy debates about community care and
older people are therefore not confined to the UK but are taking place
upon a much wider stage (see Scharf and Wenger, 1995; Challis *et al.*,
1994).

WHAT IS COMMUNITY CARE?

With the implementation of the community care reforms in 1993, it is easy to assume that community care was 'invented' or 'created' in 1993. In fact, this is a term which has been in use amongst policy makers for a considerable period. The precise origin of the term remains obscure. Bulmer (1987) observes that the first official use of the term was in 1957 and related to the field of mental illness. Development of the policy of community care during the late 1950s in Britain was fuelled by a reaction against the provision of care for the long-term chronically ill in communal or institutional settings. Institutions were perceived as inhumane, therapeutically ineffective, and, perhaps most importantly, expensive. In the field of long-stay care for older people, Townsend's book 'The Last Refuge' (1957) carefully documented the appalling conditions that older people resident in these settings had to endure. In contrast to the almost inevitable failings of long-stay provision, community care is seen as being both more effective and efficient as well as a more appropriate way of providing care for those who require support on a long-term basis (Means and Smith, 1994).

What does community care really mean? Walker (1982) observes that the term community care implies support for the person by their friends, family and neighbours, an emphasis on non-institutional types of care, the provision of domiciliary statutory services and appropriate measures to prevent (re)admission to institutional forms of care. However, whilst the terminology has remained constant, the meaning of the term community care has undergone a subtle transformation over the decades, which has profoundly altered the reality of the policy. Bayley (1973) first suggested the useful distinction between care in the community and care by the community. Care in the community implies the use of statutory resources provided in clients' own homes. This manifestation of community care implies a significant input by state services. Care by the community is associated with the mobilization of resources from within the community such as voluntary organizations and informal carers such as friends, neighbours and kin. In this guise, the main responsibility is seen as being taken by the community, with statutory services being used only in extreme circumstances. This distinction was formally recognized by the government in the 1981 White Paper 'Growing Older', with the statement that '. . . care in the community must increasingly mean care by the community' (DHSS, 1981, p. 3). These multiple meanings and interpretations give the term community care a lack of precision and clarity. This makes it possible for political parties of all persuasions to argue in favour of this policy.

The distinction introduced above implies two distinct models of community care. First there is the notion of the community using its own resources to provide care via family and friends as well as voluntary and locally based formal services, and second the idea that the community's resources will be supplemented by external sources, e.g. national government. Increasingly in Britain, statutory services are seen as being used as the last resort in the care of older people; the care of older people is being placed firmly within the domain of the family and the informal sector. We will return to the issue of informal carers later in this chapter.

THE ESSENTIAL ELEMENTS OF COMMUNITY CARE

Although the precise meaning of the term has altered over the years, it remains possible to isolate several key features that define community care. As noted earlier, in its original manifestation, the term was used to mean care outside large institutions such as hospitals or long-stay facilities. A second key element is the provision of services and care in the client's own home (or in as homely a setting as possible). Third is the idea of providing care in as normal i.e. non-institutional, a setting as is possible given the needs of clients. Fourthly, there is emphasis on the involvement of members of the community in the care of those with long-term care needs. As indicated above, the balance between these different elements has varied over time and between the type of client group.

RECENT COMMUNITY CARE POLICY DEVELOPMENTS

Overall, there has been a broad political and social consensus over the past 40 years about the appropriateness of community care as a social objective, especially for the care of older people. However, the set of policies has not been seen to be very effective. Consequently, the policy of community care has been subject to recent rigorous scrutiny by a series of government reports: that by the Audit Commission (1986), the House of Commons Social Services Committee report (1985) and the Griffiths report (1988), which resulted in the 1989 White Paper 'Caring for People' and the 1990 NHS and Community Care Act. These critical reports are not reviewed in detail here (see Means and Smith, 1994, for a comprehensive review). Instead, we concentrate on isolating the key issues which resulted in the introduction of the NHS and Community Care Act and the eventual introduction of the community care legislation in April 1993.

It was the 1986 Audit Commission review that first drew attention to the 'perverse incentive' which had resulted in a growth of funding for institutional forms of care provision whilst there was no comparable development of community care funding. Following a minor change in the rules for supplementary benefit (now income support) provision, older people claiming supplementary pension could enter private residential or nursing home care, with the full cost being met by the state. This resulted in an enormous growth in the number of private homes and a huge increase in the bill to the Exchequer. Tinker *et al.* (1994) report that the private sector provided 17% of non-NHS long-stay care places in 1980; by 1991, this had increased to 51%. Consequently, the government 'capped' the amount of money they would pay in private care fees for benefit claimants. This example illustrates how one branch of government, through a minor change in welfare benefit regulations, developed a policy in almost total opposition to the policy of community care being pursued by the health and social service agencies.

The Griffiths review (1988) may be seen as a follow-up to the report by the Audit Commission (1986) and the spiralling cost of social security payments to those in private residential/nursing home care noted above. The review was published in March 1988 as a Green Paper 'Community care: agenda for action' and resulted in the November 1989 White Paper 'Caring for People'. The new system came into operation in April 1993, two years after the implementation of the NHS reforms and creation of the internal market in health care.

This White Paper is based on the assumption that, for most people, community care is the 'best' form of care available. The ideology under-pinning this report promotes the ideals of the family as the main source of care and the home as the appropriate place to receive such care. The three main principles inherent in the policy of community care, and which are at the heart of the Griffiths review, are as follows:

1. the recipients of community care should be enabled to live as normal a life as possible in their own homes or in a homely environment in the community;
2. appropriate services should be provided to those who need them most;
3. users should be given a greater say in how they live their lives and the services they need.

The theme of user and carer empowerment is very strong within the entire framework of community care.

Not all the recommendations of the Griffiths review were included in the eventual NHS and Community Care Act. Detailed descriptions and analysis of the main differences are available elsewhere (Baggott, 1994; Means and Smith, 1994). However, as recommended by Griffiths, local authorities were given the responsibility of being lead agency in the development and implementation of community care. This means that, in the provision of community care for older people (and indeed other client groups), local authorities are responsible for:

1. assessing the needs of elderly people for social care (including residential and nursing home care) in collaboration with other appropriate agencies;

2. developing an 'appropriate' package of care designed to meet the assessed needs of older people within the resources available, with the intention of fitting services to people not vice versa as had so often been the case;
3. securing the delivery of appropriate services by the development of a mixed economy of welfare provision, using the private, voluntary and public sectors, with local authorities being expected to make maximum use of the private and voluntary sector and become enabling authorities rather than monopolistic providers of care;
4. publishing clear plans for the development of community care services which outline the authority's intentions for each financial year.

There are three main general policy objectives enshrined in the community care legislation. First, there is a generalized concern with the need to ensure that appropriate services are provided to those who need them, i.e. a concern with the effective targeting of resources to those deemed 'most in need'. Second, there is the imperative to take into account seriously the views of those using services and to provide them with greater choice. Third, there is the requirement to provide care for clients in their own homes whenever possible, with a stress on providing care in as normal a setting as is possible given the client's needs. Hence the review is very clear that 'the family' or a family-type environment is the best way of meeting the needs of individuals.

IMPLEMENTATION OF THE 1993 REFORMS

How effective have the community care reforms been in achieving their goals? Means and Smith (1994) point to the climate of political and financial uncertainty within which local authorities have had to implement the new community care legislation. Furthermore, implementation has been hampered because the new community care legislation came very shortly after the complete overhaul of the system of child carer law enshrined in the Children Act 1989. Given the short time which has elapsed since the implementation of the community care reforms and the difficult circumstances under which it has been introduced, how much progress has been made in its implementation?

Perhaps the central feature of the new system is the introduction of needs-led assessment and care management. The implicit criticism of the previous system was that it fitted people to a narrow range of inflexible and very traditional services which did not meet people's needs and were organized for the benefit of providers rather than users. However, the path towards care management is not without its problems, and there has been only limited progress towards the development of needs-led assessment. To date, there has been an emphasis on defining eligibility criteria and assessment structures, with only a very modified version of needs-led assessment in place. Whilst most authorities have established teams and care management structures, these are not yet fully operational.

The progress towards the development of a 'mixed economy' of social care provision has also been slow. It is an important part of the community care legislation that local authorities move towards an enabling rather than providing role. Hence, there is a clear imperative for local authorities to separate out the roles of the provision and purchase of services.

FACTORS INFLUENCING THE DEMAND FOR COMMUNITY CARE

Before moving on to consider what services are currently provided to older people, it is necessary to briefly consider some of the factors that influence the need for community care services by older people. At the 1991 census, 16% of the population were aged 65 years or more (OPCS, 1993). Of special concern for those concerned with the provision of community care services is the number of very old people, those aged 85 and over, in the population. At the 1991 census, there were 890 000 people aged 85 or more in the UK, and it is predicted that there will be a 50% increase in this to 1 349 000 by the year 2021 (Tinker et al., 1994). Whilst it is true that a considerable percentage of the very elderly live active and independent lives into advanced old age, increasing age does bring with it an increased probability of living alone, ill-health and use of health and social services.

Although living alone is not a problem in itself, it does imply the restricted availability of people to provide care. Indeed, those with limited social networks are at increased risk of using statutory services and of admission to long-stay care (Wenger, 1994). Overall, about 30% of those aged 65 or more live alone, and the prevalence of solo living is greater amongst women than men and increases sharply with age. Almost two-thirds (60%) of those aged 85 or more have a chronic health problem, 20% have difficulties with self-care activities (e.g. washing, dressing) and 60% have problems with domestic care tasks such as housework, shopping or cooking (Goddard and Savage, 1994). These are crude prevalence rates and do not recognize that the experience of ill-health in later life is strongly related to social class (Victor, 1991b) and that rates of ill-health may be higher amongst members of minority communities (Blakemore and Boneham, 1994). The prevalence of major mental health problems also increases markedly with age. It is estimated that the prevalence of severe dementia doubles for every five-year increase in age, such that amongst those aged 85 or more it is about 20% (Jorm et al., 1987). Assuming that future generations of older people show similar patterns, then the ageing of the 'older' population implies a considerable additional demand for community care services (and indeed health services).

PROVISION OF COMMUNITY CARE SERVICES

The previous sections have described very briefly the development of community care policy and the new system. However, as is readily apparent, the very recent introduction of this new pattern of provision means that few data are available about how the service is functioning. In order to consider how community based services are used by older people, we have to use data about utilization provided from routinely available sources. As has already been alluded to, support in maintaining older people at home comes from both the formal sector (i.e. agencies of the state) and the informal network of family and friends. This section considers the contribution of the formal sector to the maintenance of older people within the community. In a later section, we will consider the role of the informal sector.

Formal services, as has been noted earlier, may be provided by a variety of different agencies including health authorities, local authorities, voluntary agencies and the private for-profit operators. In this section, we will review current expenditure on community care and consider the use made by older people of the main community care services. It is worth emphasizing at this juncture that to achieve the staged policy objective of maintaining older people at home for as long as possible involves agencies such as those concerned with housing and income support as well as those traditionally thought of such as health care and 'social services'. The scope of this chapter is limited to 'traditional' community care services. However, the contribution of housing and income support policies in achieving the policy goal of community care should not be underestimated.

HOW MUCH DO WE SPEND ON COMMUNITY CARE?

Given the large number of agencies potentially involved in the provision of community care, this is a difficult question to answer with any accuracy. According to estimates compiled by Robins and Wittenberg (1992), total public expenditure on health and social services for older people amounted to £11 350 million in England in 1989/1990. This represents about half (47%) of the total public expenditure in these areas. Per capita expenditure increases markedly with age, so that the average expenditure for each person aged 85 or more is almost £4000 per year. This is an underestimate as it does not include expenditure on pensions or other important areas such as housing.

UTILIZATION OF HEALTH SERVICES

Hospitals play a vital role in the provision of medical care for all members of the community, especially older people. For older people, hospitals are perhaps the service that they use most extensively. In 1990/1991, 45.5% of acute beds were occupied by those aged 65 or more (Tinker *et al.*, 1994). The proportion of the population reporting a hospital in-patient stay increases with age. For the older age groups, men have a higher rate of hospital admission than women. For those aged 75 or more, 20% of men and 16% of women reported an in-patient stay in hospital in the previous year (Goddard and Savage, 1994).

Over the last decade, there has been a significant reduction in the number of acute hospital beds available – by 27.6% in England (Tinker *et al.*, 1994). However, over the same period, there has been a massive increase in the throughput of patients treated. Tinker *et al.* (1994) report that, between 1981 and 1991, the number of patients treated per bed each year increased by two-thirds. This increased utilization has been achieved by significant reductions in the length of time people spend as in-patients and by the growth of day case treatment. However, the average length of stay in hospital for older people is usually longer than that for a young person with a similar medical condition. This reflects the multiple pathology which is often a feature of older people presenting with specific medical conditions. Very aggressive in-patient treatment regimes may result in 'sicker' patients being discharged back to the community, with a resultant increased strain on community care services.

DISCHARGE FROM HOSPITAL BACK TO THE COMMUNITY

For many patients, irrespective of age, admission to an acute hospital constitutes only one phase of their medical career. Many patients need continuing care, follow-up or rehabilitation. A constant theme in research concerned with the hospital care of older people is discharge from hospital back to the community. Discharge is, perhaps, the wrong term to use. This implies a severing of relationships when many will need continuing care; perhaps the term 'transfer' is a more accurate representation of the concept involved.

Research consistently has demonstrated that the transfer of older patients from hospital to the community can be problematic, with older people sent home without adequate arrangements having been made for their continuing medical and community care (see Marks, 1994, for a comprehensive review). Some medical specialities, especially geriatric medicine, are much better than others at arranging effective transfer. This problem centres on effective communication between hospital, community and local authority services. It remains unclear how the new community care changes will expedite or hinder such communications. However, it is still the case that some older people remain in hospital for longer than is necessary because of the difficulties in organizing and providing appropriate community care services (including long-stay residential and nursing home places).

DELAYED DISCHARGE AND INAPPROPRIATE USE OF ACUTE BEDS

The most appropriate way of providing health care for older people within the hospital sector remains a point of contention. Should older people be treated by a specialist age-related service or should they be cared for within the mainstream? The absence of any rigorous evaluative work makes it difficult to come to a scientific judgement. However, even if an age-related service is established for those older people with acute medical problems, it seems likely that older people will remain high consumers of surgical services and other specialist areas of modern medicine.

Alongside the debates about the most appropriate method of caring for older people are concerns about the 'blocking' of acute beds by older people who no longer need the facilities provided by an acute setting but who, for other reasons, cannot be discharged. Such older people are inevitably given the pejorative label 'bed blockers', which implies that it is the older person's fault that they cannot be discharged. This is highly inaccurate as it is almost always the case that people cannot be discharged because we cannot supply the appropriate services for them.

A number of studies have sought to define methods of empirically identifying 'inappropriate' patients, describing their characteristics and the reasons why such patients could not be discharged. Research in inner London reported that 19% of older patients (i.e. those aged 65 or more) were defined by medical and/or nursing staff as 'bed blockers'. This estimate suggests that 8% of acute beds were being 'blocked' by those patients (Victor et al., 1993). However, inappropriate bed use is not specific to older patients. Victor et al. (1993) reported that only half of all patients identified as inappropriate were aged 75 or more. Why are patients described as being inappropriately placed in an acute unit? Victor (1990) reports that, from a study in inner London, the single most important reason cited was the need for nursing/institutional care (81%). Comparatively few older people were remaining in hospital because of problems in providing community-based services.

Whilst London appears to have perhaps the biggest problem with the supply of long-stay care, it is also an important issue throughout the rest of the country. Those older patients identified as being inappropriately placed within an acute unit almost always had a very real need for non-acute care. Indeed, their health characteristics highlight the types of problems which often occupy the interface between acute and community care. Typically, patients identified as 'inappropriate' present problems such as incontinence and dementia which are likely to present considerable nursing care problems (Victor, 1990).

PRIMARY HEALTH CARE

Primary health care is perhaps one of the key services in achieving the objective of community care: the maintenance of older people in their own homes for as long as possible. Through the annual health checks of all those aged 75 or more on their lists, general practitioners have a key role in the surveillance and monitoring of older people. However, they are also important in making referrals to hospital and community-based services. According to the 1991 General Household Survey (Goddard and Savage, 1994), 56% of those aged 65 or more consulted their general practitioner in the three months before interview (see Table 9.1). It is estimated that approximately 75% of those aged 65 or more will visit their family doctor at least once a year (Victor, 1991a).

COMMUNITY NURSING SERVICES

District nursing services, and, to a lesser degree, health visiting services, are important for older people as part of the framework of primary health care services. Overall, about half (54%) of visits undertaken by district nurses were to those aged 65 or more, compared with 10% of health visitor contacts (Victor, 1991a). In 1991, approximately 5% of those aged 65 or more were in receipt of district nursing/health visiting services. Utilization rates increase significantly with age. For example, 2% of those aged 65–69 are in receipt of district nursing/health care compared with about 15% of those aged 85 or more.

Whilst the percentage of the population aged 65 or more receiving community nursing doubled between 1972 and 1985, the situation for health visiting remained constant. The role of health visitors with older people remains unresolved. Research has suggested that health visitors have a major role to play in screening and assessing older people (Vetter et al., 1984), clearly activities which are at the heart of community care. Health visitors are seen by their fellow health professionals as the group most suited to undertake this activity (Tremellen and Jones, 1989). The same study revealed that at least half of the health visitors surveyed saw the focus of their work being the 0–5-year-olds, which probably reflects the balance of their training, where the emphasis is on pre-school children. However, given the proven effectiveness of health visitors working with older people, it might be appropriate to strengthen their training in this area.

Table 9.1 Use of selected health and social care services by those aged 65 or more (%): Great Britain, 1991

	65–69		70–74		75–79		80–84		≥85		All ≥65	
	M	F	M	F	M	F	M	F	M	F	M	F
In last month												
district nurse/health visitor	2	2	2	4	6	9	10	11	11	21	4	7
home help (local authority)	2	2	3	6	7	14	14	22	26	32	6	11
home help (private)	2	2	2	3	2	4	8	9	15	11	4	4
meals on wheels	1	0	1	2	3	2	7	9	9	10	2	3
In last 3 months												
doctor	53	50	55	54	60	60	62	62	68	56	57	55
social worker	2	2	1	2	3	4	3	4	8	7	2	3
chiropody	6	16	11	25	18	31	27	37	35	48	14	27
dentist	15	14	13	15	12	10	8	8	1	7	12	12
optician	9	12	9	10	11	12	13	13	10	12	10	12

Source: adapted from Goddard and Savage (1994), tables 65 and 62.

PERSONAL SOCIAL SERVICES

Despite the emphasis in the community care legislation moving local authorities towards being organizers of care, they still remain significant providers of care. The key services provided by local authorities include home care (home help) services, day care, social work, meals services, occupational therapy and home aids/adaptations. It is evident that local authority services are received by only a minority of older people. Even amongst those aged 85 and over, who certainly constitute the most frail and vulnerable members of the older population, 9% receive meals, 29% receive a home help and 7% have seen a social worker. Coverage of these services in the very old population remains strictly limited. Victor (1991a) reports that, amongst those living alone, 19% were receiving home help services, as were 32% of those defined as severely disabled.

ASSESSMENT AND MANAGEMENT OF COMMUNITY CARE

The data presented earlier about the receipt of community-based health and social care services by older people largely relate to the situation before implementation of the reforms in 1993. As there are few nationally available data, it is not possible to comment on the effectiveness of the reforms. However, it is pertinent to raise some issues that are of considerable importance in the new regime. These are assessment, care management, the role of users, and quality of life.

The cornerstones of the 1993 reforms are the needs-led assessment of individuals and the resultant systems of care management. These topics merit a whole chapter to themselves and here we can only raise some of the key issues. According to Means and Smith (1994), there are three issues to be addressed; assessment of users' needs, negotiation with users of an appropriate care package to meet the identified needs within the resources available, and the implementation and monitoring of the care package. The obvious criticism of previous systems here is that previously users had been fitted into 'existing' services rather than looking at users' needs and then finding appropriate services. Progress in achieving involvement of users and carers has been slow (Allen et al., 1992). Local authorities have concentrated on developing assessment structures and eligibility criteria. The lack of standardized instruments being used in community care assessment schedules is worthy of note. Progress towards developing care management is limited because of continued debates about who should undertake this role, who should hold the budget, and whether there should be a separation between assessment and the subsequent management of the care package.

Promoting choice by users and carers was a key objective of the community care reforms. Again progress towards this ideal has been limited. There is no easy answer to the question 'what is user empowerment?'. However, at its most basic, this concept implies that users will be given more power over decisions involving their welfare. If users are given more power, service providers will lose power. Furthermore, there is potential for conflict between the views of users and carers. Involvement of users and carers in their own needs assessment remains very limited as does their role in developing the community care plans that all local authorities have to develop.

It is a key premise of the move to community care that it will enhance the quality of life of recipients, especially when compared with those who are receiving care in institutional environments. There are few data to support (or refute) this proposition. Small research projects testing the utility of care management in Thanet and Gateshead (Challis and Davies, 1986) reported an 'improved' quality of life amongst those who received care management. However, these schemes may be criticized because of the highly restricted nature of the way the samples were derived. Direct comparison, using reliable and valid instruments, of the quality of life of older people in institutions with their contemporaries in the community is clearly an important area to research. However, for a very dependent older person who is likely to receive community care, we may speculate that community care may replicate in their own homes all the negative features of an institution, such as lack of control over their daily lives.

THE INFORMAL SECTOR

Just as community care was not 'invented' in 1993, neither was the informal provision of care for older people 'invented' in the 1980s. It seems highly likely that it has always been the informal sector (family, friends and neighbours) who have provided the bulk of care to those with long-term health problems. This expectation was enshrined in the 1930 Poor Law, which stated 'It should be the duty of the father, grandfather, mother, grandmother, husband or child of a poor, old, blind, lame or impotent person, or other poor person, not able to work, if possessed of sufficient means, to relieve and maintain that person not able to work' (quoted in Means and Smith, 1994). However, it was in the 1980s that a now significant body of research identified the true extent of the informal care sector and carefully determined the characteristics of those who provided such care, who they provided it to and how much care was provided. This section explores the contribution of the informal sector and considers the nature and characteristics of those who provide informal care.

The provision of care to older people is divided between the formal and informal sectors and the contribution of the informal sector is recognized in recent policy development. Indeed, carers are now entitled to a community care assessment in their own right. However, given the large number of carers, this has significant resource implications even if no services are supplied after the assessment.

WHAT IS THE INFORMAL CARE SECTOR?

The informal sector may be defined as care provided by family, friends and neighbours that is not organized via a statutory or voluntary agency. The informal sector has always been the main provider of help to older people, especially with the personal and household tasks which are required to maintain them in the community. This statement is still applicable to the present time, contradicting the powerful myth that older people are neglected by their family and that the main burden of caring for older people falls on the state.

THE EXTENT OF INFORMAL CARE

The extent of the contribution of the informal sector may be estimated from the 1985 General Household Survey which made a special study of this topic (Green, 1988). This survey revealed that 15% of women and 12% of men defined themselves as carers. Although this is almost certainly an underestimate, it means that at least 6 million adults in Britain are carers. The majority of informal carers, 75%, are looking after a person aged 65 and over, 1.4 million adults provide care for more than 20 hours per week, and 3.7 million have sole responsibility for the care of their dependents. The key role of informal carers is recognized in the Griffiths White Paper which states '. . . the reality is that most care is provided by family, friends and neighbours'.

THE CHARACTERISTICS OF CARERS

Who is a carer? As with other social groups, informal carers are not a homogenous group. Several important subdivisions of the informal caring population may be made. The first relates to the relationship between carer and dependant. This largely distinguishes between spouses, who are likely to be men or women, and daughters (in law). The second distinction is whether the carer lives in the same household as the dependant. These distinctions have implications for the type of care provided, the support services required and the stresses and problems associated with caring (Parker and Lawson, 1994).

Where the carer and dependant are resident in the same household, there is little difference in the gender of the carer. This situation describes an elderly spouse looking after their marriage partner. However, non-resident carers are predominantly female and aged 45–64. This group is dominated by daughters (in law) (Arber and Ginn, 1991).

This reflects the 'hierarchy of obligations' proposed by Finch (1989). She suggests that informal care is organized around four central tenets.

1. The marital relationship is of primary importance so that the spouse is the first source of care for married people.
2. The parent–child relationship is the second source of obligation. Adult children are a principal source of care for elderly parents and parents the main source of care for disabled children.
3. Those who share a household are major care providers; an adult child who shares the parental home is more likely to provide care than siblings living away from home.
4. Where there is a 'choice' between male and female relatives as to who becomes the carer, then it is the female relative who usually becomes the carer.

THE RELATIONSHIP BETWEEN FORMAL AND INFORMAL CARE

Clearly the contribution of state services in monetary terms is, as we saw earlier, highly significant but not as significant as informal contributions. The value of the work undertaken by informal carers is difficult to estimate with precision. However, if we ascribe a nominal value of £4 per hour to the work undertaken, then informal carers undertake work to the value of £15 599–24 041 billion per annum. This is considerably more than that expended by the formal sector and does not include such factors as opportunity costs, i.e. loss of earnings, and reduced quality of the life for the carer.

Another way to look at the relative contributions of the formal and informal sectors is to look at the sources of help for older people. For 77% of older people in the community who need help with mobility or self-care tasks, this help is provided by family. Similarly, for help with domestic care tasks, 92% of older people report help from their family. Overwhelmingly, it is the informal sector that provides help with the sort of mobility, personal and domestic tasks which help to keep older people at home.

THE SUPPLY OF INFORMAL CARE

There are debates about the supply of informal care by families in future decades. It seems unlikely that there will be changes in the supply of care between spouses. However, there are debates about the possible future role of children in providing care. The notion of family care provided by daughters assumes a specific model of family life, most notably a stable nuclear family with a non-working female at home able to provide care. Divorce, decreases in family size and the increased labour market participation of women raise questions about future supplies of informal care.

CARERS AND COMMUNITY CARE

What impact has the new community care legislation had on carers? As we are still in the early days of the implementation of the changes, it is difficult to come up with a definitive statement. However, research based on a sample of members of the Carers National Association (Warner, 1994) highlighted the problems carers had in obtaining assessments for their dependents. Current legislation will entitle carers to assessment in their own right but the resource implications of this are immense. The report also highlighted that even the very low expectations that carers had from community care had not been met and that 79% reported that community care had 'made no difference' to them or the services they were receiving for their dependent.

CONCLUSION AND POLICY IMPLICATIONS

The recent implementation of the community care changes has several key themes. There is an emphasis that services should be responsive to local needs. The philosophy is that services should be moulded to fit the needs of clients rather than vice versa. The key question of how such needs are to be measured and evaluated is not tackled by the government in the policy document. A central concern is that patients/clients should be treated as consumers and the notion of choice is paramount. The development of a mixed economy of provision is posited as a way of improving the quality and quantity of services. By service providers competing against each other, service quality will be improved. This is an assertion of faith rather than a carefully evaluated conclusion based on available evidence. Community care for older people will ultimately be judged a success (or otherwise) by the impact the reforms have on the level, range and quality of services provided to older people (and their carers) at a local level.

REFERENCES

Allen, I., Dally, G. and Leadt, D. (1992) *Monitoring change in social service departments*, Policy Studies Institute, London (for the Association of Directors of Social Services).

Arber, S. and Ginn, J. (1991) *Gender and later life*, Sage, London.

Audit Commission (1986) *Making a reality of community care*, HMSO, London.

Baggott, R. (1994) *Health and health care in Britain*, Macmillan, Basingstoke.

Bayley, M. (1973) *Mental handicap and community care*, Routlege and Kegan Paul, London.

Blakemore, K. and Boneham, M. (1994) *Age, race and ethnicity*, Open University Press, Milton Keynes, UK.

Bulmer, M. (1987) *The social basis of community care*, Unwin Hyman, London.

Challis, D. and Davies, B. (1986) *Case management in community care*, Gower, Aldershot.

Challis, D., Davies, B. and Traske, K. (eds) (1994) Community care: ambition and imperative – an international agenda, in *Community care: new agendas and challenges from the UK and overseas*, Areana, Aldershot, pp. 1–10.

Department of Health and Social Security (1981) *Growing older*, HMSO, London.

Finch, J. (1989) *Family obligations and social change*, Policy Press, Cambridge, UK.

Green, H. (1988) *Informal carers, OPCS General Household Survey Series no. 16*, OPCS/HMSO, London.

Goddard, E. and Savage, D. (1994) People aged 65 and over, in *General Household Survey No. 22, Supplement A*, OPCS/HMSO, London.

Griffiths, R. (1988) *Care in the community: agenda for action*, HMSO, London.

House of Commons Social Services Committee (1985) *Community care, HC13–1 session 84/85*, HMSO, London.

Jorm, A., Korten, A. and Henderson, A. (1987) The prevalence of dementia: a quantitative integration of the literature. *Acta Psychiatr. Scand.*, **76**, 465–79.

Marks, L. (1994) *Seamless care or patchwork quilt?*, Kings Fund, London.

Means, R. and Smith, R. (1994) *Community care: policy and practice*, Macmillan, Basingstoke.

Office of Population Censuses and Surveys (1993) *Persons aged 60 and over, CEN 91 TM PEN*, HMSO, London.

Parker, G. and Lawson, D. (1994) *Different types of care, different types of carer*, HMSO, London.

Robins, A. and Wittenberg, R. (1992) The health of elderly people: economic aspects, in *The health of elderly people: an epidemiological overview (companion papers)*, HMSO, London, pp. 10–19.

Scharf, T. and Wenger, G.C. (eds) (1995) *International perspectives on community care*, Avebury, Aldershot, UK.

Tinker, A., McCreadie, C., Wright, F. and Salvage, A. (1994) *The care of the frail elderly in the United Kingdom*, HMSO, London.

Townsend, P. (1957) *The last refuge*, Routledge and Kegan Paul, London.

Tremellen, J. and Jones, D.A. (1989) Attitudes and practices of the primary health care team towards assessing the elderly. *J. R. Coll. Gen. Pract.* **39**, 142–4.

Vetter, N.J., Jones, D.A. and Victor, C.R. (1984) The evaluation of health visitors working with elderly people in general practice. *BMJ*, **288**, 369–72.

Victor, C.R. (1990) A survey of the delayed discharge of elderly people from hospital in inner city district. *Arch. Gerontol. Geriatr.* **10**, 199–205.

Victor, C.R. (1991a) *Health and health care in later life*, Open University Press, Milton Keynes, UK.

Victor, C.R. (1991b) Continuity or change? Inequalities in health in later life. *Ageing Soc.* **11**, 23–39.

Victor, C.R., Nazareth, B., Hudson, M. and Fulop, N. (1993) The inappropriate use of acute medical beds in an inner London DHA. *Health Trends*, **25**(3), 94–7.

Walker, A. (ed.) (1982) *Community care*, Blackwell and Martin Robertson, Oxford.

Warner, N. (1994) *Just a fairy tale? Community care and carers*, Carers National Association, London.

Wenger, G.C. (1994) *Understanding support networks and community care*, Avebury, Aldershot, UK.

The physician's role in long-term care 10

The number of elderly people in institutional care has been steadily increasing during recent years and is set to rise still further well into the next century. Hidden within this plain statement of fact is a sea change: the major transfer of long-term nursing care from NHS hospitals into private, charitable or voluntary accommodation. The change has had a major impact on doctors who look after residents in institutional care, i.e. the consultant physicians in geriatric medicine and general practitioners. As a result some consultants now have little or no commitment to long-term care or those who receive it. In 1994, a British Geriatrics Society survey found that, of consultants responding to the survey, only 45% spent time each week concerned with long-term care, and now the proportion is likely to be even smaller. For general practitioners, there may well have been an extensive and perhaps unwelcome expansion in the number of frail older clients to be cared for by their practice. Although the approach to care may differ between consultants and general practitioners, many issues present common areas for debate and discussion.

THE ROLE OF THE CONSULTANT/PHYSICIAN IN LONG-STAY CARE

There are several reasons why consultants in geriatric medicine should continue to take an active interest in continuing care patients. Firstly, although consultants are less likely to take the lead role in continuing care, medical input will still be important to individual patients and for the facility as a whole and should not be neglected. Secondly, consultants remain responsible for the overall clinical management of the patients. Thirdly, the consultant needs to supervise the day-to-day medical cover, which may be provided by an interested local general practitioner.

Fourthly, consultants may also need to be involved in decisions surrounding treatment or non-treatment issues, questions of living wills or even euthanasia (see Chapter 4). Grimley Evans (1987) has pointed out that doctors are required, trained and expected to take such decisions and accept responsibility for the outcome. No other caring profession has a similar function. Fifthly, consultants should be involved in discussions which aim to alter the style or model of continuing care and would also be expected to take an active role in negotiations with private institutions who are tendering for continuing care previously carried out in NHS accommodation. Finally, it is only by visiting the wards that a consultant will be able to assess general standards of care as well as the morale and attitudes of staff. Lack of senior medical input may irritate staff and impair morale.

However, regular visiting of long-stay wards does present something of a dilemma to consultants. On the one hand, the consultant has clinical responsibility for the patient and therefore needs frequent contact with these wards. On the other hand, it can be very reasonably argued that, since the long-stay wards are in effect the patient's home, then they would not expect a weekly ward round from a consultant. The point is perhaps emphasized by the fact that in long-stay units there is often very little clinical change in a patient's physical condition over many weeks or months. How can these anomalies be resolved? The frequency of visits to the patients might be reduced, but the time made available used to carry out a series of audit studies considering, for example, complaints, chiropody services, use of medicines, pressure area care and wound management, nutrition and diet, and dental care. Lectures could be given to the staff as part of an ongoing educational programme. Staffing levels and staff turnover could be discussed with the nursing manager. Regular discussion meetings could be arranged with regard to discussing the ethical problems arising from long-term care and those clinical problems that require regular review and multi-disciplinary input.

THE ROLE OF THE GENERAL PRACTITIONER

The expansion in private sector provision of long-stay care has placed a seemingly ever-expanding workload of physically and mentally frail older patients on general practitioners and primary healthcare teams. Where the local hospital still has long-stay beds, it is likely that the most physically frail and those with severe behavioural problems will remain in NHS accommodation. However, where such facilities do not exist, such patients will be placed in the private sector and are likely to become the direct responsibility of general practitioners who may not have been approached when plans were first laid for the private development. The situation is intensified in retirement areas such as coastal regions, where migration of older people into the locality may have caused the provision of private nursing care to be far in excess of local needs and general practitioners may have patients in ten or more homes. Clearly therefore, there is a need for general practitioners to have particular expertise in the physical, mental, social and ethical problems associated with care of older people. Indeed, there is much to be said for them possessing either the Diploma in Geriatric Medicine of the Royal College of Physicians or membership of the Royal College of General Practitioners.

What might be the role of general practitioners in relation to these frail older people? All patients new to the practice really need to be assessed on or shortly after arrival and be subject to regular reviews, although this is not always the case (Hepple *et al.*, 1989). Such reviews could cover not only the patients' physical and mental capabilities or limitations, but also their medication (see below). The general practitioners could agree with the care staff management guidelines for conditions such as pressure sores and the maintenance of continence. Such discussions might also encompass general quality issues and may provide the basis for regular audit of care provision. Activities along these lines should be adopted by institutions and poor quality care avoided.

ISSUES COMMON TO BOTH CONSULTANTS AND GENERAL PRACTITIONERS

DRUGS AND MEDICINES

As a group, older people are more likely to be taking a greater number of medications than their younger counterparts, reflecting the increased number of medical diagnoses in the group. An epidemiological study of drug use in people over the age of 65 living in the community found an average number of 1.9 prescription items per person. However, 31% took no medication and 10% took more than five items (Cartwright and Smith, 1988). Coupled with this, older people have an increased susceptibility to drug interactions and adverse reactions (Divoll and Greenblatt, 1981; Nolan and O'Malley, 1989; Lindley *et al.*, 1992). The increased number of medical diagnoses in this frail older group increases the likelihood of adverse drug reactions (Carbonin *et al.*, 1991). Community drug usage contrasts with a much higher use in nursing homes and there is considerable published work illustrating the very high levels of prescribing in long-term care (Primrose *et al.*, 1987; Hatton, 1990), much of which appears to be a poor standard (Browne *et al.*, 1987). Nolan and O'Malley (1989) found a mean of four drugs, with a range of 0–14, prescribed per patient in Irish nursing homes, with 41% of patients taking five or more drugs and 42% of residents taking drugs with potential interactions. The use of sedation is widespread and sometimes appears to be used to 'switch the patients out with the lights'.

Regular review of therapy and the objectives of treatment is necessary to avoid iatrogenic complications. Regular monitoring of the residents receiving therapy such as diuretics or angiotensin-converting enzyme (ACE) inhibitors should be carried out. There should be a well-understood policy on which medications can be withheld in times of acute illness. The use of a local formulary will help to rationalize prescribing and assist in monitoring of drug use. It is useful if there is a limited list of medications such as simple analgesics, laxatives and enemas that can be prescribed by the nursing staff. Recommendations regarding the use of drugs in older people are contained in a Royal College of Physicians report (1984), which is currently being updated. Drug usage is also a useful audit topic, which is contained in the Royal College of Physicians CARE scheme of clinical audit in long-term care (RCP, 1992). As with all prescribing and any treatment, there should be a clear indication for medication and the potential benefits of the treatment should outweigh the potential risks. If there are any doubts, then it is best not to prescribe the drug.

MONITORING AND QUALITY OF CARE

At present, there are no nationally agreed guidelines applied to the quality of long-term care in the NHS. The National Association of Health Authorities and Trusts (1988) lists regulations regarding the registration and inspection of nursing homes, while local authority social service departments have a statutory duty to review all people placed by them into long-term residential care. Each authority can devise its own regulations and some social service department inspection units have yet to agree standards. Reviews normally consider medical illness, drug usage, accidents and social and physical functioning, as well as reviewing the environment of the resident. Many community health councils are involved in visiting long-stay wards and reporting on standards of care; unfortunately, their concern is not always followed by sensible action from the hospital authorities. In the past, the NHS Health Advisory Service had a peer review function of NHS long-term care but this has largely disappeared. As an authoritative independent figure, the doctor providing medical care can take a valuable lead in ensuring that standards of care are maintained.

ETHICAL ISSUES

The problems raised by 'living wills' and euthanasia are considered in Chapter 4.

REFERENCES

Browne, M.M., Tallis, R.C., Vellodi, C., Al-Hamouz, S. and Edmond, E.D. (1987) Contra-indicated and interacting drugs in long stay geriatric patients. *Br. J. Pharm. Pract.* **9**, 250–4.

Cartwright, A. and Smith, C. (1988) *Elderly People, their Medicines and their Doctors*, Institute for Social Studies in Medical Care/Routledge, London.

Carbonin, P., Bernabei, R. and Sgadari, A. (1991) Is age an independent risk factor for adverse drug reactions in hospitalised patients? *J. Am. Geriatr. Soc.*, **39**, 1093–9.

Divoll, M.K. and Greenblatt, D.J. (1981) Drug interactions and adverse drug reactions, in *Clinical Pharmacology in the Elderly* (ed. C.S. Swift), Marcel Decker Inc., New York.

Grimley Evans, J. (1987) The sanctity of life, in *Medical Ethics and Elderly People* (ed. R.J. Elford), Churchill Livingstone, Edinburgh.

Hatton, P. (1990) *Primum non nocere* – an analysis of drugs prescribed to elderly patients in private nursing homes registered with Harrogate Health Authority. *Care Elderly*, **2**, 166–9.

Hepple, J., Bowler, I. and Bowman, C.E. (1989) A survey of private nursing home residents in Weston Super Mare. *Age Ageing*, **18**, 61–3.

Lindley, C.M., Tully, M.P., Parmasothy, V. and Tallis, R.C. (1992) Inappropriate medication is a major cause of adverse drug reactions in elderly patients. *Age Ageing*, **21**, 294–300.

National Association of Health Authorities and Trusts in England and Wales (1988) *Registration and Inspection of Nursing Homes: Supplement* NAHAT, Birmingham.

Nolan, L. and O'Malley, K. (1989) The need for a more rational approach to drug prescribing for elderly people in nursing homes. *Age Ageing*, **18**, 52–6.

Primrose, W.R., Capewell, A.E., Simpson, G.E. *et al.* (1987) Prescribing patterns observed in registered nursing homes and long stay geriatric wards. *Age Ageing*, **16**, 25–8.

Royal College of Physicians (1984) *Medication for the Elderly*, Royal College of Physicians, London.

Royal College of Physicians (1992) *The CARE Scheme (Continuous Assessment Review and Evaluation) Clinical Audit of Long-Term Care*, Royal College of Physicians, London.

Nursing care

11

This chapter focuses on issues associated with maintaining the independence and dignity of older people living in continuous care facilities. Under this umbrella, there are several key points for discussion, such as promoting continence and managing incontinence, taking risks, understanding pain and providing relevant, purposeful activities; however, before considering specifics, I think it is important to understand the way(s) in which care has been/can be provided to older people. For me, this can be best described as the style in which nursing is delivered.

Over 30 years ago, nursing older people was described as 'largely routine work of a particularly heavy nature' (Exton-Smith *et al.*, 1962). Although some readers may find themselves agreeing with this, they may also feel able to highlight the rewarding nature of their work, which should put the needs of older men and women first and provides a culture in which old people are seen as individuals and care is provided holistically.

The challenge of nursing older people requiring continuous care is to maximize independence and minimize the reduction in well-being which Redfern (1989) feared may accompany continuing care when she stated that: 'Elderly people who find themselves ending their days in long-stay geriatric wards can so quickly decline into an apathetic state of "learned helplessness", in which any vestige of independence has long gone.' (p. 157).

The hallmark of quality care is the facilitation of 'new learning, health, happiness and fulfilment' (RCN, 1993a). The degree of success that nurses have in achieving this will depend on the style of nursing adopted by the unit and indeed by each individual nurse. This is likely to be intimately linked to how the nurse feels about growing older, about looking after older people and to what extent ageing is seen as a positive phase of life.

The literature describes various approaches to nursing older people in continuous care units. Some are unlikely to be found within present day care settings, others may be more familiar. Several years ago, Evers (1981) observed and described three types of care on eight wards for old people: the acute care, minimal warehousing and personalized warehousing. The acute care is characterized by goals related to restoring independence in preparation for discharge home and emphasizes the multidisciplinary nature of care provision. In contrast, the remaining two styles are associated with continuing periods of hospitalization and are typified by dependence rather than the active promotion of independence. Minimal warehousing is characterized by enforced physical independence, psychological dependence and minimal purposeful activity. The provision of care is rarely undertaken by multiple disciplines and falls by default, rather than design, to nurses. Outcomes such as depression, humiliation and boredom are attributed to this style. Personalized warehousing, on the other hand, is characterized by the encouragement rather than enforcement of physical and psychological independence, with the provision of some, albeit limited, opportunities for activities. Care is undertaken by members of the multidisciplinary team, although nurses are delegated the responsibility for it.

These descriptions may strike a chord with you. I include them not only to challenge your practice and indeed your attitudes to nursing older people, but also to highlight the importance of partnership between all members of the multidisciplinary team and a clear delegation of responsibility to the professional most in contact with older people living in long-stay care facilities. This professional is the nurse and therefore, by design, rather than default, nurses are the key providers and co-ordinators of care to older people needing continuous long-term care. Nurses have increasingly developed extremely specialized skills and sophisticated knowledge of the needs of older people (RCN, 1993b) and are in positions which can help residents to 'make adjustments to health changes, to use what normal capacities they possess and enjoy the satisfactions and potentialities of older age' (RCN, 1993b).

Evers (1981) concluded her work by emphasizing the need to develop an alternative style of care and described a framework in which nurses were given this authority. She called it the 'tender loving care' model and described its five key tenets as:

- promoting independence
- promoting choice
- valuing individuality
- emphasizing the enabling role of staff
- encouraging home making.

In other words, the model enables each older person to live their life in as much accordance with their wishes as possible.

I would like to consider each of these features and link them to some of the central issues related to being old and living within an institution as a home.

PROMOTING INDEPENDENCE

Promoting independence is often associated with the physical aspects of care and frequently related to functional independence. Whilst it is inappropriate here to consider every element of care associated with daily living, it is important to remember that dependence in one area is likely to affect another. This is compounded by the nature of illness in old age which is frequently characterized by multiple pathologies and related polypharmacy, making the nursing care needed by older people complex and highly skilled.

I intend to focus on four issues which impinge on the physical, psychological and social well-being of many older people and may have contributed, initially, to their need for continuous care. They are continence, mobility, pain and inclusion in purposeful activity. A fuller exposition of the nursing care required by older people in care homes is provided by Ford and Heath (1996) and interested readers are referred to that text, in particular, for details of wound care and issues related to mental health.

PROMOTING CONTINENCE AND MANAGING INCONTINENCE

Whilst growing older itself does not necessarily equate with reduced bladder and bowel control, incontinence is, for some older people receiving long-stay care, a distressing reminder of increased dependence on others.

The sensitive management of both urinary and faecal incontinence is central to preserving dignity and promoting independence for each resident requiring extra support. However, the success of this also has an impact on residents collectively as incontinence may affect the environment of care, through smell or visually (e.g. use or storage of equipment), influencing residents' and visitors' feelings about the quality of the care provided. For those who are not incontinent, the increased attention required by residents who are incontinent, or who require extra support to maintain continence may make them feel neglected and 'different'.

Several approaches are popular in the nursing management of incontinence and can provide a useful repertoire from which to select an appropriate strategy for each individual resident. Wyman (1992) emphasizes the importance of nurses in the identification, diagnosis and management of incontinence in older people, together with others skilled in this specialism (e.g. the continence advisor or physiotherapist), and discusses management strategies related to supportive interventions (pads with pants, collecting devices) and behavioural interventions. Of the latter category,

Table 11.1   Scheduling strategies (adapted from Wyman, 1992)

Strategy	Action taken
Bladder training	Scheduled voiding with gradually increasing time intervals between voidings.
Habit retraining	Scheduled toiletting which reflects resident's voiding pattern. Intervals between voiding altered as necessary.
Timed voiding	Fixed voiding pattern which remains unaltered.
Prompted voiding	Resident prompted to void at set times.
Patterned urge-response toileting	Voiding pattern determined using electronic device to detect incontinence. Toileting scheduled in accordance with results.

the most frequently used interventions include scheduling strategies and pelvic floor exercises. Scheduling strategies, identified in Table 11.1, may be used independently of each other or as part of a progressive continence improvement programme.

All too frequently, the first and only approach to managing incontinence is a supportive strategy. Smith *et al.* (1992) urge nurses to consider the alternative behavioural strategies before resorting to supportive techniques which may often be perceived as easier for both the nurse and the resident, as well as being less time-consuming. However, as a preliminary strategy, supportive management may compromise an older person's sense of independence, dignity and self-esteem.

Scheduling strategies allow individualized continence programmes to be tailored to the particular problems and routines of each person. Evaluation of the success of these approaches should be undertaken regularly and coupled with a reappraisal of the appropriateness of continuing the scheduling strategy, complementing it with supportive intervention, or relying solely on supportive intervention.

Although individual continence programmes focusing on tailor-made scheduling routines are realistically achievable, their success will depend on staff availability and resident and staff motivation. However, a reduction in incontinence, no matter how large or small, will have a marked effect on the physical, psychological and social well-being of an elderly person and is therefore worth actively pursuing.

MAINTAINING MOBILITY

Accidents, particularly falls, have a considerable impact on independence. In the past, fear of falling or accidents may have been reflected in curtailing of the activity of older people through the use of restraints. This may have been either explicit (cot sides, wheelchair lap belts) or implicit, with people sitting tipped backwards in chairs, hemmed in by furniture or excluded from certain activities (e.g. cooking or gardening). However, rather than reducing falls, some of these practices may have exacerbated them (Hogue, 1992) and be in themselves potentially hazardous, causing injury to people as they 'escape', prolonging immobility with resultant pressure sore development, and increasing the potential for incontinence. They may also have been coupled with isolation, loss of self-esteem and increased dependence (Evans and Strumpf, 1992). Consequently, they are now frowned upon and nurses feel more able to take up the challenge of creating a restraint-free environment, even though this can be time-consuming and resource-intensive.

Since all accidents have the potential to limit activity and reduce people's quality of life, preventive strategies are recommended after risk has been assessed. Several risk factors have been identified and consideration of these should be a central feature in accident prevention. Recognizing that someone is at risk and minimizing that risk are the key elements in maintaining mobility and independence.

Hogue (1992) identified four types of risk factors which may contribute to falling or reduced mobility.

1. age-related decline (e.g. visual limitations);
2. disease, either acute or chronic (e.g. cardiovascular disease, disorders of gait and balance);
3. medication (e.g. sedatives, hypnotics, tranquillizers);
4. environmental hazards (poor lighting, trailing wires, ill-fitting clothing/ shoes).

Risk needs to be assessed and minimized on an individual and collective level. Nurses have particular responsibility for this as they know residents well, can predict potential hazards and are sensitive to subtle changes in health which may increase the risk of an accident. Some general preventive points to focus on are detailed below:

1. Ensure that call bells can easily be reached.
2. Monitor changes in condition and regularly determine how change will influence mobility and risk of accident: reassessment needs to be built into this process.
3. Ensure that clothes and shoes are well-fitting and belong to each individual.
4. Minimize environmental hazards and ensure that equipment is regularly maintained.
5. Ensure that when new furniture is bought, it is of an appropriate height and facilitate sitting/lying down or getting up. Of course, this is

difficult as furnishing needs will vary between residents, so providing a variety of differing styles of furnishing may be a realistic approach. Residents can also be encouraged to bring furniture with them.

6. Consider introducing a programme of physical activity to lessen the potentially sedentary nature of life within the long-stay environment; this may minimize muscle weakness associated with inactivity and be both beneficial and enjoyable.
7. Determine the level to which residents can actively participate in transferring from place to place as well as their willingness to transfer (Heslin *et al.*, 1992).
8. Introduce rest stops by strategically placing chairs between bedrooms and bathrooms to allow rests during journeys and hence reduce accidents during movement between places (Soja *et al.*, 1992).

Risk of falling may also be associated with the need for elimination (Ross *et al.*, 1992), showing a clear link between this section and the previous discussion related to continence. Predicting the need to eliminate in people at risk of falling and offering appropriate help, at regular intervals, may minimize this risk and lead to a greater sense of independence. Building a rapport and understanding a resident's need for elimination are central to this.

In general, the nurse's role is to ensure that older people are aware of the risks of mobility and immobility and facilitate safe movement throughout the long-stay care environment in order to promote feelings of independence.

MANAGING PAIN

Pain has been described as 'whatever the experiencing person says it is and exists whenever he says it does' (McCaffery, 1972). Whilst at first glance this seems vague, it is in fact a useful way of defining the varied concept of pain. Pain is individual and is rarely exactly the same in different people, or even for an individual over time. Pain has a uniquely individual interpretation.

For residents, pain may be multifaceted. It may be manifested as physical pain, associated with acute or chronic disease, or psychological pain linked to bereavement, isolation, depression or loneliness; and can be expressed physiologically, behaviourally, verbally (Reading, 1984) or non-verbally (Table 11.2). Nurses may be challenged to interpret these expressions with, or for, residents. This is particularly relevant for those with illnesses which inhibit verbal mechanisms such as aphasia (Fordham and Dunn, 1994) or when a language is not shared.

Identification of these expressions of pain is a central skill of nursing older people and is likely to be associated with forming a rapport with

Table 11.2 Expressions of pain (based on Reading, 1984)

Expression	Manifestations
Physiological	Increased heart rate Increased blood pressure Pupil dilation Sweating
Behavioural	Holding painful area Stillness Rocking/rubbing
Verbal	Explicit statements of pain Rambling Short phrases
Non-verbal	Facial expressions: frowning or screwing up face Grunting Groaning

residents, and being sensitive to change over time, which may be subtle or overt.

The skill of recognizing changing cues can be complemented by using readily available assessment scales such as the London Hospital's pain observation chart (Raiman, 1986), which allows nurses to collect several different types of information:

1. the location of the pain(s);
2. the degree of severity (ranging from 'excruciating', scoring 5, to 'no pain at all', scoring 0);
3. details of measures to relieve pain (e.g. analgesia, massage, distraction and/or positioning).

This type of approach allows the person in pain and their carer to form a comprehensive picture of the pain, facilitating sensitive management, accurate monitoring and evaluation in both the short and the long term.

Other approaches include visual scales where residents are asked to mark the severity of their pain along a line or agree with one of a series of words describing their pain. Seers (1991) reminds us that some older people with memory/cognitive problems may find it difficult to describe pain accurately in these ways. In these instances, the knowledge and skills that nurses possess are crucial to the identification, assessment and management of pain.

The management of pain is central to the reduction of discomfort and enhancement of the quality of life for the person in pain. No matter how slight pain is, it is likely to affect independence and feelings of well-being and therefore should never be ignored or accepted as an expected or normal part of growing older. Nurses have a central role in helping a person to manage their pain.

Traditionally, pain management has been described as either pharmacological or non-pharmacological, and nurses can play an important part in both of these approaches. In pharmacological management, their role includes discussing the type of therapy with the doctor and the resident, and helping them to come to a shared decision about medication. This done, the role changes to one of ensuring medication is given and its effects monitored so that pain is relieved. This monitoring is central to promoting well-being and determining, with the resident and doctor, the therapeutic effectiveness of the medication.

Non-pharmacological mechanisms include massage, local applications of heat or cold, the use of transcutaneous electrical nerve stimulation, distraction and imagery (Fordham and Dunn, 1994). These may be used to complement drug therapy or as pain-relieving strategies on their own. Nurses may be involved, to varying degrees, in each of these approaches. Just as pharmacological interventions can vary in their effectiveness, so too can non-pharmacological strategies, and therefore careful monitoring and evaluation remain an important feature of the care given to someone experiencing pain. Seers (1991) emphasizes the need to persist with non-pharmacological techniques as these require practice to reach their full potential. This is particularly useful advice as both the nurse and resident may become disheartened if an approach does not have an immediate effect.

Fordham and Dunn (1994) remind us that pain isolates people, and this may be especially distressing for a person receiving continuous care, as pain may exacerbate already present feelings of isolation from friends, family and indeed other residents. Pain may make it hard for the person to join in activities with others, to go outside the home, or to enjoy more solitary activities such as reading, craft or gardening. Pain may compound loneliness, and therefore the nurse's role is not merely one of alleviating pain but also considering, creatively, how to help the person with pain to continue living as full a life as they wish. Nurses may find themselves becoming more involved with the person and developing the skills of companionship or 'being with' the person (Fordham and Dunn, 1994).

Establishing a rapport with the person in pain is central to developing companionship and showing understanding of the unique experience of pain for that person, making them feel that you are there for them and care how they feel. This involves the skilled use of both verbal and non-verbal communication techniques. Once this has developed and the relationship maintained, Fordham and Dunn (1994) suggest that the nurse may then be able to involve others, such as doctors, friends or specialists, in non-pharmacological interventions to manage pain.

Helping a person to manage pain is a complicated, skilled component of good nursing care. It involves developing a depth of understanding about the person who is experiencing pain, what it means to them, how it affects them and which pain-relieving strategies are useful to them. Pain has an impact on how people live their lives, the quality of their life and how others interact with them. Nurses are in key positions to influence positively each resident's experience of pain, to work in partnership with them and to find out how they want to manage pain. Simply giving out medication is insufficient if we are trying to promote independence and maintain the dignity and self-esteem of residents living in long-stay settings.

PROVIDING PURPOSEFUL ACTIVITIES

Subsequent chapters in this book emphasize the range of activities available to residents in long-stay care units. These innovative schemes highlight the importance of a variety of activities, so that the older people can choose which to take part in. Again, nurses have a central role in imaginatively addressing this issue. In larger homes, there may be others involved in or responsible for these programmes, but nurses may be able to contribute to these plans through knowledge of an individual resident's likes or dislikes, so that a programme which caters for all tastes can be designed.

Turner (1993) has described how the introduction of a formal approach to activities, led specifically by a nurse, can enhance the quality of life for a group of residents. She defined activity nursing as: 'a simple concept of therapeutic care which meets a patient's psychological and social needs through mental stimulation and individual care, structured in the form of an activity programme' (p. 1727). The activity programme is individually determined and takes into account the resident's level of functional and cognitive ability. Turner refers to it as 'a combination of stimulation, reinforcement of functional ability and, most of all, of enjoyment' (p. 1727). Included in this approach are activities related to reality orientation, reminiscence, validation and resolution. Each resident's likes and dislikes, past experiences and present abilities are initially assessed so that the programme can be tailored to their needs. Nurses may also facilitate activities which range from visits to the local library to helping a person plan a meal for friends and cook it.

However, there is no substitute for conversation, sharing experiences, getting to know residents and understanding what makes them tick. This is part of skilled nursing but may become relegated to a secondary position when the pressure of day-to-day care becomes overwhelming.

Sharing may also be difficult since all experiences cannot be shared. Older people's experiences span most of this century and may be almost inconceivable to some who have not been exposed to them. Facilitating sharing is a central component of good nursing and can contribute constructively to the process of life review which many older people find valuable in later life.

PROMOTING CHOICE

The next important element of skilled nursing care is creating an atmosphere in which residents are encouraged to choose what they do. This centres on choice over things which, as nurses, we may take for granted. These include when to have a bath, when not to have a bath, which clothes to buy and wear, what type of meal to eat, when and with whom, and whether or not to have a sherry or beer before it. All of these things are part of ordinary life but, for a person living with others in an institution, they are not ordinary – these, and the choices associated with them, are the things which contribute to making life better.

As people grow old, each individual tries to maintain the habits, preferences and lifestyles that have been acquired during a lifetime. Victor (1987) states that ageing is a 'battle to preserve favoured lifestyles'. Old people admitted to institutional care may face difficulties in maintaining a previous lifestyle because their environment, companions and activities have changed. One way of contributing to the creation of an acceptable lifestyle is to encourage choice and to facilitate choices which are related to that previous lifestyle. These may include going to church regularly, eating special foods or visiting old haunts, as well as the more usual choices highlighted in the last paragraph.

VALUING INDIVIDUALITY

This is intimately linked to choice and independence since valuing individuality and providing care on an individual basis are central to both these and to the enhancement of physical and psychosocial well-being. Caring for someone as an individual, rather than just one of a group, means that nurses can really understand what their clients want from them and how they can actively contribute to creating a better lifestyle. This may focus on any aspect of life and so involve areas often skirted around by nurses, such as dying and sexuality.

Ways of valuing individuality are linked to establishing a rapport with each resident which incorporates mutual feelings of honesty, trust and respect. To help achieve this, it may be useful to know what residents want from nurses. Recently, Ford (1994) asked four continuing-care patients what they valued in nurses. The results are fascinating and may confirm some of your own intuitive feelings about the contribution that nurses make to the quality of life of older people. Information was obtained through semi-structured interviews and then categorized into a series of themes. The themes focused on classifying the nurse, what the patients thought the role of the nurse was, how they perceived their own role, and what they felt was important in the nurse–patient relationship.

Several interesting points emerged. Patients found that they could classify nurses as experts or novices and suggested that experts acted as role models to novices and were characterized by practising knowledge-ably and intuitively. Participants classified the ideal nurse as 'organised, calm and professional . . . intuitive . . . a nurse who really cares does things differently and they are greatly valued by patients' (p. 45). They stated that 'Expert nursing makes you feel life is worth living' (p. 46) and indicated that the role of the nurse is one which includes showing under-standing, caring and friendship.

Participants felt that being a patient was associated with dependency, feelings of vulnerability and having no home of one's own. Good nursing was associated with helping them to come to terms with being a long-term patient. Although not explicitly identified, this is likely to be linked to the elements they proposed as central to the nurse–patient relationship. These were sociability (civility, humour, socializing), reciprocity (friend-ship, sharing and problem solving) and the idea of 'my nurse' (showing involvement and working towards partnership, being a confidant, showing love and caring individually for each person).

These values show that, for these older people, good nursing went beyond sound physical care. Although leading to the creation of a better life, these components of care are hard to measure and may, because of this, be undervalued in economic terms. It is central for nurses to assess these crucial elements of care more frequently.

THE ENABLING ROLE OF THE NURSE

Throughout this chapter, the enabling role of the nurse has been empha-sized. This element of the nurse's role includes forming a partnership with residents through collaborative decision-making, sharing experiences and being empathic. Such partnerships are likely to enable older residents to feel that their lives retain a sense of dignity, independence and fulfilment, and that their care is in accordance with their wishes. The skills required by nurses to facilitate this are those described in Ford's study (1994) and may be summarized as expert nursing which includes understanding, caring and friendship and which can be extended to the resident and their friends and relatives.

HOME MAKING

The results of Ford's study (1994) emphasized that some older people see continuous care as being characterized by the removal of their own home. A crucial element of care, then, is to foster a homely atmosphere and environment in which to live. This can be achieved through the creation of a physical environment where residents have their own bedroom/area that is seen as their personal space and where their privacy and ownership is respected. This area can be furnished with favourite items from their own home and may be decorated to suit their taste. Nurses can facilitate this by encouraging residents to discuss their wishes and actively plan for this before or on admission. The creation of this type of environment is detailed in later chapters.

Nurses can also contribute to the ambience of the home by creating a therapeutic environment which fosters hopefulness, self-confidence, feelings of control and dignity (RCN, 1993a). This contributes to the homeliness of the environment and helps to create the feelings of safety and comfort which residents may attribute to their previous life in their own home.

DETERMINING THE QUALITY OF CARE

In the previous version of this chapter (Denham, 1991), Pam Hibbs emphasized the value of determining the quality of care provided for residents. Assessment of the quality of care provided remains a crucial aspect of monitoring care and helping potential residents and their carers to choose one facility over another. It is therefore a vitally important area for nurses to consider.

Although there a several 'off-the-shelf' tools to measure the care that older people receive in acute settings (e.g. Senior Monitor; Goldstone and Maselino-Okai, 1986), the type of innovative care provided within long-stay facilities may require a more individual approach. This may be achieved through the process of standard setting advocated by the Royal College of Nursing (Kitson, 1986). This approach captures the dynamic nature of care and emphasizes that standards, based on sound research, require continual monitoring and review. Staff involved in giving care are those who set the standards, and there is room for resident involvement to ensure that care is provided in accordance with their wishes, thus reinforcing the ideas of collaborative decision-making, partnership and choice discussed earlier.

Monitoring the quality of care emphasizes the link between measuring care and showing how valuable skilled nursing is to older people. Only through establishing this in an accepted, measurable way will the skills, knowledge and understanding of nurses caring for long-stay residents be appropriately evaluated and acknowledged by other nurses, other professionals and, perhaps most importantly, by older people seeking environments which can provide homely, therapeutic care for the rest of their lives.

REFERENCES

Denham, M. (ed.) (1991) *Care of the Long-Stay Elderly Patient*, 2nd edn, Chapman & Hall, London.

Evans, L. and Strumpf, N. (1992) Reducing restraints: one nursing home's story, in *Key Aspects of Elder Care* (eds S. Funk, E. Tornquist, M. Champagne and R. Wiese), Springer, New York.

Evers, H. (1981) Tender loving care? Patients and nurses in geriatric wards, in *Care of the Ageing* (ed. L. Archer Copp), Churchill Livingstone, Edinburgh.

Exton-Smith, A., Norton, D. and McLaren, R. (1962) *An Investigation of Geriatric Nursing Problems in Hospital*, Churchill Livingstone, Edinburgh.

Ford, P. (1994) What Older People, as Patients in Continuing Care, Value in Nurses. Keele University, MSc Thesis.

Ford, P. and Heath, H. (eds) (1996) *Older People and Nursing: Issues of Living in a Care Home*, Butterworth-Heinemann, Oxford.

Fordham, M. and Dunn, V. (1994) *Alongside the Person in Pain*, Baillière Tindall, London.

Goldstone, L. and Maselino-Okai, C. (1986) *Senior Monitor. An Index of the Quality of Care for Senior Citizens on Hospital Wards*, Newcastle upon Tyne Polytechnic Products, Newcastle upon Tyne.

Heslin, K. *et al.* (1992) Managing falls: identifying population-specific risk factors and prevention strategies, in *Key Aspects of Elder Care* (eds S. Funk, E. Tornquist, M. Champagne and R. Wiese), Springer, New York.

Hibbs, P. (1991) Nursing care, in *Care of the Long-Stay Elderly Patient* 2nd edn (ed. M. Denham), Chapman & Hall, London.

Hogue, C. (1992) Managing falls: the current bases for practice, in *Key Aspects of Elder Care* (eds S. Funk, E. Tornquist, M. Champagne and R. Wiese), Springer, New York.

Kitson, A. (1986) Methods of measuring quality. *Nursing Times*, 82 (35), 32–4.

McCaffery, M. (1972) *Nursing Management of the Person in Pain*, JP Lippincott, Philidelphia.

Raiman, J. (1986) Towards understanding pain and planning for relief. *Nursing*, 11, 411–23.

Reading, A. (1984) Testing pain mechanisms in persons in pain, in *Textbook of Pain* (eds R. Wall and R. Melzack), Churchill Livingstone, Edinburgh.

Redfern, S. (1989) Key issues in nursing elderly people, in *Human Ageing and Later Life* (ed. A. Warnes), Edward Arnold, London.

Ross, J. *et al.* (1992) Evaluation of two interventions to reduce falls and fall injuries: the challenge of hip pads and individualized elimination rounds, in *Key Aspects of Elder Care* (eds S. Funk, E. Tornquist, M. Champagne and R. Wiese), Springer, New York.

Royal College of Nursing (1993a) *Older People and Continuing Care. The Skill and Value of the Nurse*, Royal College of Nursing, London.

Royal College of Nursing (1993b) *The Value and Skills of Nurses Working with Older People*, Royal College of Nursing, London.

Seers, K. (1991) Pain and elderly people, in *Nursing Elderly People* (ed. S. Redfern), Churchill Livingstone, Edinburgh.

Smith, D. *et al.* (1992) Reduction of incontinence among elderly in a long-term care setting, in *Key Aspects of Elder Care* (eds S. Funk, E. Tornquist, M. Champagne and R. Wiese), Springer, New York.

Soja, M. *et al.* (1992) A risk model for patient fall prevention, in *Key Aspects of Elder Care* (eds S. Funk, E. Tornquist, M. Champagne and R. Wiese), Springer, New York.

Turner, P. (1993) Activity nursing and the changes in the quality of life of elderly patients: a semi-quantitative study. *J. Adv. Nurs.*, **18**, 1727–33.

Victor, C. (1987) *Old Age in Modern Society*, Chapman & Hall, London.

Wyman, J. (1992) Managing incontinence: the current bases for practice, in *Key Aspects of Elder Care* (eds S. Funk, E. Tornquist, M. Champagne and R. Wiese), Springer, New York.

Occupational therapy for older people with mental health problems   12

INTRODUCTION

Older long-stay patients often have complex needs arising from a multi-pathology of physical, psychological and social conditions. This requires a variety of skills which are often only available in a multidisciplinary team. Membership of this team should vary according to the needs of the individual and the setting. Commonly, in long-stay care of older people, the multidisciplinary team will include a consultant, nurses, occupational therapists, physiotherapists and social workers. When working with older people, team members should agree on common principles which uphold the individual's fundamental rights to dignity, choice, independence, privacy and fulfilment.

Occupational therapists can offer a range of services to older long-stay patients. This may include assessment of the individual's level of function, planning and implementing a programme of treatment to improve or maintain functional levels, educating the individual to adopt alternative strategies for achieving tasks, the provision of aids to enable tasks to be carried out, or adaptation of the individual's environment. Occupational therapists may also use counselling skills to support a patient's relatives or carers.

The first section of this chapter explores the definition of occupational therapy. The remaining sections describe the process of occupational therapy from the methods used to make the initial assessment to the approaches used to plan, implement and evaluate treatment. A case study, which is based on the occupational therapy treatment of an actual patient (although the identity has been altered for reasons of confidentiality), is presented to demonstrate translation of the theory of occupational therapy into practice. In summary, the chapter looks at the new opportunities for developing practices that arise when working with older patients and how occupational therapists can contribute to these. The research opportunities available to occupational therapists and other members of the multidisciplinary team are also discussed.

OCCUPATIONAL THERAPY: DEFINITION

Occupational therapy uses the medium of specific, selected occupation to treat physical or mental disorders. In this context, occupation is the meaningful use of activities, occupations, skills and life roles that enables people to function purposefully in their daily life. The aim of occupational therapy is to help patients to achieve maximum independence and quality of life and encourages them to help themselves. The four operational areas are to:

- diminish or control pathology
- restore or reinforce functional capacity
- facilitate learning of skills essential for daily living
- promote and maintain health.

THE OCCUPATIONAL THERAPY PROCESS

Occupational therapists should begin by collecting data about the individual and then using their knowledge of the theoretical basis of models of treatment to analyse the data and determine which approach is the most appropriate. These models of treatment are explained in more detail elsewhere (Hagedorn, 1992). An occupational therapist should then plan and implement the treatment accordingly. Finally, the occupational therapy process must include review and evaluation.

DATA COLLECTION

In order to assist older people to become as independent as possible, the occupational therapist must first determine each individual's abilities, problems, wishes and interests. By considering the person's abilities, the occupational therapist can use these to motivate the patient to participate in the treatment programme and can ensure the abilities are used and maintained.

Typically, the data collection method will include the use of interview, standardized assessments, and observation of the individual carrying out functional tasks.

INTERVIEW

When an older person's communication skills have been affected by mental disorder, it is not unusual for the person to be missed out altogether in the information-gathering process. However, a person with dementia will often try to communicate, and it is frequently the role of the therapist to utilize communication skills to understand the individual. Occupational therapists should use their knowledge of non-verbal as well as verbal skills and pay particular attention to the posture, gestures and facial expressions of the older person who is attempting to communicate. This can be a lengthy process and time has to be allowed by the therapist to allow the interview to be conducted at the slowed pace of the older person.

In addition to obtaining information directly from the individual, therapists will also talk with carers and other people who know the person well enough to be able to contribute to the data collection process.

STANDARDIZED ASSESSMENTS

Standardized tests are used to detect impairment and are therefore used by occupational therapists to obtain a baseline level of function against which the impact of subsequent occupational therapy can be measured. Interview and observation methods are also used so that the individual's abilities are also recognized. Assessments which have been well documented as reliable and valid, and which are appropriate for occupational therapists to use with older long-stay people, are the Clifton Assessment Procedures for the Elderly (CAPE) (Pattie and Gilleard, 1979), the Middlesex Elderly Assessment of Mental State (MEAMS) (Golding, 1989) and the Allen Cognitive Level Test (Allen, 1985).

Clifton Assessment Procedures for the Elderly (CAPE)

CAPE has both cognitive and behavioural components, which can be administered separately. It provides a dependency rating scale that can be used as a basis for treatment or for indicating the level of care needed by an individual.

Middlesex Elderly Assessment of Mental State (MEAMS)

MEAMS is a screening test used to detect impairment of specific cognitive skills in older people by asking them to perform simple tasks, each sensitive to the functioning of discrete areas of the brain. It is designed to assist in differentiation between organic and functional illness.

Allen Cognitive Level Test

The Allen Cognitive Level Test assesses the individual when carrying out a specific activity. An analysis of the individual's function during the test enables the therapist to determine which cognitive level the patient is at and the therapy required to help the individual live as normal a life as possible given that the disability exists.

OBSERVATION

Observing the older person carrying out a familiar activity may reveal the person's level of ability to perform even when cognitive disability exists. In a long-stay unit, an occupational therapist will typically have an assessment department which will have a kitchen, a bathroom, a bedroom and possibly a workshop. The older person may be observed carrying out a task in these areas or the occupational therapist may accompany the person to their own home where the familiar surroundings may help the individual to relax and perform at a higher level.

An appropriate task will be selected or designed by the occupational therapist which will reflect the individual's particular interests or lifestyle and performance of which will highlight any functional or cognitive deficits. For example, a housewife may be asked to make a cup of tea and a retired joiner to unscrew a screw from a piece of wood. Performance of either of these tasks will test orientation, sequencing, memory, safety, perception and visuo-spatial skills.

In addition to observing the actual performance of the task, the occupational therapist will also have an opportunity to obtain information in an informal manner about the older person's social and communication skills.

TREATMENT APPROACHES

When the information about the patient has been collected, it is used by the therapist to formulate a treatment plan. The person's interests and past roles are taken into consideration when planning the therapeutic activities. The techniques, or approaches, to be used to implement the therapy will depend on the therapist's definition of the patient's dysfunction and more than one approach may be used to complement each other.

COGNITIVE APPROACHES

These can be used within a rehabilitative and a developmental model. In rehabilitation, the aim is to restore functional ability and the criterion for evaluation of outcome is whether function has been demonstrated to be restored to a normal, or acceptable, level. An alternative criterion is whether a satisfactory method of compensating for any residual disability has been found. The techniques used involve redevelopment of cognitive skills. For example, a person with agnosia may work with pictures to improve naming skills and would then go on to naming actual objects. Although the progressive nature of the conditions of long-stay elderly patients is such that they appear unsuitable for rehabilitative treatment, it is often possible to address the symptoms of the condition rather than the condition itself and hence improve on function.

In the developmental model, the criterion for evaluation of outcome is whether the patient has shown progression from one level to a more advanced one. The techniques that occupational therapists would use within this model would not usually aim to improve cognitive function to a higher level than the assessed baseline as often the cognitive disability itself is untreatable. Instead, therapists would use their knowledge of their patients' levels of cognitive disability to assist them to overcome functional difficulties arising from the symptoms of the condition. If the therapist suspects that the patient is functioning below his potential, she will probe for function at the next cognitive level, giving support to aid task completion until the task can be completed unaided.

BEHAVIOURAL APPROACHES

A behavioural approach is most commonly used with long-stay older patients with dementia within a rehabilitative model to reduce the challenging behaviours associated with this condition. The therapist will collect data about the behaviour in terms of the triggers, the behaviour itself and the direct consequences of the behaviour, and will then design a behaviour modification programme which aims to reduce the unwanted behaviour by reinforcing the desired alternative. This approach is very much a team one where all members work together to the same programme using the same reinforcing strategies.

In many cases, the challenging behaviour is simply an expression of need by a person who is trying to communicate through the barrier of dementia (Stokes, 1995). The therapist's programme will therefore be aimed at understanding and meeting that need so that the challenging behaviour is reduced or prevented from occurring.

INTERACTIVE APPROACHES

Interactive approaches are person-centred. Occupational therapy is grounded in an holistic approach which is based on a knowledge of social relationships and utilizes the social environment (Willson, 1983). There is currently an explosion of interest in the experience, as opposed to the symptoms, of the person with dementia. The principles behind interactive approaches were first articulated and popularized by Carl Rogers in the 1950s. Validation therapy built on these frames of reference and was the first recorded attempt to use a person-centred approach in dementia care (Feil, 1967). The importance of social interaction on the quality of dementia care and on the person's state of well-being, regardless of the extent of neurological damage, is becoming increasingly apparent. It is now possible to measure the quality and effectiveness of care within a theoretical framework of dementia care based on a socio-psychological approach (Kitwood and Bredin, 1992).

NEURODEVELOPMENTAL APPROACHES

An occupational therapist may use a neurodevelopmental approach in the treatment of a patient. The basis of this approach is that any motor output is in response to sensory input, and that, by selectively stimulating the senses, it is possible to elicit the desired response. This approach may involve introducing special environments for sensory stimulation, such as coloured lighting, music and scents, which are housed in a room kept for that purpose. Alternatively, the therapist may use items of equipment in the activity, such as objects with varying textures or weight, perfumes and oils in a personal care activity, or music appreciation. The movement from one environment to another stimulates an individual to engage in, and act out, different roles. The occupational therapist will plan activities so that the patient is enabled to experience this stimulus.

TREATMENT PLANNING AND IMPLEMENTATION

After defining the terms of reference of working with an individual, the occupational therapist is then able to use the selected approaches to plan her treatment. Traditionally, group leisure activities have been the medium chosen when working with long-stay older patients. However, because the aim of the activity is to achieve the goals of therapy and have meaning for the person, a basic living task may be more appropriate. If, in the past, an older person has not had time to engage in leisure activities, they may feel uncomfortable with that role in the present and therefore not be so motivated to participate as they may in a light domestic task. When leisure activities are planned, the therapist has to take care to ensure that the equipment is age-specific. An older person may not be motivated to take part in a game that uses brightly coloured children's toys. The decisions that the therapist will make about the therapy will include whether to use a group or an individual approach and leisure or everyday activities. The choice will depend on the needs of the individual patient.

Some treatment techniques have a specific therapeutic value. These include reminiscence therapy and reality orientation.

REMINISCENCE THERAPY

Reminiscence has many benefits. It can help people to preserve their identity, find meaning and relevance in the present, or to solve problems by reviewing past experiences. Reminiscence can also be used as a recreational and social activity and may have therapeutic value if it facilitates communication and social skills.

A great variety of media can be used to trigger reminiscence, some of this in published form. Museums, libraries and community groups are useful sources of material.

The use of a lifestory book, which can include personal memorabilia, photographs and written information, can help older people to preserve their identity, promote self-esteem and enable others to gain a greater understanding of the person.

REALITY ORIENTATION

This is a treatment method which aims to stimulate people to relearn basic facts about themselves and their surroundings. The 24 hour method of reality orientation utilizes the systematic presentation and reinforcement of relevant information. It relies on the individual being able to learn and retain new information and is therefore not appropriate for people with moderate or severe dementia. A more individualized approach to reality orientation is to stimulate an individual's senses selectively over a series of treatment sessions. The aim is to assist the older people to become more aware of themselves and their surroundings. This method is called group reality orientation but it can also be carried out on an individual basis.

A RETURN OF HOPE AND SELF-ESTEEM

The following case study describes the practice of occupational therapy, and is set out in the format used in the model of human occupation, (Kielhofner, 1985).

Dr Warren was a 76-year-old patient who was admitted to long-stay hospital when his wife felt she could no longer look after him at home. He was diagnosed as having vascular dementia and hypertension, controlled by medication. Dr Warren had expressive dysphasia and his communication difficulties undermined his self-confidence. His short-term memory had also been affected by the dementia and he constantly sought reassurance from others about his circumstances and his surroundings. Dr Warren was referred for occupational therapy evaluation of his level of cognitive function and his potential for task performance.

PERFORMANCE EVALUATION

Motor skills

Dr Warren's ability to perform motor tasks was not impaired by his hypertension. When observed carrying out everyday tasks, his anxiety level was seen to rise as his cognitive limitations affected his ability to function. It was vital to consider the effect of Dr Warren's increased anxiety on his cardiovascular system when planning his treatment.

Cognitive skills

Dr Warren was evaluated using the Allen Cognitive Level Test. He was found to have a cognitive level of 3.7 (6 is normal). This means that his main difficulty was with deciding on the order and steps needed to complete a task. This was confirmed by the therapist's observations during the cognitive assessment and by Mrs Warren's report of her husband's level of function at home before he was admitted to hospital. Dr Warren needed repeated verbal prompts to complete tasks with several stages. In addition, Dr Warren's expressive dysphasia limited his ability to communicate. He displayed his frustration by the use of expletives and facial expressions.

HABITUATION EVALUATION

Roles

Dr Warren's roles were identified by interviewing him and his wife. Dr Warren stated that he views his role as husband and family man as very important. Until his illness, Dr Warren's married life was a partnership in which he and his wife both worked and shared the household tasks, decision-making and family commitments. Since the onset of Dr Warren's cognitive disability, his wife had taken over all of these roles.

Dr Warren was a retired academic. He lectured at the local university in the department of physics until his retirement at the age of 65. His wife, who was ten years his junior, continued to work as a business woman with her own management consultancy until her semi-retirement at the age of 60. She then became a director of the business and was still vocationally engaged to some extent.

Dr Warren had two children and three grandchildren. They all lived some distance from the hospital but visited him frequently and were concerned about his well-being.

Values

The values identified by Dr Warren as important were equality and being kind and helpful to others.

Interests

Dr Warren's social activities with his wife, family and friends and his vocational activities were his main interests prior to his retirement. Since the onset of his expressive dysphasia, Dr Warren isolated himself socially and became anxious and unsure of his functional ability.

Assets

• Could initiate actions to produce an end result.
• Could follow a two- to three-step sequence.
• Could communicate needs and feelings.
• Had a supportive family.

Limitations

• Did not notice mistakes or solve problems.
• Relied on learned material.
• Could be very demanding.

GOALS AND TREATMENT

Goals

The primary goals for Dr Warren were to develop his sense of self-worth, to improve his language skills to the optimum, increase his ability to engage in social and daily living activities, and reduce his anxiety level.

Treatment

The following actions were taken to achieve these goals. To improve Dr Warren's language skills, picture cards of everyday objects were shown to him each day and he was encouraged to name them. Initially the therapist gave him verbal prompts, but these were reduced as Dr Warren's confidence and his language skills improved. To reinforce this achievement, a graph was completed with Dr Warren which highlighted the increase in the number of objects he was able to name correctly. As his naming skills using pictures improved, Dr Warren was then encouraged to generalize his refound ability to objects in the long-stay unit. The therapist then worked with Dr Warren to increase his engagement in social activities. Initially they played a simple card game together to test his memory and mental manipulation skills. Dr Warren won several times. He was then encouraged by the therapist and the nurses on the unit to participate in the card group which met twice weekly. Dr Warren voiced his enjoyment of his new activity and the social interaction this involved him in.

The therapist also worked with Mrs Warren to help her to understand her husband's assets as well as his limitations so that she could enable him to carry out simple tasks successfully. When Mrs Warren visited her husband she worked with him to compile a photographic history of their life and family. This gave them a chance to share a simple task together and offered opportunity for both reminiscence and reality orientation.

To increase Dr Warren's successful engagement in daily living activities, the therapist advised staff working with him to break down the tasks into two- to three-step activities which he could achieve with minimal verbal prompting.

Finally, although Dr Warren's anxiety levels were seen to decrease as his functional abilities improved, relaxation therapy was introduced. This was achieved in two ways. Firstly, Dr Warren joined the relaxation group which met in comfortable surroundings with reduced lighting and listened to soothing music. Secondly, one of the nurses who was also an aromatherapist gave him a weekly aromatherapy massage.

OUTCOMES

Six months after the implementation of this treatment, Dr Warren's sense of self-worth seemed to have been restored. He exhibited less anxious behaviour and was not asking for as frequent reassurance from staff. Nurses reported an improvement in his ability to carry out self-care tasks. Mrs Warren reported that she found it much easier to relate to her husband and was starting to enjoy her visits to him in hospital, although she still had difficulty reconciling herself to leaving him when she went home. When the Allen Cognitive Level Test was readministered, Dr Warren was found to have improved to a cognitive level of 4, which could be accounted for by his improved state of well-being which positively affected his functional ability.

SUMMARY

Significant changes continue to occur in long-stay care for older people. The increased awareness of the impact that a nurturing social environment can have on an individual's cognitive and physical function has brought about great improvements in the work that is being done with older people in this setting. The occupational therapist is able to contribute to this process by utilizing holistic skills to understand each person's physical and cognitive abilities and limitations within the context of their individuality. The occupational therapist therefore makes an active contribution to the overall care process by using assessments to obtain a baseline of function against which to measure the impact of any interventions. The therapist can also help to maintain the older person's active engagement by offering and suggesting appropriate activities and simplifying tasks as necessary.

As research into the needs of older people in long-stay units continues, there will be improvements in the understanding and implementation of good care practices. Occupational therapists can contribute to this research process by measuring outcomes and publishing reports of their findings. A growing number of collaborative research studies by multidisciplinary teams are taking place. The advantages of this shared approach for all professionals involved and, more importantly, to the older people who are their patients, should not be underestimated.

ACKNOWLEDGEMENT

I am grateful to Rosemary Barnitt, Reader in Occupational Therapy in the School of Occupational Therapy and Physiotherapy, University of Southampton for her useful comments on the contents of this chapter.

REFERENCES

Allen, C.K. (1985) *Occupational Therapy for Psychiatric Diseases: Measurement and Management of Cognitive Disability*, Little Brown, Boston, MA, USA.

Feil, N. (1967) Group therapy in a home for the aged. *Gerontologist*, **7**, 192–5.

Golding, E. (1989) *The Middlesex Elderly Assessment of Mental State*, Thames Valley Test Company, UK.

Hagedorn, R. (1992) *Occupational Therapy: Foundations for Practice; Models, Frames of Reference and Core Skills*, Churchill Livingstone, Edinburgh.

Kielhofner, G. (1985) *A Model of Human Occupation: Theory and Application*, Williams & Wilkins, Baltimore, MA, USA.

Kitwood, T. and Bredin, K. (1992) Towards a theory of dementia care: personhood and well-being. *Ageing Soc.*, **12**, 269–87.

Pattie, A.H. and Gilleard, C.J. (1979) *The Clifton Assessment Procedures for the Elderly*, Hodder and Stoughton, London.

Stokes, G.J. (1995) *Challenging Behaviour in Dementia*, Winslow Press, Bicester, UK.

Willson, M. (1983) *Occupational Therapy in Long-Term Psychiatry*, Churchill Livingstone, Edinburgh.

The role of the physiotherapist in continuing care

13

Within continuing care settings, physiotherapists aim to maintain optimal levels of function or minimize the rate of deterioration through a care management plan agreed with the older person and their carers. Admission to a continuing care setting will follow a period of assessment and rehabilitation. Care plans directed towards the prevention and alleviation of movement disorders will prevent a decrease in functional level following the ending of the rehabilitation phase on transfer to continuing care. Carers need to ensure that 'caring for' the older person encourages as much independent activity as possible within individual limitations.

Within their life span in continuing care, older people will have intercurrent illnesses and injuries that will make movement difficult, e.g. falls with fractured bones and sore backs, influenza with increased muscle weakness and unsteadiness. Following these episodes, functional ability can be regained by a rehabilitation care package combined with a maintenance care plan. Physiotherapists also give appropriate advice to help minimize staff injury and maximize patient comfort and safety while being handled.

Older people are entitled to monitoring and reassessment of their physical condition at intervals by the physiotherapist whatever their care setting (NHSME, 1995). The caseload demand of visiting patients in their own home or in a variety of smaller care homes has implications on the cost and provision of equitable care. Other factors which can affect the effectiveness of the physiotherapy intervention are:

- lack of space to mobilize due to poor building design;
- lack of privacy in the care setting;
- lack of continuity of care staff to oversee the treatment practice;
- lack of access to treatment modalities due to shortage of portable equipment.

The role of a chartered psysiotherapist in continuing care can be summarized (CSP, 1992a) as:

- analysis of physical ability and mobility problems;
- continual review of physical ability within an agreed timescale;
- planning and carrying out skilled treatment;
- advising on pain management;
- advising on walking aids, wheelchairs, splinting for joint stability or pain relief, seating, pressure relief cushions, footwear, prostheses, hoists;
- delegating appropriate elements of the care plan to others;
- identifying the best way for staff to help and handle residents, to avoid injury to either;
- training carers and staff to carry out care and mobility programmes;
- identifying the need for intervention by another healthcare professional;
- liaising with the manager, relatives, carers and other professionals.

ASSESSMENT OF MOVEMENT ABILITY

Physiotherapists are skilled in identifying the practical problems associated with mobility impairment. Most older people want to be able to move within a limited environment, thus meeting their basic safety needs and increasing their levels of self-esteem (Maslow, 1962). Mobility is seen as the key to independence (Squires and Livesley, 1993) and affects quality of life as well as the long-term placement of an individual. Loss of mobility may necessitate the move from residential to nursing home, and will also be a contributing factor to the four giants of frail older care: contractures, falls, incontinence and pressure sores (Isaacs, 1992).

Analysis of movement during functional activities will identify problems within the movement process which may be remediable to physiotherapy intervention. Use of standardized assessment tools will ensure that intervention programmes can be evaluated, provide a structured format for clinical decision-making, and provide information for carers (Simpson and Forster, 1993)

The General Mobility Index (Figure 13.1) (Squires *et al.*, 1987) covers six areas of functional mobility. While ability on stairs and getting up from the floor may be inappropriate for very frail older people, this functional assessment can be completed quickly and can be used as an outcome measure when target levels are set following assessment. It has also been successfully used as a communication chart (Finlay, 1994) and can identify manual handling risks for carers.

In assessing and monitoring mobility, the Timed Up and Go Test (Podsiadlo and Richardson, 1991) is a valuable tool which can be completed in the home situation. The key components of this test are valuable functional indicators of balance reactions in sitting, standing, turning and gait analysis. Through this assessment, the physiotherapist can identify movement problems, e.g. difficulty standing from a chair; specific joint/muscle pain limiting walking ability, which the older person

	C	B	A
1. In/out bed and bed mobility			
2. In/out chair			
3. Toilet			
4. Walk inside			
5. Stairs (if necessary)			
6. Up from the floor			
7. Mental score			

Please block as appropriate   **Walking aid** _____

Levels of independent performance

C   Cannot do, does not or requires skilled help to perform the activity

B   Needs some help, verbal or physical, to carry out the operation

A   Independent, needs no help from another person, may use aids if required

---

Figure 13.1   General mobility index (Squires *et al.*, 1987).

may be able to improve and thus enhance their quality of life. The limited availability of clinical information from carers requires physiotherapists to undertake a detailed physical and psychosocial reassessment at each visit. In a community situation, this can be one of the factors contributing to the increased length of time required to treat a patient in their own home.

GOAL SETTING

Following discussion with the older person and their carer(s), goals of physiotherapy intervention will be agreed (Figure 13.2). The care packages provided by physiotherapists in meeting continuing health needs will involve mainly musculo-skeletal, neurological and circulatory care, with enabling, maintenance and palliative care objectives. Where a remediable problem such as a fracture or a stroke event occurs, rehabilitation will be required. The care objectives will be met by an intervention plan, which may involve training care staff in appropriate physiotherapeutic skills, e.g.

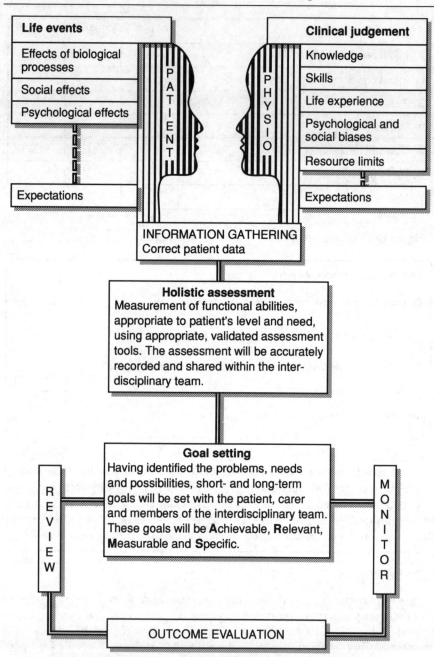

Figure 13.2   Holistic assessment and goal setting (adapted from ACPSIEP, 1991).

repetitive exercise, positioning, ambulation practice. Good physiotherapy outcomes have been shown in nursing home residents of advanced age (Chido *et al.*, 1992). Improvements in muscle strength and endurance, functional ability in rising from a chair, stair climbing and increased walking speed are all positive outcomes for older people in care settings (Fisher *et al.*, 1993). Where ambulation is not possible, wheelchair independence may improve the quality of life of an older person. With extremely disabled people, pain relief may be an effective goal to improve the quality of life. Where an older person does not require physiotherapy, their carers may require a physical health and well-being care package to prevent them suffering physical injuries while caring.

CASE HISTORY 1

Sarah, a fiercely independent 94-year-old lady living in a residential home, tripped and fell at a coffee morning 10 days previously. She has a badly bruised left leg and the care staff feel that she is staying more in her room and ask the physiotherapist to assess her.

Physiotherapist's assessment

Sarah has a very swollen and bruised left leg and can only wear her slippers after having cut the left one. She is also complaining of right shoulder pain with pins and needles in her right hand. This has bothered her for a month or so. She felt that her right hand and stick just didn't support her when she fell. She admits to having had a little urinary incontinence recently and at times she can't clear her right foot from the ground. Assessment tests found that Sarah had cervical spondylosis, trapping a nerve in her neck which was causing the problem with her right arm. She has an osteoarthritic left hip which makes her left leg 2 cm shorter than her right one, which is why she has been unable to clear her right foot at times.

Plan

1. Investigate the cause of the fall. Was it a pure accident? Did she turn her head suddenly? Did she move suddenly? Was she on any new tablets? Did she blackout at the time? What was she wearing on her feet at the time? How normal are her balance reactions? How does she feel now? Has she lost confidence walking? Why is she staying in her room?
2. Descrease the pain and pins and needles in her right arm and improve functional movements.
3. Ensure availability of good fitting footwear and arrange for a raise to

be put on to the left shoe with any necessary wedging to improve her gait pattern. Improve her balance reactions.
4. Encourage her to increase her mobility within the home by walking varying distances throughout the day. Sarah was unwilling to accept a Zimmer frame (that was for old people) but reluctantly agreed to accept two walking sticks instead of her previous one, which was too tall for her.

MAINTENANCE OF MOBILITY LEVELS

It is important to encourage older people to do as much for themselves as possible to prevent disuse atrophy. This can happen in care homes by not allowing the required time for transfers and dressing activities, as well as in an individual home by kind neighbours providing flasks of tea and sandwiches, placing the telephone and television controller at hand and using incontinence pads 'just in case', thus reducing the need to move to get a cup of tea, switch over the television, answer the telephone, or walk to the toilet. Living in one room during the winter months may economize on fuel but may also mean that the stairs are never tackled again. Attention to the environment is essential in maintaining the functional ability of older people in their care situation.

Physiotherapy and exercise are synonymous, and the benefits of exercise are widely accepted in all age ranges. Health benefits have been shown to accrue with increased physical activity by even the very old population, (Jirovec, 1991; McMurdo and Rennie, 1993; Pescatello and Dipietro, 1993). Apart from the physical benefits of improved movement, improvements in bowel and bladder function, social interaction and psychological benefits are apparent. Weight-bearing exercise has been shown to increase bone density, and weight-bearing activity needs to be encouraged throughout life to prevent osteoporosis.

Seating is an important aspect of the environment. A chair of an appropriate height and dimension for the individual will facilitate mobility and prevent excessive demands on carers for helping older people out of chairs. The use of properly adjusted spring-assisted seats may be beneficial to some patients who do not have the necessary muscle strength in their hip and knee extensors to move from a sitting to a standing position. Where special seating needs are identified, e.g. pressure-relieving cushions and wheelchairs, then these may be obtainable from the health authority.

CASE HISTORY 2

Tom, a resident in a nursing home, is being pushed to the toilet by care staff in a sani-chair to save him walking. He has recently been confused and noisy in the evenings and his general practitioner started him on a evening dose of thioridazine. Care staff complain to the physiotherapist that he is not mobilizing and just 'hangs' on them for all transfers, with the result that some care staff have injured their backs.

Physiotherapist's assessment

Tom functions best in the early afternoon as he is very sleepy in the morning. He has a poor gait pattern, with short shuffly steps. He is beginning to get hip and knee flexion contractures and has a shortened Achilles tendon on both legs. His shoes don't fit his feet any more due to ankle swelling which gets worse towards evening. He sits in a recliner chair all day and pressure sores are beginning on his ischial tuberosities.

Plan

1. Discuss with care team whether medication is making him too sleepy and contributing to his decreased walking ability.
2. Encourage care staff to sit Tom in a better position in a more appropriate chair, where his feet can be flat on the ground and his Achilles tendon can be stretched.
3. Use intermittent compression on his legs to decrease gravitational oedema and passively stretch knee contractures. Maintain control of ankle oedema by the use of support stockings applied by care staff.
4. Ensure staff are using appropriate manual handling aids for all transfers and that risk assessment forms have been completed by the management.
5. Encourage care staff to stand Tom at every opportunity using appropriate footwear, e.g. felt boots.
6. Gradually re-introduce walking a short distance in an upright posture between physiotherapist and support worker as his legs become stronger and he becomes less sleepy and more co-operative.

FALLS

Most people take calculated risks in their everyday life. For some older people, falls will be a common occurrence – the risk they take in choosing to maintain mobility. For other people, a fall may be a single incident, which requires thorough investigation into its cause and the rebuilding of confidence in their physical ability. Guidelines for treating people who have fallen are given in the fall intervention diagram (Figure 13.3).

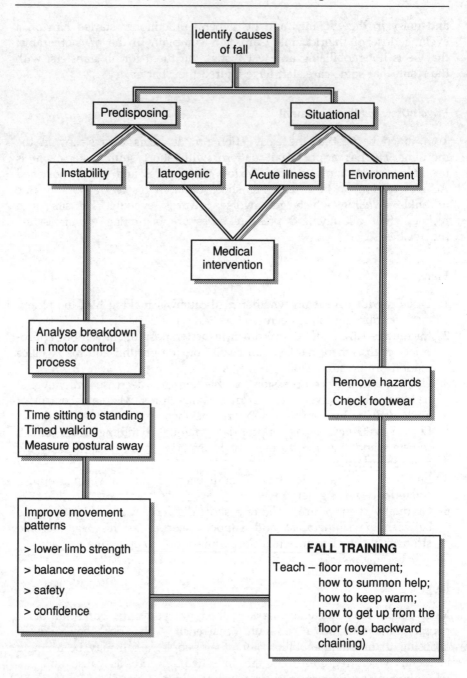

Figure 13.3   Physiotherapy: fall intervention diagram.

ORTHOTIC PROVISION

The supply of any orthoses (mechanical devices to support or correct weakened or deformed joints) will vary throughout the country. For advice on local provision, contact the local NHS Trust Physiotherapy Department or Appliance Officer.

ORTHOSES

A wide range of supports for joint stability or pain relief are available as stock or prescribable items.

WALKING AIDS

Patients will be assessed by a physiotherapist, and advice on the most appropriate aid, instruction in its use and advice on how to obtain it locally provided. People need walking aids for two reasons: (i) weight relieving, to reduce the stress on a painful or weakened joint; and (ii) to increase base area where balance reactions are diminished. In recent years, the use of wheeled rollators/mobilators has replaced standard walking frames (Zimmers), as a more natural gait pattern is facilitated and balance is not lost when lifting the frame forward. Manufacturers now produce a range of domestic frames which will pass through domestic doorways. Ergonomic consideration has also improved the design of the handles for walking sticks and it is possible to get differently shaped handles for easier grip. It is essential that the ferrules on all walking aids are checked regularly to ensure that they are safe and not worn. Walking aids should also be checked at all joints and hand grips to ensure that they are not deteriorating due to wear. Any faults should be reported to the supplier and replacement sought.

FOOTWEAR

Many older people wear inappropriate footwear which is too long, too tight, too high, too loose, or worn. Most older people are well advised to purchase flat walking shoes with either a lacing or Velcro fastening in a width suitable for them. Mail order companies are often a good source of appropriate footwear (including slippers), and the majority will check the fit of the shoe from a tracing of both feet in a standing position (DLF, 1990). If tying shoe laces is difficult, it is possible to obtain Velcro closures to replace the laces. The use of elastic shoe laces is not recommended as the shoe needs to be laced too loosely to allow the foot to be pushed into the shoe, reducing the support for the foot.

For wide, deformed feet, a wide range of stock orthopaedic footwear is now available at approximately 25% of the cost of bespoke footwear. Once suitable shoes have been found, they should be worn at all times when ambulating. Where walking is impaired, it is made more difficult in ill-fitting slippers where the foot muscles are required to hold the slipper on the foot, rather than performing their proper role in walking.

Sometimes it may be appropriate to arrange for orthotic adaptation of a shoe to alter the weight-bearing pattern, improving the gait pattern or ankle stability or reducing pain. Where there is weakness of ankle muscles, the use of a well-fitting boot (even a sports boot) can make a considerable difference to the gait pattern.

PALLIATIVE CARE

To relieve symptoms of terminal illness, the physiotherapist can assist with pain relief and the management of lymphoedema and chronic swelling, and give advice on positioning and pressure relief.

PAIN RELIEF

The skills of the physiotherapist can be used to relieve pain and discomfort. These may include massage, movement techniques, acupuncture, hot-and-cold therapy and a variety of electrotherapy modalities. Positioning and appropriate handling of the affected part will be required throughout the day. Where the aim of physiotherapy is the facilitation of movement, the reduction of pain to allow movement is an essential part of the physiotherapy intervention, to reduce the protective reflex mechanisms that are the body's reaction to pain (Figure 13.4).

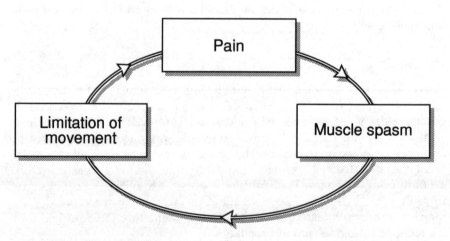

Figure 13.4 Pain cycle diagram.

LYMPHOEDEMA

An individual treatment package compiled from massage, manual lymph drainage, padded, multi-layered graduated compression bandaging, containment garments, skin care and gentle exercise can be used to control swelling.

CHRONIC SWELLING AND DEPENDENT OEDEMA

Many older people are unable to wear suitable footwear due to swollen legs. This is often due to low protein levels and a lack of exercise to ensure a sufficient venous return to the heart, not cardiac failure. Older people who have problems with swollen legs should be encouraged to:

- move around as much as possible;
- sit with their feet raised on a footstool of appropriate height to ensure the feet are at knee level with the knees supported;
- wear support stockings which fit properly: the support from the stockings increases the effectiveness of the muscle pump and grade 1 compression stockings are an acceptable form of compression for many patients to prevent the evening swollen ankle syndrome (Badger and Regnard, 1989)

POSITIONING

Inattention to good seating, lying and standing positions by carers can increase pain and lead to a fear of being handled. Appropriate positioning with particular attention to the position of the pelvis in the chair can:

- prevent the older person slipping out of the chair,
- prevent shearing forces on the ischial tuberosity when moving the older person back in the chair;
- increase the social interaction of the older person with the surrounding environment.

Chairs should:

- be of a height which allows the older person to have their feet rested on the ground, with their knees at right angles;
- be of a depth which supports the length of the femur;
- be wide enough to allow the patient access and not cause friction on the thighs;
- have a back support suitable for the shape of the older person, with cushions supplied to make allowances for kyphotic and osteoporotic spines.

Careful handling, using a palmar hold while moving limbs, will reduce the pressure on painful limbs. Passive movements of stiff and painful limbs should be carried out routinely, when moving an older person from one position to another. Many frail older people spend most of their day in a seated position with flexed spines, hips, knees and ankles. To prevent them contracting into a chair-shaped position, it is important to allow them the opportunity to stand erect whenever possible and to ensure that, when lying in bed, they get the chance to stretch hip and knee joints fully.

CASE HISTORY 3

Jane has had multiple sclerosis for many years and is now confined to a wheelchair. She lives in a private sheltered housing complex in a flat which is suitable for wheelchair living. Following a recent chest infection, she is now unable to transfer independently to her wheelchair and requires the help of two people to be lifted there from her bed. Her general practitioner has requested that the community physiotherapist see her to improve her transfering ability.

Physiotherapist's assessment

Jane has contractures of her hips and knees and has very little control of her knees. She has some spasms of her hips with internal rotation and a poor sitting position in her wheelchair. Her truncal muscles are weak, but her arms remain fairly strong and she is able to use them to groom herself, dress her upper body, write and propel her wheelchair. Transferring ability is poor as her truncal control will not allow her to sit without support. She requires the assistance of two people to transfer from wheelchair to bed, toilet and chair. Bed-to-wheelchair transfer is very difficult due to her inability to flex her trunk from a lying position. Her sacral and femoral pressure areas are at risk.

Plan

1. To alter her sitting position and reduce pressure on 'at-risk areas' by arranging a review of her wheelchair and cushioning by the wheelchair centre.
2. To reduce knee and hip flexion contractures and improve truncal strength by a programme of activities and exercise supervised by her support workers.
3. To prevent injury to support workers and healthcare staff by the provision of a mobile hoist and instruction in its use.
4. To review after two months whether truncal and leg strength will allow independent transfers.

SPECIAL NEEDS OF OLDER PEOPLE WITH MENTAL IMPAIRMENT

Older people with mental impairment can also have physical impairments such as mobility problems, acute injuries, pain and stiffness. Physiotherapists should use tactical approaches designed to overcome the communication and behavioural problems. These should include auditory, physical and memory cues to gain a functional response and have been well documented by Oddy (1987).

COMMUNICATION TACTICS

To encourage an appropriate response, approach slowly from the front, respect personal space and keep movements smooth and unhurried. It will help to use the person's name, speaking clearly (in a manner acceptable to an adult) and making eye contact.

VERBAL TACTICS

Allow plenty of time for understanding the spoken word, limiting requests to one at a time. Use words and expressions which are likely to be familiar and try to be positive, thus avoiding refusal. If necessary repeat what you say, using different words.

NON-VERBAL TACTICS AND CUES

The use of non-verbal cues will help understanding and facilitate movement. Gesture and light handling cues in the direction of movement will help to indicate where to sit, stand, turn, etc. Pictorial cues, such as 'nose over toes', can encourage the patient to transfer weight forward prior to standing and give a more specific direction than 'lean forwards'. The use of auditory cues and visual cues can also be helpful.

Handling skills which facilitate movement are taught to the carer as well as techniques to reduce the older person's fear of movement in open spaces. Specific physiotherapy techniques may be taught to the carer to mobilize joints and muscles as the older person will have memory retention problems. Steps must be taken to ensure the carer does not suffer from overload with too many tasks. It may be appropriate for physiotherapy assistants to work with the physiotherapists in the community, supporting the carers in specific movement activities.

MANUAL HANDLING

Every person caring for the physical needs of an older person will be involved in some manual handling. Increasing dependency levels will result in greater manual handling demands. The introduction of the HSE

Manual Handling Regulations placed a statutory duty on all employers and employees, in service and industrial sectors, to ensure the safe manual handling of all loads, including people as well as inanimate objects. The employer is expected to assess the risk of each manual handling manoeuvre. The employer is responsible for supplying training and equipment to reduce the risk of injury to the employee from a manual handling task. Each employee must ensure their personal fitness to carry out the task, be aware of the risk factors for each task and use the necessary equipment provided to reduce the risk of injury. Care staff who have to move patients will need training to ensure safe, efficient handling skills. The legal responsibilities of managers, staff and trainer need to be clarified prior to any adverse incidents occurring. Standards for trainers in moving and handling are available (CSP, 1994).

The increased awareness of manual handling has led to an increased demand for appropriate aids in all care situations. The risk assessment process will identify the types of aids which may be required, and the environment and the finance available will determine the model of aid purchased. The physical and mental state, together with the pattern of disability of the older person, will determine the level of support to be provided by the manual handling aid. Above all, aids must be acceptable to the older person and the carers using them, and adequate training in their use must be provided. Issues about the funding of manual handling aids will need to be addressed locally between health and social services department.

TYPES OF MANUAL HANDLING AIDS

Transfer belts and handling slings

A variety of fabric slings, webbing belts and moulded plastic slings and slides are produced by several manufacturers to reduce the amount of twisting and lifting required in moving people in bed and in lifts from bed to chair. To encourage people to move in bed, rope ladders, lifting blocks and over-bed lifting poles can be used.

Compressed air lifters

Many devices using compressed air are now on the market to lift legs into bed, sit the patient up in bed, or lift them out of the bath or off the floor.

Transfer boards and turntables

A variety of transfer boards is available to bridge the gap between two surfaces during sideways transfers. Turntables are particularly useful during an assisted standing transfer from chair to chair or chair to commode.

Wheeled shower chairs/commodes

To decrease the need for four transfers (from chair to wheelchair to toilet to wheelchair to chair), wheeled commode chairs can be used which can be placed over the toilet, with only two transfers being needed.

Hoists

Mobile hoists

An increasing variety of types and sizes is available at a wide range of costs. The limitations of the environment, the sling requirements and the carers' abilities will help to identify the most appropriate hoist in each situation. As lifting an older person off the ground is a highly risky manoeuvre, any hoist provided should be able to achieve the task. The provision of a hoist will not automatically reduce the required number of carers for the lifting task. Electrically controlled hoists may be easier to use, but a battery power supply should always be available.

Mobile seat lifts

A few pieces of equipment have been designed for people who need assistance for transferring from bed to chair or to toilet but do not require a full lift, as they are able to stand and take some weight through their bodies.

Electric overhead hoists

These are fixed ceiling- or wall-mounted hoists which are permanently sited in a building of a suitable construction. They can be used where space is restricted. In supported accommodation such as sheltered housing and residential or nursing homes, they can be of greater use to care staff than portable hoists.

For further information, refer to 'Hoists and Lifts Equipment for Disabled People' (Oxfordshire Health Authority, 1994).

ACCESSING PHYSIOTHERAPY SERVICES

The provision of physiotherapy services to continuing care residents varies widely throughout the country. With the closure of continuing care hospital beds, many physiotherapy staff were re-allocated within the acute hospital service and did not follow the patients out into the community. A survey of the availability of physiotherapy services in the nursing home sector (CSP, 1992b) found that:

- only a quarter of respondents knew of clear guidelines or a local policy regarding the provision of services in nursing homes;
- some older people resident in private nursing homes did not have access to free NHS physiotherapy services, which were enjoyed by their counterparts who still lived in their own homes, due to the lack of funding of physiotherapy posts for older care in the community;
- lack of resources restricted many NHS physiotherapy services to providing a very limited service.

While the above study considered private nursing home residents, older people living in the community may still have barriers of access to physiotherapy treatment:

- ageist referral policies may give priority to younger people who need to get back to work;
- acute problems may receive priority over chronic conditions;
- financing of services may be for specific client groups/Health of the Nation targets;
- geographical and boundary problems may exist between trusts (Hastings *et al.*, 1993).

Where physiotherapy is not available or is restricted within the local NHS trust, many officers in charge of residential/nursing homes have tried to employ their own private practitioners in physiotherapeutic activities, e.g. exercise classes, yoga, massage and aromatherapy. As physiotherapy is not a protected title, the credentials of anyone presenting as a physiotherapist should be checked. State registration with the Council for Professions Supplementary to Medicine – Physiotherapists Board is the minimum requirement for working in the health service or with general medical practitioners.

Having identified the needs of residents in private nursing, Duthie and Chesson (1994) recommend that:

- a national policy on the provision of physiotherapy services to people living in private nursing homes, along with an appropriate physiotherapy staffing level, is implemented;
- education is provided to nursing home managers and staff on the importance of activity in maintaining the health of older people and the role of physiotherapy in maintaining and improving the mobility of older people;

- the cost benefit of providing physiotherapy either through hospital outreach or community-based teams is investigated.

The Association of Chartered Physiotherapists with a Special Interest in Elderly People have collaborated with the Northern Ireland Health and Social Services Board to produce a checklist for mobility and independence in residential and nursing homes. This covers the following areas:

- access
- architecture and environment
- seating and beds
- physiotherapy provision
- health and safety
- wheelchairs
- promotion of independence
- footwear
- staff awareness.

CONCLUSION

Residents with continuing healthcare needs require access to a wide variety of physiotherapy interventions to enable them to retain as high a quality of life as possible in their later years. If lower levels of morbidity are expected in frail older people (i.e. they stay fitter longer), then preventive and rehabilitative measures must be carried out. This often requires a rapid response to the development of new problems, and these problems need to be managed by a team approach, which involves co-ordination and co-operation to ensure the delivery of the most appropriate care. Without access to a responsive and effective physiotherapy service, older people in continuing residential care will increasingly develop contractures, incontinence and pressure areas, decreasing their quality of life and increasing their dependence on staff and the health service.

REFERENCES

ACPSIEP (1991) *Physiotherapy with Older People, Standards of Clinical Practice,* Association of Chartered Physiotherapists with a Special Interest in Elderly People, London.

Badger, C. and Regnard, C. (1980) Oedema in advanced disease: a flow diagram. *Palliative Med.,* **3,** 213–15.

Chido, L.K., Gerety, N.B., Mulrow, C.D. *et al.* (1992) The impact of physical therapy on nursing home patient outcomes. *Phys. Ther.,* **72**(3), 168–73.

Chartered Society of Physiotherapy (1992a) Physiotherapy with older people in long-stay care. *Physiotherapy,* **78**(12), 904–6.

Chartered Society of Physiotherapy (1992b) *Survey of Pysiotherapy Services to Older*

People Resident in Nursing Homes, Professional Affairs Department, Chartered Society of Physiotherapy, London.

Chartered Society of Physiotherapy (1994) *Standards for Trainers in Moving and Handling Skills*, Chartered Society of Physiotherapy, London.

Disabled Living Foundation (1990) *Footwear: Disabled Living Foundation, Resource on Footwear and Disability*, Disabled Living Foundation, London.

Duthie, J. and Chesson, R. (1994) *Physiotherapy in Private Nursing Homes*, School of Health Sciences, Robert Gordon University, Aberdeen, UK.

Finlay, O. (1994) Communication chart. *Physiotherapy*, **80**(3), 172–3.

Fisher, N.M., Gresham, G.E., Abrams, M. *et al.* (1993) Quantitative effects of physical therapy on muscular and functional performance in subjects with osteoarthritis of the knees. *Arch. Phys. Med. Rehab.*, **74**, 840–7.

Hastings, M. and Squires, A. (1993) Physiotherapy staffing levels for older people: ACPSIEP recommendations. *J. Assoc. Chartered Physiotherapists with a Special Interest in Elderly People*, **July**, 16–17.

Isaacs, B. (1992) *The Challenge of Geriatric Medicine*, Oxford University Press, Oxford, UK.

Jirovec, M.M. (1991) The impact of daily exercise on the mobility, balance and urine control of cognitively impaired nursing home residents. *Int. J. Nurs. Studies*, **28**(2), 145–51.

Maslow, A.H. (1962) *Towards a Psychology of Being*, Van Nostrand, New York.

McMurdo, M.E.T. and Rennie, L. (1993) A controlled trial of exercise by residents of old people's homes. *Age Ageing*, **22**, 11–15.

NHS Management Executive (1995) *Health Service Guidelines: NHS Responsibilities for Meeting Long Term Health Care Needs*, Department of Health, Leeds, UK.

Oddy, R. (1987) Promoting mobility in patients with dementia; some suggested strategies for physiotherapists. *Physiother. Pract.*, **3**, 18–27.

Oxfordshire Health Authority (1994) *Hoists and Lifts Equipment for Disabled People*, 3rd edn, Oxfordshire Health Authority, Nuffield Orthopaedic Centre, Oxford, UK.

Pescatello, L.S. and Dipietro, L. (1993) Physical activity in older adults, an overview of health benefits. *Sports Med.*, **15**(6), 353–64.

Podsiadlo, D. and Richardson, S. (1991) The timed 'up and go': a test of basic functional mobility for frail elderly persons. *J. Am. Geriatr. Soc.*, **39**, 142–8.

Simpson, J.M. and Forster, A. (1993) Assessing elderly people – should we all use the same scales? *Physiotherapy*, **79**(12), 836–8.

Squires, A., Dolbear, R. and Smoker, S. (1987) Evaluation of physiotherapy in a day unit. *Physiotherapy*, **73**(11), 596–8.

Squires, A. and Livesley, B. (1993) The future of physiotherapy with older people: demographic, epidemiological and political influences. *Physiotherapy*, **79**(12), 851–7.

Communication and swallowing: do they matter?

14

COMMUNICATION AND NORMAL AGEING

Many people assume that old age and senility go hand in hand; that part of growing old inevitably involves memory loss and increasing physical and social dependence. This is not necessarily the case. Older people do not form a homogenous group and have as many individual differences as any other age group. However, these common perceptions lead to expectations and attitudes towards older people that can limit and disempower them. This is particularly true when related to communication (Kaakinen, 1992; Ryan, 1994). For the majority of people, growing older does involve changes in cognitive and communication skills. These are frequently portrayed as 'deficits'. However, Maxim and Bryan (1994) suggest that 'A much more positive view of the elderly is to regard cognitive processing as [simply] changing with age and to separate "normal" changes from the pathological changes associated with disease. Thus, what is "normal" for a 20 year old is different from what is "normal" for a 60 year old.' The accumulation of a lifetime's experiences does bring about benefits also, in that knowledge and use of vocabulary and grammar may improve throughout adulthood.

The most common age-related changes affecting communication are perceptual deficits in hearing and vision. Beyond these, the main changes appear to be in terms of a slowing of response times. Retrieval of information in tasks such as decision-making, generation of ideas and making associations may take longer. These changes are usually thought to be discrete, however, and may not markedly interfere with normal conversational interaction. At least until late old age, communication skills appear not to be significantly affected in themselves. Sensory deficits, and other factors such as depression, can impair both verbal and non-verbal communication, and should therefore be carefully differentiated from normal ageing and dementia.

With increasing physical dependence and social isolation, long-term residential or nursing care is an increasing option for many elderly people. The effects of such environments on communication can be profound. Lubinski (1991) suggested that both homes and institutional settings can become 'communication-impaired environments'. She outlined some common characteristics:

1. lack of sensitivity to the value of interpersonal communication as the cornerstone of effective functioning and self-realization;
2. perceived restrictive 'rules' inhibiting communication;
3. few or no communication partners of choice present;
4. few reasons to talk;
5. individuals perceiving themselves as having little meaningful contribution to their environment through communication;
6. a lack of privacy inhibiting conversation;
7. an environment with either too much or too little sensory stimulation.

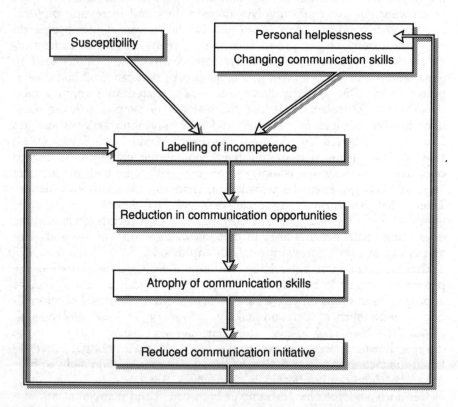

Figure 14.1 Social breakdown syndrome as applied to communication (reprinted from Lubinski *et al.* (1991), with permission).

Ryan *et al.* (1994) describe a 'communication predicament' model of ageing. In this model, 'babytalk' addressed to some older people (especially those who are frail or in a home) is seen as based on stereotyped assumptions of incompetence and dependence. This, they say, can lead to lower self-esteem in the older person and a decline in opportunities for satisfying communication (compare with Lubinski's proposals (1991) for the extension of a learned helplessness model to communication, Figure 14.1).

Kaakinen (1992), however, outlines some self-regulatory beliefs that result in limited talking amongst nursing home residents, which included such communication 'rules' as:

- ignore those perceived to be senile;
- talk to people who talk to you (therefore, residents would stop talking if placed with a non-talking resident);
- do not initiate conversation with those 'hard of hearing';
- withdraw from communication with other residents for fear of being misunderstood;
- avoid those who talk 'all the time'.

She puts these 'rules' into some context by saying that residents reflect societal mores that exist in the larger community in which they lived for most of their lives.

The physical nature of the environment can also mitigate against or facilitate communication. The effects of lighting, background noise, private and public space are considered by Lubinski (1991), who has produced a 'communication/environment assessment and planning guide'.

COMMUNICATION-IMPAIRED ENVIRONMENTS AND INTERVENTION

A reason for the low level of interactions between staff and residents may be due to the absence from nurse education of adequate communication skills training. The charity 'Action for Dysphasic Adults' has compiled a package for residential or nursing home care staff – 'Communicate' – under the supervision of trained speech and language therapists. This useful resource gives in-service training in how to facilitate communication with people with speech and language difficulties.

Careful assessment of sensory deficits, and the appropriate provision of hearing aids and glasses, is essential in ensuring that the precursors to communication are dealt with. Creating regular opportunities for meaningful interaction and communication, beyond basic health care, is essential. Small groups, led by a person skilled in interactive communication skills, are ideal. Activities that emphasize the importance of individual contributions can help to validate people's experiences and self-worth. Finally, trained volunteers have been used as conversation partners by many organizations (e.g. the Stroke Association in the UK).

COMMUNICATION AND DEMENTIA

There are many different types of dementia. The most commonly cited symptom is memory loss, with deterioration in communication not considered until later in the progress of the disease. However, extensive research over the last 15 years particularly has shown that subtle language and communication deficits may occur in the early stages of dementia. Rabins *et al.* (1982) found that almost 70% of families in their study reported communication difficulties in relatives with dementia. Nearly 75% of these saw those communication problems as significant for them as carers.

The typical pattern of communication breakdown in Alzheimer's disease appears to be in semantics (the meanings of words) and pragmatics (the use of communication in context). Other skills, such as phonology (the sounds in words) and grammar, seem to be relatively spared, at least until the late stages of the disease. Words may be forgotten or incorrect words substituted. Conversations may go off at tangents. Speech is characteristically empty of content but grammatically correct.

Kemper *et al.* (1994) found that people with dementia responded more appropriately when their spouses reduced the complexity of their language and emphasized important key words. Therefore, explanation and training in these type of skills would be valuable in reducing the frustration and helplessness felt by caregivers (Tanner and Daniels, 1990). Appendix 1 gives details of practical strategies for improved communication.

COMMUNICATION AND APHASIA

Aphasia (or dysphasia, as it is more commonly known in the UK) is a complex disorder of language. Other cognitive skills are generally preserved. It can affect the understanding of spoken and written information, and the ability of the person to put their thoughts into words and sentences. It is most commonly the result of a stroke, but can occur after head injury and brain tumours.

The severity of symptoms ranges from complete inability to speak or write, to mild word-finding difficulties or sound substitution errors. Aphasia is usually of sudden onset, can have a dramatic emotional impact on the person and those around them, and can even produce long-term stress in relationships.

A comprehensive assessment can be carried out by a speech and language therapist. This includes an evaluation of verbal and non-verbal skills, as well as emotional and psychosocial factors. The purpose of such assessment is to provide a picture of communication strengths and needs, a rationale for therapy, and a baseline for monitoring change.

Byng (1993) outlines the scope of the speech and language therapy intervention:

- an assessment of the uses of language made by the person with aphasia before becoming aphasic;
- detailed assessment of the language breakdown and remaining strengths in communication;
- an attempt to treat the language disorder itself;
- support in coping with changed communication skills;
- encouragement in the use of all other potential means of communication, e.g. gesture, drawing, pointing;
- enabling the person to use what remaining language they have to its best effect;
- help with using their changed communication skills in everyday real-life settings;
- education of those around the person with aphasia in how they can change their approach to communication to ease frustration.

To that list should be added education of the person with aphasia and their family about the cause and nature of aphasia, and counselling about the distress and role changes it brings.

The effectiveness of speech and language therapy intervention in aphasia has been questioned. However, more recently, many published studies have shown that specific language gains can be made in spoken language (e.g. Marshall *et al.*, 1989), in understanding language (Byng, 1988), and in reading and writing (de Partz, 1986).

Interestingly, the effect of age on the prognosis for recovery in aphasia is not felt to be significant (Basso, 1992). Furthermore, the length of time after acquiring aphasia is not necessarily a key determinant of how people can respond to therapy. Improvements in communication have been reported after intervention months or even years after onset of the aphasia (Poeck *et al.*, 1989).

The focus of therapy needs to be a broad one, with attention also paid to developing functional communication where the language system is impaired, training conversational partners to facilitate communication, and the use of volunteers to support and encourage people with dysphasia. Recently, self-help groups have been created, run by people with aphasia for people with aphasia (supported by Action for Dysphasic Adults). These resources can also be used for the aphasic person in long-term care as a bridge to the community and an affirmation of their value as individuals, despite their communication problems.

COMMUNICATION AND DYSARTHRIA

Dysarthria is a disorder of speech that results from disturbances in muscular control – weakness, slowness or lack of co-ordination – of the speech mechanism due to damage to the central or peripheral nervous system or both. Speech movements may show abnormal speed, range, strength or co-ordination. It may occur alongside dysphasia or dysphagia or in isolation. As dysarthria is not a disorder of language, it does not affect the person's ability to read, write, formulate sentences or understand what is said to them. It can be caused by a variety of medical conditions. The most common causes of dysarthria in older people are cerebrovascular accident and Parkinson's disease.

Dysarthria is an umbrella term for six different types of dysarthria, each presenting with specific speech characteristics. It can affect any of the following areas of speech activity in a variety of combinations and with varying severity:

- breathing pattern for speech
- oral and facial muscles
- muscles of the throat
- intonation and pitch

Table 14.1 indicates some of the more frequent dysarthric features found in a variety of comon neurological diseases.

Table 14.1   Symptoms of dysarthria

Aetiology	Symptoms
Cerebrovascular accident (stroke)	Slurred speech Hypernasality Poor breath support for speech Reduced pitch and volume control
Parkinson's disease	Monotonous sounding speech Variable rate of speech Difficulty with initiating speech Breathy voice and poor volume
Motor neurone disease	Slow, slurred speech Hypernasality and air escape Reduced volume
Multiple sclerosis	Slow and laboured speech Strained/strangled voice Low pitch and little variation Hypernasality

DYSARTHRIA AND CLINICAL MANAGEMENT

Speech and language therapy intervention primarily seeks to reduce or achieve maintenance of the level of disability rather than restore normal speech. However, for some patients, great gains can be made in restoring the affected parameters and achieving excellent intelligibility. Studies reporting on treatment efficacy are in their infancy but there are a number of well-documented case studies which reveal positive treatment outcomes (Netsell and Daniel, 1979; Keatley and Wirz, 1994). Other patients may never regain functional intelligibility and may therefore need to use a communication aid system or a communication aid to augment their speech. Others still may have adequate intelligibility but reduced volume, making their speech indistinct. In this instance, a voice amplifier, which is extremely easy to use, may be helpful to restore volume to a desirable level for communication. The choice of aid may vary from a straightforward communication chart through to a dedicated communication aid using notebook computer technology. The choice will depend on a multiplicity of factors, including the exact nature and severity of the patient's speech problem, their specific communication needs, the likely course of the disorder (i.e. stable or deteriorating) and the demands of their environment.

Finally, mention must be made of the adverse effects of certain medications on speech. Xerostomia – the decrease or absence of salivary secretions – can cause difficulties with speech, mastication and swallowing. Table 14.2 lists the types of drugs that may be responsible for producing or exacerbating the symptoms of xerostomia (Soon, 1992). However, this list is not exhaustive, and where there is doubt it is useful to discuss the problem with a pharmacist or the doctor.

Table 14.2   Drugs that can cause xerostomia

Type of drug	Examples
Anticholinergics	Propantheline
Antihistamines	Diphenhydramine, dimenhydrinate
Antipsychotics	Thioridazine, chlorpromazine, haloperidol
Psychotropic	Lithium carbonate
Antidepressants	Amitriptyline
Anti-Parkinson's	Benztropine
Anti-anxiety	Hydroxyzine, diazepam
Anti-hypertensives	Reserpine, methyldopa
Diuretics	Frusemide, hydrochlorothiazide

DYSPHAGIA

Dysphagia (difficulty with swallowing) is a common and increasing problem among the older population. Dobkin (1991) found that 10% of acute hospitalized older people and 30% of those in nursing homes presented with dysphagia. It is therefore an area of great concern when caring for long-stay older patients.

Normal oral intake for nutrition requires fine neuromuscular control of structures in the oral cavity, pharynx, larynx and oesophagus in order to hold and prepare food prior to swallowing and for safe transport to the stomach.

NORMAL SWALLOW PROCESS

The swallowing reflex is a complex and highly co-ordinated activity involving an intricate neural network from the frontal cortex to the salient

Table 14.3　The normal swallow

Stage	Procedure
Oral	Liquids held and food reduced to a texture appropriate for swallowing by: • lip closure to keep food in the mouth; • adequate facial tone to maintain closure of the anterior and lateral sulci and moving food to the tongue midline to faciliate chewing; • jaw motion to chew food; • lateral tongue motion to control food in the mouth and mix it with saliva; • lowering and engorging of the soft palate to prevent premature spillage into the pharynx; • upward and backward propulsion of the tongue moving the food towards the pharynx; • initiation of the swallow reflex in the region of the faucial arches
Pharyngeal	Closure of the soft palate against the pharyngeal wall to prevent nasal reflux Elevation and upward movement of the larynx and hyoid bone Closure of the epiglottis and vocal folds to prevent aspiration Relaxation and opening of the cricopharyngeal sphincter
Oesophageal	Bolus passes down oesophagus to the stomach propelled by peristaltic waves

musculature. The swallowing process can be divided into three component stages:

- oral
- pharyngeal
- oesophageal.

The oral stage is voluntary and controlled by cortical centres in the brain, whereas the pharyngeal and oesophageal stages are involuntary and co-ordinated by centres in the brainstem. Table 14.3 identifies the key components of the normal swallow.

SWALLOWING PROCESS AND AGEING

It is important to note that normal ageing has an effect on swallowing. The effect of these changes will not be evident before the age of approximately 80 years. Several studies have documented the changes brought about by the ageing process (Feinberg *et al.*, 1990; Donner and Jones, 1991; Shaker and Lang, 1994):

- altered tongue position and movement;
- changes in lip position perhaps leading to habitual drooling of saliva;
- decrease in production of saliva possibly leading to xerostomia;
- decrease in senses of taste and smell;
- overspill of liquid to pharynx prior to swallowing; this can usually trigger a swallow and avoid significant airway penetration;
- increased need to chew food more thoroughly;
- reduced movement of the hyoid bone and larynx, possibly leading to aspiration;
- the laryngeal surface epithelium becomes less sensitive to aspirated material and this, associated with loss of the protective gag reflex, may explain why silent aspiration seems to occur more often in older people;
- decrease in co-ordination between the oral and pharyngeal stages.

These factors may be excaberated by problems with dentition, i.e. absent/ poorly fitting dentures. It is therefore not surprising that eating and swallowing can be difficult even for normal older people. In addition, changes in pulmonary function that occur with ageing may decrease cough effectiveness, diffusion capacity and oxygen saturation.

THE EFFECTS OF DISEASE ON THE SWALLOWING PROCESS

A common cause of neurogenic dysphagia in the elderly is a cerebrovascular accident (stroke): 75% of all strokes occur in people over 65 years old. Acute and chronic swallowing problems in stroke patients are associated with many complications, including dehydration, malnutrition, aspiration, pneumonia and even death. Other common neurological

Table 14.4 Indicators of dysphagia

Stage	Indicator
Oral	Difficulty with controlling saliva Food seeping from mouth, including dribbling of liquids Pocketing of food in cheek Avoidance of certain foods and consistencies
Pharyngeal	Coughing/spluttering before, during or after eating or drinking Weak reflexive cough; weak spontaneous cough Food sticking in throat Nasal regurgitation of food or drink Wet/hoarse voice

disorders may give rise to dysphagia are the progressive diseases such as Parkinson's disease, motor neurone disease and Alzheimer's disease, and demyelinating diseases, e.g. multiple sclerosis.

DYSPHAGIA AND CLINICAL MANAGEMENT

Dysphagia can be recognized by the symptoms mentioned in Table 14.4. Its management should ideally take place within a multidisciplinary team framework with each professional contributing their specific skill and expertise. This enables the overall management to be holistic and enables information to be integrated. Referrals are made to the speech and language therapist by the medical team for assessment, diagnosis and management of the swallowing disorder. Assessment involves:

• a detailed medical history;
• a case history including the patient's description of the problem;
• a bedside swallowing examination that incorporates an orofacial and cranial nerve examination;
• clinical trials of various food consistencies (if cough reflex and swallow reflex adequate);
• maybe a radiographic study such as videofluoroscopy to determine the presence and extent of aspiration and the effects of various therapeutic strategies.

From the information gathered, a diagnosis and detailed profile of the dysphagia can be documented and management strategies devised. If oral intake is not possible immediately, a non-oral feeding regimen should be recommended until adequate swallow function recovers.

A common mistake in assessment of the swallowing function is the importance placed on the gag reflex. It should be noted that there is no causal link between an absent or diminished gag reflex and the presence or otherwise of dysphagia (Dilorio and Price, 1990; Bleach, 1993; Lugger, 1994).

DAILY MANAGEMENT STRATEGIES FOR DYSPHAGIA

Numerous techniques and strategies useful for assisting the dysphagic person when eating are documented in the literature. The following are general guides for daily management.

Guidelines for eating in normal older people

1. Provide an environment conducive to eating. Limit distractions and allow the person time to eat. If the person feels hurried or distracted, ability to concentrate on the act of swallowing is diminished.
2. Be aware of the importance of regular oral hygiene. Check this before a meal and clear out any food residue left in the mouth after eating.
3. Encourage the person to wear their dentures whenever possible providing they are a good fit.
4. Position the person upright with head and shoulders slightly forward.
5. Choose foods and fluid (in association with the person) of suitable consistencies. Some foods may be more difficult than others, e.g. meats.
6. Make sure the person is sitting as upright as possible when eating and for half an hour afterwards.
7. Be aware of the following which may indicate difficulty with eating:
   - loss of weight
   - hunger
   - excess of oral secretions
   - respiratory problems
   - coughing and choking
   - refusal to eat
   - dehydration.

Guidelines for those with dysphagia

1. Follow the guidelines in the swallowing programme if one has been provided by the speech and language therapist and those outlined above.
2. Be aware of any sensory neglect or visual problems – make sure they can see the food.
3. Head posture – make sure their head is in the midline front to back and is not tilted backwards. Encourage the person to tuck their chin into their chest as this helps to reduce the risk of aspiration.
4. Place food on the unaffected side of the tongue, allowing the patient to sense where the food is, decreasing the likelihood of aspiration.

5. Encourage the person to take two swallows per mouthful.
6. Encourage the person to cough after several swallows.
7. Observe the person after eating for:
   - coughing and choking
   - change of colour
   - sounds of respiratory difficulty – wheezing or gurgling
   - wet or gurgly-sounding voice quality
   - gasping
   - rapid heart rate
   - pocketing of food in the mouth.
8. Keep a record of the patient's oral intake.

If a person is suspected of having difficulty with swallowing or demonstrates any of the symptoms outlined in Table 14.4 or above, a referral should be made to a speech and language therapist for assessment.

REFERENCES

Basso, A. (1992) Prognostic factors in aphasia. *Aphasiology*, **6**(4), 337–48.

Bleach, N. (1993) The gag reflex and aspiration: a retrospective analysis of 120 patients assessed by videofluoroscopy. *Clin. Otolaryngol.*, **18**, 303–7.

Byng, S. (1988) Sentence processing deficits: theory & therapy. *Cognitive Neuropsychol.*, **5**, 191–201.

Byng, S. (1993) Hypothesis testing and aphasia therapy, in *Aphasia Treatment: World Perspectives* (eds A.L. Holland and M.M. Forbes), Chapman & Hall, London.

Dilorio, C. and Price, M.E. (1990) Swallowing: an assessment guide. *Am. J. Nurs.*, **7**, 38–41.

Dobkin, B.H. (1991) The rehabilitation of elderly stroke patients. *Clin. Geriatr. Med.*, **7** (3), 507–23.

Donner, M.W. and Jones, B. (1991) Aging and neurological disease, in *Normal & Abnormal Swallowing – Imaging in Diagnosis and Therapy* (eds B. Jones and M.W. Donner), Springer-Verlag, New York.

Feinberg, M.J., Knebl, J., Tully, J. and Segall, L. (1990) Aspiration and the elderly. *Dysphagia*, **5**, 61–71.

Kaakinen, J.R. (1992) Living with silence. *Gerontologist*, **32**(2), 258–64.

Keatley, A. and Wirz, S. (1994) Is 20 years too long? Improving intelligibility in long-standing dysarthria – a single case treatment study. *Eur. J. Dis. Commun.*, **29**(2), 183–201.

Kemper, S., Anagnopoulos, C., Lyons, K. and Heberlein, W. (1994) Speech accommodations to dementia. *J. Gerontol.*, **49**(5), 223–9.

Lubinski, R. (1991) Environmental considerations for elderly patients, in *Dementia & Communication* (ed. R. Lubinski), B.C. Decker Inc., Philadelphia, PA, USA.

Lugger, K.E. (1994) Dysphagia in the elderly stroke patient. *J. Neurosci. Nurs.*, **26**(2), 78–84.

Marshall, J., Pound, C., White-Thomson, M. and Pring, T. (1989) The use of picture–word matching tasks to assist word retrieval in aphasic patients. *Aphasiology*, **4**(2), 167–84.

Maxim, J. and Bryan, K. (1994) *Language of the Elderly*, Whurr Publishers Ltd, London.

Netsell, R. and Daniel, B (1979) Dysarthria in adults: physiologic approach to rehabilitation. *Arch. Phys. Med. Rehab.*, **60**(11), 502–8.

Orange, J.B., Molloy, D.W., Lever, J.A. *et al.* (1994) Alzheimer's disease: physician–patient communication. *Can. Family Phys.*, **40**, 1160–8.

de Partz, M.P. (1986) Re-education of a deep dyslexic patient: rationale of the method and results. *Cognitive Neuropsychol.*, **3**, 149–77.

Poeck, K., Huber, W. and Willmes, K. (1989) Outcome of intensive language treatment in aphasia. *J. Speech Hear. Disord.*, **54**, 471–9.

Rabins, P., Mace, N. and Lucas, M. (1982) The impact of dementia on the family. *JAMA*, **248**, 333–5.

Ryan, E.B., Hamilton, J.M. and See, S.K. (1994) Patronising the old: how do younger and older adults respond to baby talk in the nursing home? *Int. J. Aging Hum. Dev.*, **39**(1), 21–32.

Shaker, R and Lang, I.M. (1994) Effect of aging on the deglutitive oral, pharyngeal and esophageal motor function. *Dysphagia*, **9**, 221–8.

Soon, J.A. (1992) Effects of drug therapy on oral health of older adults. *Can. Dent Hygiene/Probe*, **26**(3), 118–20.

Tanner, B.B. and Daniels, K.A. (1990) An observation of communication between carers and their relatives with dementia. *Care Elderly*, **2**(6), 247–50.

APPENDIX 1

COMMUNICATION STRATEGIES FOR PEOPLE WITH SPEECH AND LANGUAGE PROBLEMS

Body language

- Use calm facial expressions, body movements and posture; becoming angry or over-excited can alarm and confuse.
- Get the person's attention first before talking, e.g. call out their name, bend down if he or she is in a wheelchair.
- Touch lightly on the hand to regain attention and to reassure, but do not touch the person until your presence is known.

Conversation

- Taking time out for conversation is important.
- Focus on information exchange rather than the person's accurate use of words.
- Explain what you are doing as you are doing it, and use gesture and pointing to supplement, if needed. For example, in helping with dressing, point out the clothes and mime the movements required as you talk.

- Learn and use the person's personal history to make conversation meaningful and relevant.
- When starting a new topic, give background information to help focus the person's attention.
- Use statements that maintain and extend the conversation, e.g. 'That sounds very interesting. Tell me more about it.'
- Signal to the person when you are about to change the topic, e.g. 'Now let's talk about . . .'
- Try not to interrupt the person; it can be confusing and cause them to forget what they wanted to say.
- Use clear signals that specify exactly what you misunderstood, e.g. 'I don't understand what . . . means'.
- If you are unable to get the person to understand, acknowledge the problem and change the topic, e.g. 'I'm sorry I don't understand . . . shall we talk about . . .?'
- If the person repeats sentences to the point that it bothers you, acknowledge the perceived intent behind the statement, and change the topic.

Language

- Limit use of pronouns, e.g. he, she, they, this, that. Use proper nouns (i.e. names) instead.
- Use explicit statements e.g. 'Swallow one pill after breakfast', rather than 'Remember to take your pills'.
- Limit use of colloquialisms, such as 'Just hop into bed', as they can be interpreted literally.
- Use familiar vocabulary; limit the use of technical terms and jargon.
- Minimize lengthy and elaborate explanations.
- Limit the number of open-ended questions. They may provide too many choices, e.g. 'Where is your pain?'
- Use questions that require a 'Yes' or 'No' answer, e.g. 'Do you have any pain?'
- Place modifiers after nouns, e..g 'Do you have any pain . . . is it sharp?'
- Modify a question to provide choice, e.g. 'Do you have any pain . . . is it sharp . . . or dull?'
- Place important information at the beginning of your sentence, e.g. 'You must be tired after your day out' rather than 'Going out for the day must have made you tired.'

Speech

- Use pauses and stress words to highlight information, e.g. 'Would you like tea . . . or coffee?'
- Speak slowly and clearly, without raising your voice.

Environments

- Quiet locations will enhance communication. Talking above the television/radio or other background noise is not conducive to conversation.
- Be sensitive to the person's need for privacy. Try not to discuss things of a personal or intimate nature in front of others.
- Be aware of the effects of lighting and positioning of furniture in communal spaces in encouraging or inhibiting conversation, e.g. poor lighting can make it difficult to lip read and pick up other important facial expressions.

Memory

- Act as a memory jogger for the person; you cannot assume that they will search their own memory. Summarize and prompt in order to facilitate memory retrieval.
- Minimize the effects of poor memory on communication by giving written instructions, one small step at a time (including symbols, drawings or photographs if reading is difficult), and giving ample time for the person to respond verbally.

Perceptions and attitudes

- Watch your use of 'secondary baby talk', i.e. exaggerated pitch and loud voice, terms of endearment, e.g. 'good girl' and non-verbal behaviours that suggest a lack of respect and the person's dependency and incompetence, e.g. patting or stroking hair.
- Work through your own views of older people, recognizing that any feelings of resentment, anger or disgust will show through your language, facial expression and body language, and will affect the person.

Adapted from Orange *et al.* (1994)

APPENDIX 2

Referral to speech and language therapy can usually be made via a general practitioner. Some speech and language therapy departments can organize domiciliary visiting and training packages for care staff, if needed.

USEFUL ORGANIZATIONS

The Royal College of Speech and Language Therapists,
7 Bath Place, Rivington Street, London, EC2A 3DR;
tel: 0171 613 3855; fax: 0171 613 3854

Action for Dysphasic Adults, 1 Royal Street, London SE1 7LL;
tel: 0171 261 9572

The Stroke Association (Dysphasic Support Scheme),
CHSA House, Whitecross Street, London, EC1Y 8JJ;
tel: 0171 490 7999; fax: 0171 490 2686

Nutritional care

15

INTRODUCTION

Does it matter what the elderly eat? Nutritional deficiencies do occur in long-stay care. This is often caused by lack of knowledge, inexperience, inadequate planning and sometimes even indifference. Furthermore, older people admitted for long-stay care vary in how well nourished they are: studies have shown that those from acute hospitals may be undernourished compared with those who have been living at home (Nelson *et al.*, 1993).

Aspects that need to be considered include:

- the nutritional state of the person prior to admission;
- the nutritional needs of the individual in long-stay care;
- planning the menu to meet their needs;
- preparing and cooking the food so that maximum nutritional values are retained;
- not serving the food before residents are ready;
- making sure the amount on the plate is right for each individual;
- checking on a regular basis such aspects as the person's weight, appetite, type and quantity of food eaten etc.

The nutrients in food are often less well absorbed as age increases and also certain drugs can interfere with such absorption. Some residents in long-stay care, despite appearing to eat well, remain very thin and underweight. The reason is not fully understood. In some instances, all the meals are eaten and the person appears to be satisfied. However, the total energy value of the food eaten may be less than previously consumed at home, if all snacks etc. are taken into account. It is therefore helpful to make sure that extra snacks are readily available.

Exercise may be a major problem. The amount and type of exercise in long-stay care may be very different from the resident's previous habits.

This can affect appetite, as well as other health issues. It is easy to plan or obtain advice about simple activities involving physical movements.

NUTRITION FOR OLDER PEOPLE

HOW IS THE NUTRITIONAL WELL-BEING OF RESIDENTS ASSESSED?

There are three ways to assess nutritional well-being.

Weight

Weight is one of the most important indicators. Weight should be noted on admission and checked at least once a month. The weighing should be done in the same type of clothing and at the same part of the day. A weight change of more than 2 lb (1 kg) over a month needs investigating.

Standard body mass index charts are normally used and they give an indication of underweight or overweight. The index is based on the individual's weight divided by their height squared (weight/height^2). The figures obtained are interpreted as follows (Garrow, 1981):

- less than 20 – underweight
- 20–24.9 – desirable
- $\geqslant 25$ – overweight

Appetite

If all the meals of a well-planned, carefully cooked and attractively presented menu are eaten, there should be no cause for concern. However, if this is not the case, further investigation is needed. By careful observation of the amount and type of food each resident consumes, it is simple to isolate a problem that has not previously been noticed. Specific points to look for are difficulty in chewing or swallowing, speed of eating, whether help is required with feeding, etc. It may simply be due to badly fitting false teeth! However, this can lead to malnutrition.

Recording

Where there is a change in weight, one of the first actions is to record how much of the food is eaten. This can be done by using a food frequency chart, such as the one produced by Nutrition Advisory Group for Elderly People (British Dietetic Association). Keeping such a record will highlight problems. For a 'problem' eater, it may be helpful to consult your local dietitian.

WHAT DO OLDER PEOPLE NORMALLY EAT?

The last major study on the eating habits of older people was carried out in 1979 (DHSS, 1979). A further study started in 1995. This is investigating the dietary patterns, in relation to nutrition and health, of a wide sample of older people, both at home and in residential care.

HOW DO WE KNOW WHAT IS NEEDED?

The current recommendations for the energy (calorie) and nutrient needs of people in the UK were published by the Department of Health in 1991 (Table 15.1) (DoH, 1991). In addition, a Working Party reviewed the nutrition of older people, and their report was published by the Department of Health in 1992 (DoH, 1992). This report discusses, for the first time, the particular nutritional needs of those over 65 years old.

Energy needs of older people are slightly lower than those for younger adults. In most instances, activity decreases with age, so also the need for energy. However, irrespective of age, all adults need the same amount of nutrients. It is therefore necessary for the food providing the energy (calories) to be 'nutrient-dense': this means that the quality of what is eaten is particularly important.

Table 15.1 Average daily requirements[a] of nutrients for older people (DoH, 1991)

	Men		Women	
	65–74	⩾75	65–74	⩾75
Energy (kcal)[a]	2330	2100	1900	1810
Protein (g)	53.3		46.5	
Thiamin (mg)	0.9		0.8	
Riboflavin (mg)	1.3		1.1	
Niacin (mg)	16		12	
Vitamin B_{12} (μg)	1.5		1.5	
Fotate (μg)	200		200	
Vitamin C (mg)	40		40	
Vitamin A (μg)	700		600	
Vitamin D (μg)[b]	10		10	
Calcium (mg)	700		700	
Iron (mg)	8.7		8.7	

[a]Energy is expressed as estimated average requirements (EAR). The remaining nutrients as reference nutrient intake (RNI).
[b]Supplements are required for the housebound to achieve the vitamin D RNI.

HEALTHY EATING – HOW RELEVANT IS IT?

Food and health policies have been introduced in many health authorities to promote good health. In addition, a National Food Guide, 'The Balance of Health' (based on the government's 'Eight Guidelines for a Healthy Diet') was produced as part of the Health of the Nation campaign by the Health Education Authority in 1994.

The eight guidelines for a healthy diet extracted from 'The Balance of Health' are:

- enjoy your food
- eat a variety of different foods
- eat the right amount to be a healthy weight
- eat plenty of foods rich in starch and fibre
- don't eat too much fat
- don't eat sugary foods too often
- look after the vitamins and minerals in your food
- if you drink alcohol, keep within sensible limits

All these points apply to most adults of any age. Fit and healthy older people can follow the guidelines quite safely. However, the guidelines are inappropriate for those who are frail, ill or housebound. This is because some of these recommendations can affect the bulk and palatability of foods.

To encourage healthy eating, there is a National Heartbeat Award scheme for caterers and an increasing number of hospitals and residential homes have earned this award. To apply for an award, the establishment must have non-smoking catering and dining areas, comply with strict hygiene requirements and have a healthy choice of food on the menu. Details can be obtained from local environmental health units.

WHICH ASPECTS OF HEALTHY EATING ARE APPROPRIATE FOR OLDER PEOPLE?

Enjoying food, eating a variety of different foods and aiming at a healthy weight are all relevant.

'Eat plenty of foods rich in starch and fibre'

Increasing fibre (non-starch polysaccharides) increases bulk in the diet. The addition of bran is no longer encouraged because it can interfere with the absorption of some minerals. Instead, fibre can be increased by using high-fibre bread, cereals, brown rice, wholemeal pasta, fruit (fresh, dried, tinned or cooked) and vegetables. The result is improved bowel function, which helps prevent constipation and conditions such as diverti-culitis.

This is sound advice for those with a healthy appetite, but when appetite is affected for whatever reason, the total energy intake is more important.

'Don't eat too much fat'

The consumption of too much fat has been linked to coronary heart disease and it is recommended that the amount of fat in the diet be reduced. This applies particularly to cooking fats, butter, margarines, fatty meats and rich creamy products.

For a healthy and active 65-year-old person with a good appetite, this recommendation can be followed. However, for an underweight and frail person and those over 75, this may not be appropriate because foods containing fat are valuable sources of other nutrients.

'Don't eat sugary foods too often'

Too much sugar can lead to weight gain and it can also damage teeth and gums. Sugar does not contain nutrients, it only supplies energy. It is safe to reduce the amount added to drinks. Lowering the amount of sugar in puddings, cakes and biscuits can affect palatability and, as these items provide a number of other nutrients, their consumption should not be discouraged in older people.

For those with weight gain problems or diabetes, sugar should not be used in cooking. Alternative sweeteners can be used and other desserts, such as fruit, provided. For older people who still have their own teeth, receding gums and less saliva can result in teeth decay and gum disease. In such cases, a reduction of sugar in the diet, coupled with good dental hygiene, is beneficial.

OTHER HEALTHY EATING ADVICE

Salt

A high salt consumption has been linked to high blood pressure. However, salt is important for taste and palatability (particularly for older people whose taste buds are less receptive) and so care should be taken not to decrease salt too much. If there is a medical reason for reducing salt intake, then additional herbs and spices should be used to enhance the flavour of the food.

NUTRIENTS THAT REQUIRE PARTICULAR ATTENTION

Some nutrients are particularly important for older people.

VITAMIN C

Low intakes of vitamin C lead to poor wound healing and to bleeding, especially from the gums. Vitamin C is found mainly in fruits and vegetables. It is not stored by the body and hence these foods need to be eaten daily. The vitamin is easily lost from food as it dissolves out in water and is destroyed by cooking. For this reason, vegetables should not be left standing in water but should be cooked as soon as prepared, for as short a time as possible, just before the meal.

The following are good sources of vitamin C: citrus fruit and juice (oranges, grapefruit, mandarins); blackcurrant juice/drink; raw tomatoes; green vegetables, lightly cooked; potatoes, especially jacket potatoes and chips as they are not cooked in water and hence retain more of the vitamin. If instant potato powder is used it is essential to use one which is fortified with vitamin C. Frozen vegetables are generally a good source of vitamin C but dried vegetables (unless fortified with the vitamin) contain little vitamin C. Fresh fruit or fruit juice should be consumed at least once a day and vegetables, fresh or frozen, should be eaten at least twice a day.

IRON

There are many reasons why older people may become anaemic. This may be due to haemorrhoids, diverticulitis, hiatus hernia, peptic ulcers, malabsorption, a depressed appetite, or a reliance on a limited selection of convenience foods.

Good sources of iron are red meats such as beef, lamb, corned beef, black pudding, liver and kidney, or derivatives such as pâté, liver sausage; dark green vegetables, peas, beans, lentils; dried fruit such as apricots and prunes; wholemeal bread and flour; eggs. Vegetarians rely mainly on pulses, bread and cereals for their sources of iron.

VITAMIN B_{12} AND FOLATE

A deficiency of either vitamin B_{12} or folate leads to megaloblastic anaemia. Whilst B_{12} deficiency may be due to diet, it is more commonly due to lack of absorption.

Vitamin B_{12} is only found in foods of animal origin: milk, meat, fish, cheese and eggs. Strict vegetarians will therefore be at greater risk of becoming deficient in the vitamin.

The main sources of dietary folate are liver, kidney and green leafy vegetables. However, folate is destroyed by prolonged cooking.

A link between deficiency and dementia has been reported (Melamed *et al.*, 1975). Further work needs to be done to see whether depression and apathy may be due to B₁₂ and folate deficiencies.

CALCIUM

Dietary intake of calcium when young establishes bone mass. In later years, the intake of calcium is still important, although this will not improve bone mass. Lack of bone mass can result in osteoporosis, which makes bones more susceptible to fractures. An adequate level of vitamin D is important to ensure that calcium is actually absorbed and used by the body.

Sources of calcium include milk; yoghurt; cheese; white flour (fortified); some vegetables.

Prolonged bedrest also results in a loss of bone mass and exercise is very beneficial in helping to remineralize the bones thus affected.

VITAMIN D

A deficiency of vitamin D leads to osteomalacia, where there is a lack of calcium deposited in the matrix of the bone. This results in 'soft' bones. Vitamin D is mainly obtained from the action of sunlight on the skin – specifically, the ultraviolet rays which are much stronger in summer sunlight than in winter. An exposure of 15–30 minutes a day on arms, hands and face will lead to an adequate amount of vitamin D being produced. Every opportunity should be taken to encourage older people to take advantage of the sunlight. For those unable to be outside, special glass designed to allow the passage of ultraviolet rays can be used in windows.

Diet alone will only contribute a small amount of vitamin D. Foods which contain vitamin D are limited. They are: oily fish; eggs; liver; butter (to a very minor extent); margarine which is fortified by the addition of vitamins A and D. Vitamin D is added to some breakfast cereals, but it is uncertain how well it is absorbed from this source.

The Department of Health recommend an intake of 10 µg per day (DoH, 1991). This is very difficult to achieve without the benefit of sunlight. For housebound people additional vitamin D intake should be considered. This can be as a daily supplement by mouth, or as six monthly injections during the winter and early spring (DoH, 1992).

FLUIDS

Liquids are essential for the well-being of any person and it is important that older people have sufficient to drink at all times, not only at meals.

Insufficient fluids may be taken simply because they are not readily accessible or the drinking cup or glass cannot be held firmly.

Older people are often reluctant to take fluids if they have incontinence problems, particularly at night. Adjusting the times when fluids are given to the earlier part of the day could be more appropriate.

At least eight cups or glasses of liquid should be taken daily. These can be tea, coffee, milk, water, fruit juice or mineral waters.

MENUS, MEAL TIMES AND MEAL SERVICE

When, how and what we eat are habits of a lifetime. Meals are one of the most familiar routines of our lives and help to give some focus to the day. Moving into residential care, where these decisions are taken by others, is difficult to adapt to.

Meals need to be spaced out carefully during the day as older people may find it tiring to consume too much at one time and snacks between meals are helpful.

Breakfast is usually a popular meal. Ideally it should not be too early and should be available over a period of time. Lunch is usually the main meal of the day. Afternoon tea is not really necessary as it is usually rather near to the evening meal. However, a drink during the afternoon can help with fluid intake. The time of the evening meal may be a problem due to staff availability, but it should not be before 5 p.m. Suggested mealtimes are:

- Breakfast   8.00 a.m. to 9.00 a.m.
- Mid-morning drink/snack   10.00 a.m. to 10.30 a.m.
- Lunch   12 noon to 1.00 p.m.
- Evening meal   5.30 p.m. to 6.30 p.m.
- Late evening drink/snack   8.00 p.m. to 9.00 p.m.

MENUS

A framework or skeleton menu is needed and meals should be planned well in advance, covering two to three weeks at a time. Wherever possible, residents' suggestions for dishes should be included. The cook should be encouraged to talk with residents about the food and to find out which dishes are popular. It is educational for the cook to check on 'plate waste' following meals, thus widening the understanding of what is needed. If a major part of a meal is left uneaten, replacement must be considered. Presenting food in a different way can help: plain milk may not be liked, but hot chocolate drinks, custard, or yoghurt may be popular. Plain, simple and well-cooked meals such as stews, Lancashire hotpot, roast meats etc. are much more popular than convenience foods.

In a small unit it is possible to know residents' likes and dislikes, but it is still important for them, or even relatives, to take part in a simple choice of food on the day.

When planning meals, the availability of cooking staff needs to be taken into account. If there is just one cook working in the first part of the day, the evening meal may have to be left ready. However, cook–chill and frozen foods, and microwave ovens, help to provide an appetizing meal with little labour needed rather than relying on cold meals or sandwiches.

BASIC FOODS TO BE INCLUDED IN THE DAY'S MEALS

- ½ to 1 pint of milk a day taken in drinks, on cereals and in puddings: more can be included for someone with a poor appetite
- 2 oz (60 g) cooked weight of meat ⎫
- 4–5 oz (110–140 g) cooked weight ⎪ two helpings from these foods
  of fish ⎬ should be included daily
- 2 oz (60 g) of cheese ⎪
- 1–2 eggs ⎭
- for vegetarians use 3 oz (85 g) lentils, peas or beans or 1 oz (30 g) nuts instead of meat, fish, cheese or egg
- bread, potatoes, rice, breakfast cereals: one or more of these should be included at each of the three meals
- two helpings of vegetables (or salad foods) each day
- fresh, tinned or dried fruit, either as it is or in puddings
- 1 small glass natural fruit juice
- at least eight cups of fluid – tea, coffee, soup, water or fruit juice each day.

CATERING SYSTEMS

There are three main catering systems used in long-stay units:

- conventional cooking;
- cook–freeze: cooked dishes may be purchased ready frozen or cooked and frozen on the premises using special freezing equipment, held in freezers and reheated to the correct temperature in special ovens;
- cook–chill: food is cooked, then chilled in a purpose-built unit under careful quality control. It is held at 0–3°C for a maximum of five days. The food must be kept chilled at this temperature until reheated quickly, and correctly timed, in ovens or special food trolleys. These meals need to be consumed immediately after heating and clear instructions should be provided by the caterers on handling cook–chill foods.

With 'cook–chill' and 'cook–freeze', proper cooking practices and quality control can provide good nutritional food, provided procedures are adhered to and monitored regularly (DoH, 1989). They also enable flexibility in the use of staff and can be a useful adjunct to conventional cooking.

MEAL SERVICE

This is about serving the person and not the plate! Ideally the food should be served at the table. If meals are plated away from the dining area, clear instructions about the needs of each resident must be available and used.

It is a good idea to serve the main protein dish (meat, fish, egg, cheese) directly on to the plate and to have dishes of vegetables and potatoes on the tables. This gives an element of choice and decision (with guidance) for the resident. Alternatively, a mobile hot trolley can be used. Gravy and other sauces should be available separately as the moistness of a meal and precisely where the gravy is placed on the plate is an individual preference.

Small meals with a second helping available are preferable to 'pile-it-high' as a single helping. If the meal is pre-plated and served on a tray, the positioning of the dishes on the tray is important. The food to be consumed first needs to be centrally situated – it is not unknown for trays to arrive with the dessert in the middle, which will then be eaten first leaving no appetite for the main course! Ideally, the dessert should not be served until the main course has been finished.

For those with failing eyesight, time spent by carers explaining the meal – possibly by relating the position of the food items to the face of a clock – can make the meal much more enjoyable.

For all meals, familiar accompaniments can make a big difference – vinegar with fish and chips, mint sauce with lamb, horseradish with beef.

Liquid needs to be provided with every meal – water or juice.

Feeding aids

Non-slip place mats, or suction pads, can help hold the plate in position. The handles of cutlery can be difficult to grip for those with arthritic hands: slip-on rubber handles or grips help. Plate rims or plate guards stop food sliding off the plate and some china companies make attractive designs of deep plates with lips. Beakers or cups with a slanted base or two-handled cups are helpful. Flexi-straws help those who are unable to hold a cup on their own to be more independent. Such aids are often a better solution than a feeding cup with a spout. These aids can be purchased from the Disabled Living Foundation or similar local organizations.

Preparation for the meal

It is important to ensure that residents are comfortably prepared for their meals and that feeding aids are to hand. Remember that, however the meal is being served, the residents may be totally reliant on the nurse/ carer for what they eat, how they eat it and the amount eaten.

FACTORS THAT AFFECT FOOD CONSUMPTION

RESISTANCE TO CHANGE IN EATING HABITS

Long-held beliefs about food are difficult to change. Some foods are considered 'acid', some 'binding' – for example eggs. A specific problem with older people is 'hanging on' to advice. Sometimes advice for a complaint given years ago is treated as 'gospel' for ever and a day. Such restrictions not only cause monotony, but can also lead to lack of intake of certain nutrients.

LACK OF TASTE

With ageing, there is a progressive loss in the number of taste buds on the tongue. Those that are lost initially are the ones at the front of the tongue which detect sweet and salty tastes, whilst those which detect bitter and sour tastes increase. This alters sensitivity to the tastes of food which therefore needs to be well-seasoned and flavoured.

Poor oral hygiene also masks taste and a reduced ability to smell the aroma from food makes it seem less appetising.

DENTITION

All too often, the state of the teeth and dentures – well-fitting or not – can be a problem. Gums have usually hardened in older people so that most textures of food can be masticated: it is loose teeth and ill-fitting dentures that are the problem!

Instead of serving sloppy food it is best to ensure that meat is tender and large pieces are cut up: even dessert apples can be eaten if sliced.

SWALLOWING PROBLEMS

A stroke can cause facial weakness which leads to poor lipseal: this results in difficulties keeping food, liquid or saliva in the mouth, and hence troublesome dribbling.

Changing the textures of food and liquids may help. Chilled thickened drinks may be managed more easily than hot thin drinks. Liquids can be thickened by adding products made for this purpose: a dietitian can advise.

Moist foods with a firm consistent texture should be tried. Differing textures in one dish are hard to swallow, for example cornflakes and milk, soup with pieces in it, dried fruit in cakes, dry biscuits with tea (dunking in the tea helps). When a soft or puréed meal is needed, care should be taken to see that the food value of the meal is not affected by thinning with water or gravy. A food processor is useful for adjusting textures without having to add additional liquid.

Puréed/soft meals need to be presented attractively. They should be served as separate items in small containers, rather than on a large plate. This will keep the different foods separate and should give a colourful meal. Alternatively, a ring of puréed potato on the plate with the puréed meat in the centre helps with presentation.

Body positioning is very important for people with swallowing problems: they should be upright with the head tilting slightly forward. The advice of a speech therapist can be very helpful for swallowing problems.

RESPIRATORY PROBLEMS

Emphysema, bronchitis and other breathing problems may affect the ability to eat. It may therefore be necessary to supplement the meals with extra milk-based drinks.

DEPRESSION, APATHY AND CONFUSION

These conditions can lead to a lack of interest in food and poor appetite. Alcohol, such as a glass of sherry before a meal, may be a worthwhile stimulant.

DEMENTIA

In some cases, the memory may be so poor that the person affected may not remember whether or not they have eaten. Help may be needed in prompting them when their attention wanders while eating, and, if they are restless and unable to sit for long periods, it may be necessary to give them food which they can eat while walking around under staff supervision, such as sandwiches and finger-type snacks. In this case, nourishing supplementary drinks are necessary to ensure that sufficient nutrients are consumed over the day.

Where residents are unable to feed themselves, constant help and observation of the difficulties is essential. Being fed is not pleasant, as the recipient is not in control of the amount of food or the speed at which it is given. Great patience is needed and the person doing the feeding must give their full attention to the person being fed. To try to feed more than one person at a time is very degrading and unsatisfactory for all of the recipients.

INTERACTION OF DRUGS AND NUTRIENTS

FOOD INTAKE AND ABSORPTION OF DRUGS

The presence of food in the stomach may delay the absorption of medicines and therefore some medication must be taken before food, for example oral hypoglycaemic drugs for diabetes mellitus.

The absorption of calcium (from milk and milk products) may be reduced by some drugs, for example ferrous sulphate (often prescribed for anaemia) and tetracycline. This is why milk and milk products should not be taken until two hours after the drug has been given.

EFFECTS OF DRUGS ON APPETITE

Certain drugs will increase appetite. These include: sulphonylureas (tolbutamide, chlorpropamide, glibenclamide); phenothiazines (such as largactil); benzodiazepines (such as Valium, Librium); anabolic agents (such as Durabolin); insulin; alcohol.

Other drugs decrease appetite, for example: biguanides (metformin, phenformin); indomethacin; digitalis; glucagon; cyclophosphamide.

EFFECTS OF DRUGS ON FOOD NUTRIENTS

Drugs should be checked with care for an interaction with food nutrients. Some examples of such interactions are:

- thiazide diuretics with sodium and potassium;
- anticonvulsants with vitamin D and folic acid;
- antacids with phosphate;
- purgatives with potassium and vitamin K;
- corticosteroids with protein metabolism.

VEGETARIANS

Usually vegetarianism is based on religious or moral grounds. However, some people become vegetarian because some foods are difficult to eat or simply not liked.

TYPES OF VEGETARIAN DIETS

A vegetarian diet excludes not only animal flesh (beef, lamb, pork, poultry etc.) and processed meat foods, but also animal products such as lard and gelatine. Most vegetarian diets also exclude fish and fish products. Some vegetarians go further and even avoid the hard and soft cheeses that incorporate rennet.

A vegan diet is very strict and excludes all animal-derived foods. Milk and milk products such as butter, margarines with milk fats added and cheeses are therefore not eaten. Instead the diet is based on cereals, vegetables, pulses (peas, beans and lentils), fruits, nuts and seeds.

Three common versions of a 'vegetarian' diet are

1. a lacto-vegetarian diet which excludes all meat, fish and egg products but does permit the consumption of milk and milk products;
2. the lacto-ovo-vegetarian diet which is similar to the diet above except that eggs and egg products are eaten;
3. a 'partial' vegetarian diet which is used by some people as 'healthy' and excludes some meats, particularly red meats, but includes poultry and fish.

The main nutritional concern with regard to older people on vegetarian diets is that they get sufficient iron, zinc and vitamins D and B_{12}. It is advisable to ask the local dietitian for advice on the nutritional adequacy of these diets and whether any supplements are necessary.

RELIGION AND FOOD PREFERENCES

ASIAN DIETS

The three main Asian religions found in this country are Islam (the religion of Muslims), Hinduism and Sikhism, and there is a wide diversity between these three. There is also a wide cultural diversity between older Asian immigrants and the younger generation born and brought up in this country. This can add to difficulties for older Asians in adapting to long-stay care as they have been brought up in a culture of the extended family caring for the older generation. All have dietary constraints which must be adhered to.

One sect of Hindus (Jain) will not eat foods that have involved the taking of life. They are therefore vegetarian, avoiding all meats, fish, cheeses (made with rennet) and eggs. Milk and yoghurt are included in their diet. Other sects of Hindus will not eat beef, or any beef products such as cheese made with rennet. They will eat lamb, chicken white fish, milk and yoghurt.

Muslims will not eat pork or pork-based products (bacon, ham, pork luncheon meat and sausages). All meat must be ritually slaughtered (known as Halal). Kosher meat is acceptable to many Muslims. Ramadan is a major festival, and during the month of Ramadan all Muslims must fast from dawn to sunset. The date varies each year according to the Muslim callendar. Special exemption from fasting during this period is allowed for chronically ill people who could be adversely affected.

Sikhs are less strict in dietary laws than Hindus and Muslims and it is often up to the individual what they may not eat. Beef and pork are usually excluded, but lamb, chicken and fish will normally be eaten.

JUDAISM

Orthodox Jews are not permitted to eat pork (or any products of the pig, such as ham, bacon or sausages). They may eat beef, lamb, chicken, turkey and duck provided the animals have been ritually slaughtered and strictly prepared. It is then known as 'Kosher'. Fish (apart from shellfish), cheese and eggs are acceptable. Milk and dairy products must not be eaten at the same meal as meat. Kosher margarines (containing no milk products) are available. Care must be taken to ensure that puddings served after meat dishes do not contain any milk or cream.

It is possible to obtain Kosher meals ready-made or frozen. These have been ritually prepared and cooked.

Some Jewish people are less strict over their food requirements, eating fish and chicken dishes from the general menu, but avoiding other meats not prepared to Jewish laws.

MEDICALLY PRESCRIBED DIETS

Where a special diet has been prescribed for a resident, it is usually possible to adapt the menu to meet the dietary requirements.

OVERWEIGHT PROBLEMS

It is not easy to lose weight as activity decreases. However, simple changes can be made to meals to reduce calorie intake:

- replace full-cream milk with semi-skimmed milk;
- use artificial sweeteners instead of sugar in drinks or on cereals, and use low-calorie fruit squashes and mineral drinks;
- replace fried food and pastry with grilled, baked or steamed food;
- replace puddings and sweet desserts by fresh fruit, fruit tinned in natural juices, diet fruit yoghurt, egg custard or milk pudding with artificial sweetener;
- restrict starchy foods (bread, potatoes) to just one slice or two small potatoes at each meal, with only a small amount of butter or margarine.

Snacks, sweets, chocolates and biscuits may be a problem. A piece of fresh fruit, a cracker biscuit with cottage cheese, or salad foods may help to allay hunger. A hot drink may also be used in place of a snack.

Weight loss will be slow, but even achieving a halt in weight gain can be beneficial. Increasing exercise, wherever possible, is also important. If a stricter diet is required for medical reasons, a dietitian should be involved.

DIABETIC DIETS

Most older people with diabetes are treated using a 'no added sugar' diet. Those on oral hypoglycaemic agents or insulin may need their diet to be individually planned by a dietitian. People with diabetes who are overweight and treated by diet with no medication should normally follow the same advice as given above for people who are overweight.

A 'no added sugar' diet for those who are not overweight means avoiding all food and drinks with sugar added, such as jam, marmalade, honey, syrup, sweetened puddings, cakes and sweets, chocolates and sweet biscuits. However, bread, potatoes, pasta and cereals can be eaten in normal amounts, and wholemeal products are recommended to increase the fibre content, which has a beneficial effect on blood sugar.

If the person is on insulin or oral hypoglycaemic tablets, any foods containing carbohydrate (bread, potatoes, rice, desserts) in the planned diet that are not eaten should be replaced with a drink or other suitable food. The dietitian can supply a suitable list.

Useful information on the care of diabetes can be obtained from the British Diabetic Association.

LOW-FAT DIETS

Visible fat must be removed from meat and rich sauces. Creamy dishes should be avoided. Foods must be grilled, baked or steamed instead of fried. In addition, substitute:

• milk: use skimmed only
• butter: use a low-fat spread
• cream soups: use consommé or plain vegetable soups
• fatty meats (pâté, sausages, corned beef): replace with lean meats, chicken, turkey
• fish: avoid oily fish (sardines, herrings, mackerel etc.) use white fish, e.g. cod, haddock, plaice
• cheese: use low-fat cottage cheese or low-fat curd cheese
• ice cream: use sorbets or jellies.

Avoid pastry, pies, egg yolks, malted milk drinks and chocolates.

A low-fat diet is lower in calories than a normal diet. This should be compensated for by increasing the amount of bread, potatoes, cereals and sweet food provided. If a low-fat diet is given for more than three months, supplements of fat-soluble vitamins (A and D) will be necessary.

HIGH-PROTEIN DIETS

These may be required if the person is poorly nourished, or has an increased need because of infections, poor wound healing or pressure sores. It is vital to ensure that the food being eaten provides sufficient energy for the individual's daily needs, otherwise any extra protein given will be used to make up the energy deficit. If appetite is small, meals need to be concentrated in energy by the addition of sugar, butter, cream etc. to dishes. Where the appetite is good and all the food is consumed, then additional protein can be added. For example, each of the following contains 7 g protein:

- 1 glass of milk
- ⅔ oz (20 g) skimmed milk powder
- 3 fl oz (85 ml) evaporated milk
- 1 oz (25 g) meat, chicken or fish
- 1 egg

Protein intake can be enhanced by desserts with a milk basis, served with custard or evaporated milk, or an egg added. Where appetites are small, extra drinks, such as milk shakes, or milk with additional milk powder added, can be given. Supplementary 'fortified' drinks can also be used.

FORTIFIED DRINKS (SUPPLEMENTS)

Supplementary drinks are useful where extra nourishment is necessary. Milk can be 'fortified' by adding 2 oz (50 g) skimmed milk powder to each pint of whole milk. This enriched milk can replace ordinary milk in drinks and in cooking. Alternatively, products such as Complan (H.J. Heinz Co Ltd) or Build Up (Nestlé UK Ltd) are available. Some manufacturers make 'sip' feeds which come in a range of flavours. For those who cannot take milk, enriched fruit juice is an alternative. In certain cases of malnutrition, these 'sip' feeds can be obtained on medical prescription.

Following the above guidelines should make meals more enjoyable and beneficial for residents, resulting in an improved state of health and feeling of well-being.

REFERENCES

Department of Health and Social Security (1979) Nutrition and health in old age. Report on Health and Social Subjects No. 16. HMSO, London.
Department of Health (1989) Chilled and Frozen. Guidelines on Cook–Chill and Cook–Freeze Catering Systems. HMSO, London.
Department of Health (1991) Dietary reference values for food energy and nutrients for the United Kingdom. Report on Health and Social Subjects No. 41. HMSO, London.
Department of Health (1992) The Nutrition of Elderly People. Report of the

Working Group on the Nutrition of Elderly People of the Committee on Medical Aspects of Food Policy. Report on Health and Social Subjects No. 43. HMSO, London.

Garrow, J.S. (1981) *Treat Obesity Seriously*, Churchill Livingstone, Edinburgh.

Melamed, E., Reches, A. and Herschko, C. (1975) Reversible central nervous system dysfunction in folate deficiency. *J. Neurol. Sci.*, **25**, 93–8.

Nelson, K.J., Coulston, A.M., Sucher, K.P. and Tseng, R.Y. (1993) Prevalence of malnutrition in the elderly admitted to long-term-care facilities. *J. Am. Diet. Assoc.*, **93**, 459–61.

FURTHER READING

Davies, L. (1981) *Three Score Years . . . and Then?* Heinemann Medical Books, London.

Department of Health and Social Services (1986) *Health Service Catering – Nutrition and Modified Diets*, HMSO, London.

Henley, A. (1979) *Asian Patients in Hospital and at Home*, King Edward's Hospital Fund for London, London.

Hill, S.E. (1990) *More than Rice and Peas – Guidelines to Improve Food Provision for Black and Ethnic Minorities in Britain*, The Food Commission, London.

Nutrition Advisory Group for Elderly People (NAGE) (1990) *Eating Through the 90's. A handbook for those concerned with providing meals for older people*, British Dietetic Association, Birmingham.

APPENDIX

USEFUL ADDRESSES

British Diabetic Association, 10 Queen Anne Street, London W1M 0BD.

British Dietetic Association, Elizabeth House, 22 Suffolk Street Queensway, Birmingham B1 1LS (for NAGE publications).

Centre for Policy on Ageing, 25–31 Ironmonger Row, London EC1V 3QP: information service and publications include catering and nutrition in residential homes.

Disabled Living Foundation, 380–384 Harrow Road, London W9 2HU.

Health Education Authority, Hamilton House, Mabledon Place, London WC1 9TX.

Furniture and equipment

16

The physical environment has a pervasive effect on the well-being and activities of residents in long-stay settings. The thoughtful provision of appropriate furnishings, equipment and décor can not only improve the lives of older people living in nursing or residential homes or long-stay hospital wards, but may also enhance the working conditions of the staff. A well-designed and equipped unit will also benefit visitors, some of whom may have physical disabilities themselves.

In recent years, many long-stay wards have been closed and most formal care for physically dependent older people now occurs in nursing homes and residential homes. Some hospitals do provide excellent long-term care facilities, and the development of teaching nursing homes may act as a spur to better research into the optimum environment and equipment for older people. Many nursing homes provide an excellent ambience, although some fall short of the ideals and a few still exhibit the saddest features of old-style institutional care (Age Concern, 1990).

THE HOMELY ENVIRONMENT

A long-stay home should provide as normal a social experience as possible. An ideal environment is sensitive to the needs and abilities of each resident (Holder, 1987). The old people in such homes retain their values, identity and individuality. Respect for autonomy is reflected in the photographs and ornaments which adorn the person's own room. They have brought in pieces of their own furniture. A personal toilet and shower give humanizing space, elevating the status of the resident to that of a private individual. Each person has a key to their own room. The cupboard is also lockable. There is opportunity for sexual expression (the bed may be wider than a standard single bed). Residents will be able to open and close windows and alter the heating controls in their bedrooms. There is not only somewhere to be private but also places to be sociable:

to chat, play games, go out into the garden. Equipment, furniture and design features make an important contribution to the individuality, autonomy, privacy and fulfilment of old people.

PRINCIPLES AND CONTRADICTIONS

The physical environment helps to determine whether a long-stay facility is a good place to live or work or visit. Homes are not quasi-hospitals; although they have an important treatment function, there is more emphasis on care and enabling people to enjoy their lives as much as their condition allows. There is no place for standardized chairs of uniform height, placed centrifugally with their backs to the walls. Small groupings of chairs are more home-like and help foster social interaction. However, we must be careful not to deny autonomy by social engineering: people may want the opportunity not to be sociable and many sometimes prefer to sit alone, quietly. Bright colours, flowers, pictures and domestic table-settings all reinforce the feeling that this is home.

The architectural constraints of older buildings may militate against some of our objectives. Home owners may not have enough capital to install lifts (especially with suitable modifications for wheelchair users and those who are blind or deaf); they may not be able to afford those aids and appliances that can do so much to foster well-being and independence. Similarly, the needs of a totally dependent stroke victim who cannot move without assistance and is severely demented are not necessarily the same as those of someone who is wheelchair-mobile or a person who is physically independent but frail and fearful of living alone.

Other recommendations that might benefit an individual may not be good for the whole household or may clash with safety requirements or the need for cleanliness. For example, chairs with fabric covers are less 'institutional' in appearance than plastic-covered ones, yet the latter are easier to clean. A locker that is firmly placed on the floor is less likely to move if someone holds onto it when they feel unsteady, but the absence of castors makes the job of cleaning underneath the locker more difficult. A bed may be of the right height for the nurses to attend to the patient but the wrong height for the patient to stand up easily from a sitting position. A shiny vinyl floor is easily washed down but the shimmering appearance may make it appear slippery and thus impair gait. If people fall onto a hard floor, they may be more likely to hurt themselves. Carpets are preferable, but they tend to retain smells and can cause difficulties of propulsion to wheelchair users. People may wish to smoke in their own rooms, but if clothing catches fire and the door is locked from the inside, there may be a delay in reaching the unfortunate resident.

We must therefore be flexible and pragmatic in our choice of equipment and modifications but ensure that the resident's individuality and dignity are afforded the utmost respect.

ENVIRONMENT, FURNITURE AND PERSONAL CARE

The physical environment can help to create a congenial habitat for disabled older people by meeting their requirements for dignity, safety, orientation, comfort, activity, social interaction and mobility.

PERSONAL MAINTENANCE

Mirrors are important for grooming and help to maintain dignity and pride in one's appearance. A full-length mirror in the room should be complemented by a mirror above the sink. Wheelchair users will benefit from mirrors that are set at a lower height.

The sink should be accessible and of optimum height, and if necessary have levered taps, which are easier for those with impaired manipulative dexterity. Brushes with rubber suckers attached to the handles enable fixation to sinks: this makes the brushing of one's own dentures easier for those who can use only one arm. A reminder to half fill the sink with water before cleaning dentures will help prevent breakage should the dentures be dropped.

Sockets for plugs should be easy to reach. If they are too low or too high, the resident may over-reach and fall. Alternatively, they may be denied the opportunity of using the hair dryer, electric razor or other electrical gadgets. The plugs may be difficult to pull out of the sockets: a simple adaptation – a plastic handle attached to the plug – makes this task easier for those whose grip is not strong.

SAFETY AND SECURITY

The individual's bedroom door should be lockable from the inside. The key should have a large, grippable surface. Handles that are round are more difficult to turn; those with sharp edges can cause trauma. Lever handles are best; hexagonal ones may suffice. The door must be wide enough to allow wheelchair access. Visitors should ring the bell to request access and staff should not invade privacy by entering the room unannounced. High-pitched bells will not be heard by some people with sensorineural deafness. Those who are profoundly deaf will benefit from a system whereby lights flick on and off in time with the door chimes.

A wardrobe and personal chest of drawers give a room individuality, although this may not be realistic in more cramped accommodation. The bedside locker should be lockable and no-one should open it without the resident's permission. It should be reachable from a wheelchair and easy to open. Photographs and bric-a-brac can be exhibited on the top. Dentures, hearing aids, spectacles and other personal items can be kept in drawers. If the locker is the only place for storage, it must be larger than the models used in acute and rehabilitation wards. The locker should have rounded edges and reduce the risk of injury should someone fall against it.

Fires can be tragic. Burns usually occur because of fires caused by cigarettes, matches and other smoking materials. Those who are confined to a wheelchair or easy chair are most at risk from serious burns. The use of fireproof aprons might be considered. It may be prudent to ensure that, when people smoke, they do so only in certain parts of the home.

Burns also occur when people fall and become trapped next to radiators or hot pipes. Radiator guards can reduce the chances of this and low-surface-temperature radiators should be considered. Scalds still occur in baths in long-stay settings: mixer valves that ensure that the tap water never becomes too hot are important design features.

Fire alarms may be of too high a pitch to be heard by those who are hard of hearing. Deaf people will not know there is a fire unless there is a visual alarm system.

The floor surface is a potential hazard. Raised thresholds in doorways can cause the unwary to trip. Raised edges of carpets and loose mats may do the same, although this does not seem to be a common occurrence. A floor surface of vinyl which looks like cork might be considered: it does not look shiny, and helps prevent a hospital-like atmosphere. Steps and stairs must be well illuminated. The edges of stairs should be highlighted to provide contrast for those with visual impairment.

Carpets are the preferred floor covering in long-stay settings. They give a homely feel to a room, have non-slip characteristics and may result in less injury if someone falls. Wall-to-wall carpeting is better than loose mats; carpets inserted into recesses in the floor can present problems to wheelchair users and are best avoided. The biggest problem with regard to the use of carpets is with incontinent patients. Carpets made of non-absorptive nylon, acrylic or polyester fibres can be cleaned more easily. Prompt attention to cleaning may help prevent a uriniferous odour.

If someone falls or feels ill, they should be able to ask for help easily. Pull cords in the toilet, bathroom and bedroom can be useful, but cannot always be reached if someone has fallen. A portable trigger should be offered to those at risk: necklace alarms are not much favoured, but brooch or bracelet triggers may be more acceptable. Once activated, these transmit calls to the staff office.

ORIENTATION

Bedroom doors should be personalized by an identification plaque, placed at a height where it can be seen by smaller people with kyphosis and those in wheelchairs. The occupant's name and room number should be in large, easily read letters and numbers. There might be a photograph of the resident on the plaque.

Toilets should be clearly signposted and labelled, perhaps with a picture of a lavatory. This is particularly helpful for those residents with dementia and also non-demented newcomers to the home.

Signposting is perhaps more important in hospitals than nursing homes, but larger homes often benefit from well-designed, clear, unambiguous signs.

Orientation boards are supposed to help those residents whose sense of time is impaired. They have recently been criticized: in day hospitals and geriatric wards, the information on the day, date, weather and season is often incorrect (Seymour, 1993). Unless someone updates them accurately, these boards are of questionable usefulness. Moreover, they may reinforce the notion of a second childhood and do nothing for the esteem of the residents or the image of the home.

AMBIENCE

The noise of radios, televisions, telephones, and people chattering can be disturbing. The provision of a loop system for those who use hearing aids and soundproof walls may be helpful in reducing noise pollution and maintaining the well-being of everyone in the home.

Temperature affects comfort. A thermostat in the bedroom, which the resident can easily reach and modulate, gives autonomy as well as helping to provide physical comfort.

The smell of a long-stay home can give a positive or negative first impression. Frequent toileting, attention to personal hygiene and the judicious use of incontinence aids can all be helpful. The development of carpets which did not hold the aroma of urine would be an important advance.

Illumination can help improve safety on stairs. In the bedroom, there should be an overhead or table light near the bed. The room light should be controlled from the bed as well as from the doorway, so that people do not put themselves at added risk by walking across the room in darkness.

Windows should be easy to open and close. In older buildings, sills are too high: those in chairs can see only sky. Balconies allow the opportunities to sit in the sun or tend to plants.

INTERACTION

The home should provide a congenial social environment. Facilities for games (pool, billiards, darts), TV and radio, and a writing desk should be available. Tea-making facilities in one's own room allow for encounters that are more personal, which mean so much to people in long-term care.

Ideally, people should have their own telephones. If only communal phones are provided, they should be in an area where private calls can be made. There should be at least one telephone low enough for wheelchair users (the dialling details should also be placed at a lower level). Phones with amplifiers are easily installed.

Garden furniture should also be enabling: benches and seats of the appropriate height, with arm rests, will allow people to chat out of doors.

ACCESS AND LOCOMOTION

Wheelchair users, whether residents or visitors, must be carefully considered. Places in the car park designated for these people should have ample space on either side of the car to allow access for the disabled person and the wheelchair. There should be a firm ramp, with rails on each side, leading to the entrance.

Automatic doors are preferable as manual doors often present difficulties, especially if handles or doorbells are too high or the door is sprung or cumbersome.

Lifts are not often designed with disabled people in mind. There should be space in them for a powered wheelchair. The doors should have an in-built delay so that older disabled people have plenty of time to get into and out of the lift. A fold-down chair in a corner can be a boon to someone who is weary or unwell. The lift buttons should be of a height that those in wheelchairs can reach.

Corridors should have grab rails along their length. Chairs and benches should be placed at intervals along wide, long corridors so that people can stop and sit down for a breather or a chat.

Easy chairs are not always easy to get out of: they may be too low, or the seating angle may put the occupant at a mechanical disadvantage. If the resident brings a favourite armchair into the home, then considerations of personal preference and comfort should over-ride ergonomic factors. However, much thought should be given to the design features of the range of chairs provided for residents and visitors. Chairs should not be bought unless nurses and therapists have been consulted first.

The ideal chair should be comfortable and stable and the occupant should be able to sit down in and rise up from it easily. Adequate pressure relief is more difficult to achieve in a chair than a bed. The seat should be firm; low-pressure cushions may be needed by those who spend long periods sitting in chairs.

If a seat is too high, the occupant's legs will dangle and may become oedematous. If the seat is too low, it is harder to rise successfully from the chair: the joint and muscle forces used in rising from a high chair are 20%

less than from a low seat. In one study, increasing the chair seat height from 17 to 21 inches resulted in a doubling of the percentage of successful rises.

If armrests are too low, they will inhibit rising from the chair; if they are too high, the person's shoulders will become hunched when sitting in the chair. The armrests should extend forward far enough to give leverage, which is helpful to those with proximal muscle weakness.

High backs give support to the neck while transferring. Some people with Parkinson's disease initiate a rocking movement to assist getting up: a stable chair back can be helpful. The ideal chair back should support the full length of the user's back and slope gently backwards.

Sheepskin covers are comfortable, absorb moisture (while remaining dry), and reduce shear injuries. They are also easy to wash. Synthetic sheepskins are less satisfactory.

An ejector cushion or chair could be considered for those people with very weak quadriceps.

BATHING AND TOILETING

Toilets in hospital wards are often too small for physically disabled people. They are poorly signposted and badly designed (Travers *et al.*, 1992). A personal toilet is the ideal. There should be grab rails next to the toilet. Higher toilet seats should be provided for those who have difficulty rising unaided. Toilet paper should be dispensed from 'pull-out' containers: it is difficult to tear off a piece of tissue if one has a paralysed or broken arm. Those with arthritic hands may have difficulty flushing the toilet unless carefully designed handles are provided. Commodes may offer convenience but are not much liked: they cause embarrassment, are a source of smells and cleaning them is an unpleasant task.

Baths are of two types: domestic and assisted. Domestic baths are either metallic (cast iron or sheet steel) or acrylic. Metal baths are less likely to be damaged by bath aids; some acrylic baths cannot accommodate those bath seats that wedge into the tub. Thermostatically controlled mixer taps reduce the risk of scalding. Wall hooks and shelves allow ease of access to soap and shampoo. Getting into the bath can be facilitated by a platform step at the side of the bath and by bath rails, boards and seats.

Bathrooms are hazardous places and special care must be taken to incorporate safety features. The floor must not be slippery. Optimally sited grab rails can allow independent and safer bathing. Bath mats need to be replaced every few months, before the pads which give them a secure purchase to the bottom of the bath stop working. People may slip and fall in the bath and have difficulty summoning help. Carefully placed alarm cords are therefore essential.

Assisted baths can be helpful to frail or disabled older people. Walk-in baths are particularly helpful if the patient is obese or has poor balance. The bath is fixed to the floor. The patient walks or slides in and the door is sealed by a pneumatic compressor. The patient must be warned by the attendant about the rising level of water. These baths help to reduce the strain on the attendants' backs. Adjustable baths can be moved up and down: for example, the patient may find it easier to get into the bath at a low level. Once inside, the bath is raised to the level which is optimum for the bathing assistant. Other adjustable baths can tilt backwards, allowing water in the foot-well of the bath to run over the patient's trunk.

Walk-in showers with seats are greatly appreciated. The traditional belief that older British people prefer tub-baths and reject the idea of showers is questionable.

NURSING EQUIPMENT

So far we have focused on enabling equipment and aspects of furniture design and décor that allow independence and autonomy. Some long-stay petients are heavily dependent and it is important that wards and nursing homes are suitably equipped so that these people receive the highest standards of care. Proper equipment is also necessary to make nursing safer and less burdensome. We consider two types of equipment: bed aids and hoists.

BED AIDS

Beds and mattresses should allow for mobility, comfort and safety.

Mobility

Just as chairs of different heights are needed, so a selection of beds should be available. Beds of adjustable height are useful: they reduce the risk of back strain in nurses and allow the patient the opportunity to get in and out of bed without being helped. Most falls in nursing homes occur in bedrooms. Some occur because the brakes on the bed wheels or castors do not work properly.

Mobility in the bed can be facilitated by simple gadgets. A trapeze or monkey pole – a device suspended from an upright at the head of the bed – enables patients to pull themselves up off the mattress. This may relieve pressure and is also helpful during some nursing procedures. A rope ladder tied to the bottom rail of the bed can allow the person to move from a lying to a sitting position without help.

Much ink has been spilt on the subject of cot sides or side rails. In some countries (e.g. the USA), they are put in place as a matter of course. In fact, they do not prevent falls, although they may confer a feeling of security to patient and staff and may be useful to help pull oneself up the bed. The very name 'cot sides' reinforces the concept of a reversal to childhood. Side rails should be used sparingly and thoughtfully; they should be used to improve movement in bed and afford protection, not as physical restraints.

Comfort

Duvets are light and give more freedom of movement than blankets. Bed cradles keep the pressure of bed covers off ischaemic, ulcerated or paralysed legs. Support pillows and carefully adjusted backrests are useful in providing a comfortable sitting position in bed. Cantilevered tables, which allow room for the knees to flex, allow people to enjoy meals and drinks in bed.

People confined to beds (or chairs) are at particular risk of pressure sores. These are particularly common in the context of an acute illness. Sometimes, sores are caused by people being placed on unyielding surfaces such as hard seats, metal trolleys, operating theatre tables. Only occasionally are they the consequence of poor nursing. Low-pressure surfaces may augment skilful nursing care. Surveys have revealed the heterogeneous nature of mattresses used. Net beds, which suspend the patient on netting between parallel bars, seem barbaric and have largely been abandoned. Water mattresses are very heavy, require a long time to be filled and emptied, and make turning the patient difficult. The sound of water is not always appreciated by the patient. Unheated water mattresses can result in hypothermia and sometimes those with heating controls go awry, causing over-heating. Alternating-pressure air mattresses, which provide a constantly changing support surface, are liked by staff. Some patients find the noise of the motor annoying. These mattresses do not have a good history of reliability and may give a false sense of security to nursing staff. Padded mattresses containing polyester fibres seem to be of little value in preventing sores. Foam mattresses, with a composite foam core and a stretch cover (which is permeable to water vapour), are flame-retardant, relatively cheap and better than standard hospital mattresses. Although mattresses that are supposed to prevent pressure sores are vigorously promoted by manufacturers, few have been carefully evaluated in laboratory studies or clinical trials. Until information on efficacy is forthcoming, individual mattresses cannot be confidently recommended.

Safety

Old mattresses that have become torn or permeable to water can be a reservoir of pathogenic organisms, including methicillin-resistant

Staphylococcus aureus. Mattresses that are soiled, stained or damp should therefore be condemned. Some designs of side rail can trap fingers and cause lacerations.

HOISTS

Hoists help to move people to a different position in bed, ease transfers and facilitate bathing and toileting. They can be ceiling- or floor-mounted, fixed or mobile, powered or manually operated.

A typical hoist consists of legs with castors, a strong vertical pole, and a sling which is attached by straps to a spreader bar. The castors make movement over carpets difficult; vinyl surfaces are less resistant. The home must be designed so that toilets, bathrooms and bedroom doors can admit a hoist; there should be somewhere to store it when it is not in use.

Using a hoist is time-consuming. The operator must first assess the patient (weight, size, locomotor impairments), apply and position the appropriate sling and ensure that the sling is comfortable. Hoists can initially be intimidating to the operators, who should have received instruction from an occupational therapist or the manufacturer. They can also cause anxiety to the occupant: it is good idea to include the experiences of hoisting and being hoisted in the training of nurses, therapists and doctors.

What hoists gain in manoeuvrability they lose in stability: the patient's confidence may be undermined if they are swung about in the sling. The most troublesome physical problem of being in a hoist is the discomfort under the knees that results from the edges of the sling bunching up and digging into the skin. Bath hoists often have a seat rather than slings and therefore the patient feels safer. These hoists can be fixed to the head or side of the bath. At least 11 fixed cm of space is required for the legs of the hoist to go under the bath.

The material and design of slings are central to the physical comfort of the occupant. Those made of PVC are easy to clean and dry but tend to stick to the skin and cause sweating. Canvas slings are not very flexible and the raised edges can be hazardous. Nylon and cotton are mostly used. If slings are used to hoist someone into and out of a bath, net mesh slings are best, as these allow the water through.

Multi-purpose slings can support the legs individually or together and are best for helping someone into and out of bed. They are not good for toileting: here slings that go under the resident's arms are favoured, as they allow access to the perineum and clothing. However, these hoists are less supportive and must be used with care if the occupant has shoulder pain or arm weakness.

It is important to match the individual sling with a hoist from the same manufacturer. If there is interchange, and a hoist-related accident occurs, the insurance indemnity will not be valid.

REFERENCES

Age Concern (1990) *Left Behind? Continuing care for elderly people in NHS hospitals. A review of Health Advisory Service reports*, Age Concern England, London.

Holder, E.C. (1987) A consumer perspective on quality care: the resident's point of view. *Dan. Med. Bull.*, **5**, 84–9.

Seymour, R.M. (1993) Reality orientation boards: a recipe for disorientation? *J. Am. Geriatr. Soc.*, **41**, 193–4.

Travers, A.F., Burns, E., Penn, N.D., Mitchell, S.C. and Mulley, G.P. (1992) A survey of hospital toilet facilities. *BMJ*, **304**, 878–9.

APPENDIX

HELPFUL ORGANIZATIONS

Disabled Living Foundation, 380/384 Harrow Road, London W9 2HU (tel: 0171 289 6111). A national information service providing free details of equipment. They also have a large range of items on display and provide helpful advice.

Disabled Living Centres (look in your local telephone directory for the one nearest to you). Demonstration and advice centres. Do not usually sell equipment, but advise where it can be purchased. Give telephone as well as personal advice: it is best to book an appointment before you visit.

Disability Information Trust, Mary Marlborough Lodge, Nuffield Orthopaedic Centre, Headington, Oxford OX3 7LD (tel: 01865 227592). Produces an extensive series of books entitled 'Equipment for Disabled People' which give facts and comments on disability equipment. Current titles include 'Hoists and Lifts'; 'Wheelchairs'; 'Personal Care'.

Disability Scotland, Princes House, 5 Shandwick Place, Edinburgh EH2 4RG (tel: 0131 229 8632). A national disability organization for disabled people and their helpers. It provides training, advice, information and publications.

Education and creativity in long-term care

17

Both education and creative process have been shown to be effective media that offer purposeful activity. They structure that experience which leads to the development of capacity and is adjusted to changing abilities. At each step in the process, the person is motivated to respond; this develops the capacity to learn, to become more skilful, to make something original to the maker: briefly, to change. Most subjects can be studied and many creative media can be explored in long-term care. The determining factor is the teaching. The activity most commonly instituted is art (drawing, painting, and collage), while French, current affairs, cookery, music and drama, poetry and play-reading, and local history have also been instituted, with various degrees of success. All programmes have features that are instructive.

EARLY EXPERIMENTS

Poetry writing has been initiated in both a New York nursing home, and in England, at Redhills, a 104-bed hospital for the elderly in Exeter, Devon. The hospital supplements art and music therapy with poetry writing, initiated by Margaret Valk (1980) who uses the methods of Kenneth Koch (1977). A group of four to nine patients aged between 70 and 90, all in wheelchairs, meets once a week for an hour. Mrs Valk and another volunteer set a theme – perhaps 'wishes' or 'sleep' – and those patients who can use notebooks to record their poems, while others dictate to one of the volunteers. An essential part of the procedure is to read aloud what each has written, and for a volunteer to comment on some aspect. The results are of great interest. A selection of the poems has been published by Redhills Hospital and they show simplicity, beauty and sincerity. Mrs Valk suggests that the use of poetic language can 'enable people to look at things around them in a fresh light' (Kirkham, 1981). The importance of this, in the restricted circumstances of long-term care and for a disabled person in a wheelchair, cannot be overestimated. Koch himself established a group of similar age in a New York nursing home, (Koch, 1977; Valk, 1980), although here the number in the group was much larger (25) and also inspired projects in other settings of older disabled people. There were usually four people acting as facilitators for each group. He notes that his poetry writers seemed to have more animation and more confidence; they had more to say to others and they spoke more clearly. Their eagerness to express their thoughts replaced vagueness and, for some, even silence.

A class in French conversation was begun in a hospital for older people in East Anglia, UK, and, although it continued for only three months, it produced some interesting comments from the participants. The group met twice a week for about an hour, with an experienced teacher of French. The six participants were chosen by the consultant mainly because they were likely to benefit. One of these students, Mr H (who was 83, suffering from osteoporosis, degenerative joint disease and postural hypotension, and had a past history of diabetes controlled by diet) said, when interviewed:

> I am alone in the world. Very grateful to be here. I enjoy being with other classmates – look forward to the break in the routine. The class has gone well. I enjoy most the gradual build-up from the beginning of the book. Like the feeling of learning more and more. Between lessons I read the book again. We use phrases in passing one another in the ward.

Another student, Mrs L (aged 72, with spastic paraplegia, mitral valve disease and bilateral cataracts), said:

> I enjoy the class very much. Would like to get on quicker, have a lesson every day. I can't see, so I don't see the right place, but I am getting used to it now. Wish I could make notes on the lessons. The teacher brings a tape recorder, and that's very good. We look forward to the lessons. We'll be sorry when the holidays come. I would like a lesson on something else on the other days. It gives our brains something to do.

A programme of teaching local geography and history was instituted by an occupational therapist with older patients in a large urban hospital. The choice of subjects was determined by the educational background of the therapist. Again, this was a small group, and only one session a week could be provided because of pressure on the therapist's time. Her comment after several weeks indicated that 'the project . . . showed up the great need to provide stimulation and help to a specific group of patients who tend to sink into the shadows on an acute ward and become institutionalised.' I have described this project in detail previously (Jones, 1983).

Six patients who participated in an art class in an outer London older patient hospital were reassessed by the medical staff three months after classes began. The participants had previously had two classes a week in drawing, painting and modelling in a room separate from their wards, the teacher being a local education authority tutor of the community education service. An 83-year-old lady in this class, Mrs H, was completely chairbound, suffering from severe arthritis and a slight stroke, and was accordingly in a very poor state before the art class began. She was indifferent to her surroundings, had difficulty in propelling her wheelchair and was frequently incontinent by day and night. She scored 5 out of 10 on Hodkinson's (1972) mental test; she knew neither the name of the hospital nor that of the Queen. Three months into the classes medical staff reported:

> Marked physical improvement. Where previously needed two nurses to propel her wheelchair, now wheels herself about unaided. She is still chairbound, but now only requires minimal help with dressing and feeding, and is much more co-operative with staff. Washes herself, cleaner in her habits, completely continent. . . Brighter mentally. Most dramatic improvement noticed by all staff, and her daughter, who says she is brighter and easier to talk to. Mental test score 7 out of 10.

Of course one swallow does not make a summer, and it is well known that there can be many reasons for improvement. The classes might just have coincided with a spontaneous uplift in the patient's condition, and may not have been a principal contribution to it. It happens that every single one of the patients in that art class showed significant improvement in their physical and psychological states, although none as striking as that of Mrs H (Jones, 1980a).

A larger-scale programme, in music and movement, was evaluated (Jones, 1983) in two hospitals where very severely deteriorated patients were cared for in wards for older people. There were two periods of activity each week conducted by a trained and able teacher, provided by an organization of artist–teachers, known as SHAPE. Reports were made at intervals, over four months, by senior nurses and paramedical staff. Some of the patients showed sustained improvements in cognition or information-processing, in emotional state and interaction, in self-care, or activities of daily living and mobility and in a few striking cases, in continence, single and double. One 95-year-old woman demonstrated some of these features. She had had a cerebrovascular accident, and suffered severe dysphasia. Before the educational programme began, she had not sat up since being in hospital; after it, she always did and swung her legs out of bed. She had never washed her hands or face herself in hospital;

now she sometimes did. She now always fed herself, a previously rare event, and was more sociable and co-operative.

If a new drug were to achieve such results, we should urgently want to investigate its use and effects. Educational intervention has shown enough promise to warrant such serious attention as every educational experiment in a ward or hospital for older people that has been reported has shown positive outcomes (Naylor and Harwood, 1973).

These early studies demonstrate much about 'the development of human capacity.' They go much further, however, in the way that they illuminate the nature of experiences in long-term care. A short account of some of the classes and their outcomes has been published previously (Jones, 1980b). The final section of this chapter, on implementation, provides some illustrations of current practice in planning and provision.

THE CONTEXT

These approaches are not a panacea – there is no magic. It is really a question of augmenting, and in some cases changing, the nature of the patient's experience. In so doing, we seem to change the quality of life for the older patient. Because of the extent to which this can be achieved, the process of enhancement warrants consideration. I have described previously how educational programmes can be instituted (Jones, 1977). This practical guide is amplified with special attention to creativity towards the end of this chapter.

The psychological effects of a lack of stimulation in unvarying surroundings are well known, as are the physical and psychological effects of lack of exercise: 'disorganisation, loss of intellectual ability and concentration, and declines in co-ordination' (Ornstein and Sobel, 1989). One might also add boredom. It is not difficult to understand why many settings for older people have had an aura of hopelessness, helplessness, apathy and their accompaniments. Where there has been no attempt at positive active intervention, it is extraordinarily difficult for staff to secure job satisfaction and sustain morale.

INDIVIDUALS AND CHANGE

There are many ways of changing such a situation positively. The whole-hearted adoption of educative programmes is but one. Clients should be regarded in a whole sense, as persons with a history, and with individual needs, expectations, goals and desires, however frail or disabled they may have become.

The hierarchy of human needs set out so comprehensively and lucidly by Maslow (1970), and familiar to most people in the caring professions, provides a useful starting point for analysis of needs:

- physiological
- safety
- love and belongingness
- esteem (for the self, and from others)
- self-actualization.

It is very easy to dismiss the needs for love, self-esteem and self-actualization, in fact barely to consider them at all. However, if a client in care is to be regarded as a whole person, these needs must be considered, even if they are not manifest. In fact, it may be that the more withdrawn and passive the client appears, the more their psychological needs should be considered.

'Caring' in every aspect of life has been shown to induce dependence, with its attendant apathy and inertia. Seligman (1975) shows how, when our needs are met without our having to exert ourselves, awareness of helplessness and the danger of a lapse into depression result. Fortunately, the provision of educative and creative opportunities has been shown in many settings to have extremely beneficial features that help to meet the needs in question.

THE EFFECTS OF EDUCATION

Engaging regularly in the educative process has many effects. There are obvious changes in the clients who take part, and, perhaps not so obvious, changes in staff attitudes and behaviour.

PHYSICAL OUTCOMES

The physical outcomes are various. At a basic level, there is the sheer encouragement to move parts of the body, such as the arms and hands in painting, or the motor co-ordination of a cortical kind that is called for when we handle an object. All these are of great importance in restoring and maintaining the health of the body, its joints and muscles, to the extent that is physically possible. There is the added and vital factor of locomotion.

Educational activity requires the use of the body for manipulation, even to turn the pages of a book, use a pencil, or, in the case of poetry speaking or playing the recorder, use of the facial muscles and vocal chords, as well as the respiratory organs (rib cage, diaphragm etc.). The activities also invite the person to take part, to get to the scene of action, and to alter posture from time to time. There is nothing like the incentive of enjoyment and interest to tempt a person to move – to make an effort. The key is motivation. If the activity is satisfying, whether it is poetry speaking or painting, the person participates in this by using their body. Such participation is use, and it is lack of use which destroys.

One finding that has been reported for at least one of the educational programmes (Mulford, 1979) is that the participants' eyes are brighter. This is certainly not a trivial outcome. Lowen (1976) holds that bright eyes are a good sign of the state of health. Eyes can reflect interest in the surrounding world (if it is worth looking at and participating in) and can easily become dull through disuse. Thus the eye brightness that accompanies educational programmes, although a small detail, has considerable significance.

The restoration of continence as a by-product of an educational activity is an intriguing possibility. Mulford (1979) reports on the outcome of a large-scale programme in a psychogeriatric hospital which initiated art, craft, drama, music and communication studies, with a number of different classes. She says of the participants, 'they have become more alert (and). . . there has also been some improvement in continence during the daytime. . . personal appearance (has) become more important'. While the observations about alertness, continence and appearance are, as we shall see, fairly certainly related to each other, let us concentrate on the note regarding continence. This is consistent with the experience of Mrs H (mentioned earlier in this chapter) who became 'completely continent' having been frequently incontinent by day as well as by night.

In the study reported previously (Jones, 1983), four patients out of 28 showed an improvement in continence with respect to urine eight weeks into the educational programme, while two of these showed a similar improvement in continence with respect to faeces. After a further 11 weeks, three of the four had sustained this amelioration, and six further patients enjoyed a restoration of continence. Thus, nine out of 28 participants had improved continence with respect to urine, and six had become more continent with respect to faeces. It is of great importance to those planning education programmes to note that a much more significant improvement in the state of patients was apparent after 19 weeks than occurred after eight weeks. I have discussed this fully in a previous publication (Jones, 1983), and Sutherland (1976) has described the psychological aspects of incontinence.

SOCIAL OUTCOMES

The social outcomes are extremely important. There is not much social life in the average communal setting for older people. Why do people not talk in such circumstances? First of all, the clients have not normally chosen their location or their companions. It can be reasonably argued that they are in much the same circumstances of disability and needing care, and are so much of an age as to give them a good deal in common.

Consequently interaction should flourish, but often it does not. In this silent setting, one is driven to the conclusion that, in the absence of variety and stimulation, what can be said in the midst of routine has been said, and that it is very little. A second factor is lack of privacy. After all, the tradition of keeping yourself to yourself for fear of getting involved or your personal privacy being invaded by the people next door is a tenacious feature of even domestic life for many. The long-term reality is to be surrounded by strangers who are daily and hourly witnesses to one's physical frailties, and to one's social exchanges with family and friends where these exist, where there is no wall and no front door. Under such circumstances, there must be some new agent, an extra factor that will penetrate the wall of silence that replaces the physical partitions we all need from time to time.

Any event that breaks the routine can act as a catalyst. The significant factors in education, as opposed to other similar events, are that the patient must respond, move, give attention, act, and, more particularly, respond in the company of others who are doing likewise. The experience is satisfying, and it is shared. In learning and creative situations, the events are (a) under the control of the participants, freely chosen and controlled, and (b) shared physically and psychologically. There is the need, and frequently the opportunity to communicate with the teacher and fellow students. It is important to note the change of role from a dependant to student or artist. In such a new psychological, and if possible, different physical environment, social interaction is not only possible and encouraged, but necessary, as when students co-operate in a group activity. Through co-operation, the sharing, absorption and concentration that feature, and which can only be described as joy, there is an overflow of energy, the very need to communicate, to comment, to observe. As an accompaniment to sharing an activity, there is the strong tendency to identify with one's fellows, and thus to converse, and the social interaction need not be confined to the class.

Ernst *et al.* (1978) have shown that physical, social and emotional isolation are key intervening variables that 'disclose functional symptoms of disorders.' They argue that 'treatment. . . countering isolation will alleviate or reverse symptomatic disorders whether or not brain pathologies. . . are present.'

It is not only communication and instruction that are encouraged by a shared activity. A small but significant change to a neater appearance has been noticed in many participants. So much in our everyday lives depends on our meeting with others whose opinion we value. It is only when we are separated from their company that we notice the tendency to let ourselves go, e.g. a man perhaps does not shave every day or does not dress till late. While long-stay residents are rarely alone, the improvement in their appearance and self-care when they engage in a shared satisfying activity probably indicates that they are then in a group, which is perceived as different from being in communal residence.

PSYCHOLOGICAL OUTCOMES

The psychological outcomes are of the very greatest importance and may be divided into two kinds, cognitive and affective. The division is one of convenience, made for the sake of analysis. People will of course act and react as a whole, not as a collection of parts.

Cognitive change

The cognitive changes that accompany educational activity include improved memory, alertness, sense of identity, concentration, and a better grasp on reality (Jones, 1980a, b). Even the most superficial acquaintance with long-term care indicates that these changes are of the very greatest significance. So often the opposites are observed: forgetfulness in various degrees, lack of interest in surroundings, and a lack of self-initiated activity, concentration or conversation. All these features may of course be described as symptoms of 'dementia' or of other disorders, some of which may be treated. On the other hand, they are common in long-term care and may indeed come to characterize it. Besdine (1978) points out that many of these symptoms, often described as 'dementia', are treatable, if properly investigated. In some, these symptoms may be alleviated by the opportunity to participate in a satisfying and progressive activity, not merely being 'stimulated' but being expected to respond.

Improvement in memory is a main feature of learning, because learning something of interest holds the attention. Most poor remembering, and this applies to all of us, is the outcome of poor attention. What we attend to we recall. We are equipped to notice differences, and to become immune to sameness – the bases of a theory of boredom. Engaging in a novel activity, noticing, giving attention and adjusting our responses to the changing stimuli, whether visual, aural, kinaesthetic or proprioceptive, are manifestations of attention to something outside ourselves which tempt us to remember the acts and sensations involved. Practice in remembering assists the recovery or at least the maintenance of memory. It is the reverse, having nothing worthy of our attention, that causes the damage. Remembering and attending are closely intertwined. Thus, education can help in this attempt to normalize life in long-term care.

There is a big difference between lack of contact with the outside world as a temporary withdrawal, and the almost continual daydream or inertness so common in the long-stay setting. Reverie, the opportunity to fantasize, to erect a barrier between one's consciousness and a dull or irritating environment filled with companions who find the environment of similar character, may be protective. All then conspire, however silently and unwittingly, to make a grey, predictable and routine setting for those in it. It may be an adaptive response which leads to its own form of disorder when it becomes habitual. This lack of contact with reality and its very frequent accompaniment, incontinence, comes to characterize long-term care, however false the picture may be in individual terms.

Educational enterprises directly attack this syndrome. When successful, and this varies greatly between individuals and settings, the results can be dramatic, as in the case of Mrs H above (Jones, 1980a). Having something interesting to attend to, interacting with other residents and the teacher, producing a tangible end-product, communicating with others, a communication needing thought, and having an enjoyable and satisfying event to anticipate make inroads into the drift from reality, from one's fellows, and indeed from one's self. No wonder a patient's ability to remember is prone to improvement when they re-learn the satisfaction of concentration, and their grasp on reality improves when reality itself becomes worthy of attention, when, above all, stimulation is met by self-initiated response.

A word about stimulation is perhaps appropriate at this point. Many staff members, noting the boredom, the routine and the dullness of many patients in long-stay, come to the conclusion that stimulation is lacking. In a sense this is absolutely correct. However, the results of providing this stimulation are often disappointing, because beyond a temporary flurry of excitement, the patients seem to be no more stimulated or lively than before. I refer to the 'conversations' that staff or visitors may initiate, the sing-song a visiting pianist attempts to start, the youngsters from a local school who provide a lively entertainment, or the games that a well-meaning occupational therapist's aide may inaugurate. None of the activities are to be decried. They are worthy attempts to divert, occupy and stimulate. What these situations lack, in my opinion, is the opportunity for the patients to respond in a meaningful, constructive, distinctly human way.

To respond in this human sense is to go beyond reflex or reaction; it is to act, to recognize, to become conscious of sensation, to become aware of one's own contribution, of one's participation. When we talk of patients needing stimulation, what we should really be describing is the need for responding, although not all clients will want or be able to respond in the degree described.

A report from the Royal College of Physicians points out that 'there is need for research into the fundamental causes of dementia and also into agents which are effective in symptomatic control' (RCP, 1981). Professor Grimley Evans points out that people are now reaching old age with better brain function than in the past. This may be due to education among other factors and 'may have important implications for the future of dementing diseases' (Grimley Evans, 1991). Even more important is that, in his opinion, 'better brains can compensate longer for the effects of Alzheimer's'.

In their survey of more than 7500 men and women in Rotterdam, The Netherlands, Ott *et al.* (1995) showed that the risk of dementia after the age of 55 decreased in those who had had more advanced education in their youth in comparison with those who had lower educational levels. The risk factor for dementia was 2.3 in the former group compared with 4.0 in the latter.

Orrell and Sahakian (1995), commenting on the Ott study and reviewing a number of cognate researches, suggested that education might protect against the degeneration of neurones or that the onset of dementia might be delayed because education had improved neural networking so that 'when neurones died, others could carry out similar functional tasks, so minimising signs of functional and cognitive impairment'.

It seems to be the case that stimulating opportunities in later life for education and creative activity generally can have protective cortical effects. The provision of an appropriately stimulating environment may prove to be among the agents effective in symptom control. Such provision may even affect those defects in cholinergic neurotransmission and the cerebral blood supply that can result in cortical deterioration and intellectual decrement.

Routtenberg (1978) has further suggested that 'the pathways of brain reward may function as the pathways of memory consolidation. . . When something is learned actively in the brain, reward pathways facilitate the formation of memory.' Neuronal function itself can aid cerebral blood flow; Ingvar (1976) provides abundant evidence that the blood flow in non-anoxic brain tissue is controlled mainly by the functional activity of the neuron. Davison (1978) states that problem-solving increases the blood supply to the pre-motor and frontal regions of the brain. Thus education, by increasing cortical exercise, may postpone cortical deterioration, and not only through verbal or symbolic activity, as in literature or mathematics, but also through the problem-solving involved in physical games. Games with a soft ball, or aiming at targets, involve motor co-ordination and attentional processes that exercise appropriate areas of the cortex and nervous system. Physical activity of purposeful kind involves the brain as well as the rest of the body.

Affective change

While most people would agree that education and creative process have a great deal to do with the cognitive aspects of life, with learning, thinking, knowing, remembering, understanding and information-processing in general, it is possibly not so obvious that they have much to do with the affective, emotional and motivational facets of persons. To be stimulated in such a way that we respond constructively, creatively, with interest, curiosity and the motivation to repeat or to continue the process, as in the act of true creative learning, has emotional affective concomitants worthy of analysis. So many levels of emotional motivational response may be involved that we need to particularize.

When we learn we change: that is a basic fact. However, we do not only change in the sense that we now know something we did not know before, e.g. studying Spanish, or can do something that we could not do before, e.g. learning to knit. To learn anything is to demonstrate to ourselves, and often to others, that we are capable of learning, that we have the capacity. We see ourselves in a new way. Our self-concept changes to include this component: 'I am capable of speaking Spanish, or knitting a jumper, or mending a fuse.' The recognition of our own ability is reassuring. Thus, depression born of the perception of helplessness (Schulz, 1976, 1980) can be held at bay. Csikszentmihalyi (1975, 1992) has demonstrated the joy derived from the exercise of skill which extends us but does not over-extend us (he suggests that the latter causes anxiety) and which is the opposite of a constant diet of activity or non-activity that makes no call on our potential skilfulness. He suggests that the lack of demand on our abilities is at the root of boredom.

Healthy and productive diversions from the self seem to occur when a person is active, mentally and physically, in contemplation, appreciation or attending to a scene or event outside. To become involved in an outside activity in which one participates fully is the best cure for the disorders engendered by self-preoccupation, and such absorption lies at the root of the therapeutic uses of educational activity.

Any activity that improves the mood state is valuable in the light of the factors which tend to depress it: bereavement, isolation, physical disorders, and many other stressors. So much may be taken for granted. New understanding of mood, behaviour and bodily reactions is providing a strong rationale for positive, enjoyable activity. This is founded in research on psychoneuroimmunology (Maier et al., 1994). Any activity that fosters a feeling of competence or self-efficacy has been shown by Bandura (1989) to have the utmost positive effect on the immune system, making it more active and therefore more effective in its resistance to infection. It can be shown that the chain of causality from behaviour to health itself passes through the mood state of the individual (Seligman, 1990).

IMPLEMENTATION

In this section there is a brief summary of methods together with an account of current and promising programmes. A fuller guide to mounting educational programmes has been given previously (Jones, 1991). The programmes described following this summary will yield much practical detail also.

Four stages to mounting programmes are:

- gaining commitment;
- teaching and facilitating;
- meeting the needs of the clients;
- choice of arena.

GAINING COMMITMENT

The utmost care is required in planning an educational or creative programme. Since this always involves change of various kinds, the support of all concerned must be sought. Their understanding and whole-hearted commitment are essential, and no more so than at the top of the organization, including the consultant in a geriatric ward, the senior officer in a residential home, and the warden in sheltered housing or a day centre for older people. With that commitment, much is possible; without it, no programme can be wholly successful. Consultation and agreement at every relevant level are essential.

TEACHING AND FACILITATING

Some programmes and some settings may require outside facilitation by experienced and/or qualified professionals. Such experience may already be found internally. One feature of the last ten years has been a gratifying recognition by providing bodies that this area of work is not a marginal side of the quality of life of clients but a significant factor in its enhance-ment. As a result, many residential homes and some geriatric wards benefit from the integral leadership of able educationists and activity organizers.

There are no limits, in principle, to what can be provided in a variety of settings. It is the existence of able and willing facilitators that is the key, and they can be teachers, care staff, occupational therapists, or indeed anyone with a specific knowledge, whether in embroidery or Gujerati, and the enthusiasm to share this with others. This has been demonstrated in local authority residential homes by Jackie Ackroyd, who is a social services training officer in the outer London borough of Barnet (Ackroyd, 1995). Each of the ten residential homes for older people in the borough has been assigned an activity co-ordinator, as has a day centre with a similar clientele. These staff, in a new management role, have been given intensive training in relevant areas, such as overcoming common ageist prejudices about the capacities of older people, careful assessment of client's experience and interests, and planning a wide programme to cater for some of these very varied interests. A very important outcome of these appointments has been initiation of the explicit commitment of interested care staff, at every level, to sharing their own interests with their clients on a systematic basis. The results so far have been very encouraging, with good implications for the morale and status of care staff as well as the quality of life of clients. The opportunity to study for national vocational qualifications is being considered for this occupational group.

MEETING THE NEEDS OF THE CLIENT

We know that learning, the beginnings of mastery, is not only useful, as shown above; it is enjoyable. Multiplying the sources of satisfaction and enjoyment experienced in long-term care needs no justification. And if the abilities of the clients are doubted, the words of Jerome Bruner (1963) should give encouragement: '. . . the foundations of any subject may be taught to anybody at any age in some form.' This message should underlie discussion about the suitability of any educational or creative programme.

Gibson *et al.* (1992) taught a mixed group (average age 78), of mainly frail residents in a private nursing home, the elements of using computers to write their life histories, in 20 sessions of two hours, with two or more tutors at each session. There were striking improvements in general health and in attitudes to information technology. She claims that the strength of motivation was a more important factor in accounting for success than was physical disability. Although there may be gross cognitive pathology, as in severe dementia, the patient's response to educational programmes should not be pre-judged. The rewards are so great that premature exclusions are unjustifiable. It is often the case that the least promising client in terms of ability to learn may benefit most.

THE ARENA

The location for a programme obviously depends on its nature, and on what space is available, perhaps for the accessibility of wheelchairs. However, an important question is whether the clients can or should move to a central location, which is convenient for organization, or whether the facility should be brought to the clients. In the latter case although there may be some distraction by others, exposure of the activity can promote interest and be inviting to peers and, importantly, to staff. The commitment and enhancement of staff roles is a welcome concomitant of the provision of worthwhile educational programmes.

EXAMPLES

A comprehensive programme in a housing trust

An enlightened housing trust in outer London with several residential homes as well as blocks of sheltered housing has the benefit of an arts and education officer on its staff. As a result, the residents have access to a very full and varied programme of activities, including not only entertaining sessions such as concert outings and film shows, but such features as current affairs discussions and poetry reading. Within a novel project in health alternatives such as reflexology and aromatherapy, there is, significantly, a programme of visiting speakers in the health area, including nutrition, mental health, and maintaining a positive image. This project is in the process of evaluation.

A creative programme in long-term care

This novel departure has involved a partnership between a team developing a process called Building Community through Arts and a variety of long-term care settings such as a residential home, a nursing home, a sheltered housing scheme, clients in their own homes and a day centre. This has involved both the private and public sectors. Funding for the programmes has come from a variety of sources: from the training and public relation budgets of client organizations, from charities and from commercial sponsorship, which has included the training and participation of company staff.

The preliminaries of such a programme include extensive discussion and briefing of all concerned. The programmes are designed in detail only after all the initial participants, clients, carers, sponsors and volunteers have discussed the scope of the process and decided on the issues they might like to address. These might be issues of isolation, depression, staff motivation, confidence, interpersonal skills and disability awareness depending on the circumstances of the participants.

The idea of community is that of a group of people sharing a significant aspect of their lives in a joint pursuit. Such a group is interdependent and thus dynamic: what affects one member affects all. Sharing and interdependence do more than facilitate a joint task: they have profound psychological effects: friendship, belonging, being known and acknowledged.

Once all the initial participants, clients, carers, managers, sponsors and volunteers, have taken part in planning the project, then the detailed designing of the workshops begins. Highly motivated teachers committed to sharing their own fields and making their worlds accessible are essential. In the initial stages of a programme, professional artists design approaches to artwork that accommodate participation on a wide variety of levels.

Each level, including the first one of 'I'm just looking, thank you', provides opportunities for enablers to draw participants out, and training manuals and leaflets are specially designed for each project. Once the original parti-cipants have become confident in the art process being explored, they receive training in basic enabling skills from a management trainer and practise role plays with each other, before going on to introduce more people, people with different roles, clients and carers, into the project.

By adopting this approach, it not infrequently occurs that a patient or resident may end up 'teaching' or 'enabling' a member of staff or a carer. This role reversal has proved very powerful for both sides, causing partici-pants to see themselves and each other differently. Staff have gained non-intrusive insights into the lives of those in their care while the potential effects on the 'enablers' are particularly interesting especially when they are recipients of 'care'. They now provide care for others. Giving, which is the essence of enabling, has been described by Erich Fromm (1975) as 'the highest expression of potency. In the very act of giving I experience my strength.'

The communication and sharing between old and young, people in wheelchairs and those taking their mobility for granted, residents in care homes and people in their own homes, and professionals from different fields and company employees are themselves a learning and stimulating experience.

THE CHANGING PERSPECTIVE

A transformation in the lives of some residents in long-term care, in residential homes, geriatric wards, and, for some, in their own homes, has been demonstrated as possible and certainly desirable. If educational and creative opportunities are imaginatively provided on a regular basis, the results for many are indeed powerful, and if this is carried out whole-heartedly and with the support of all concerned at every level, it is not only beneficial to the clients, it has benefits for the staff.

A new kind of development is in the offing. A radical plan for the conversion of a long-stay setting into a residential college for older people, as I proposed nearly two decades ago (Jones, 1978) now seems much more likely to be adopted by imaginative providers. All the necessary features are now *in situ* in some locations.

The new thinking about education, creativity and the quality of life offers promise to us all.

ACKNOWLEDGEMENTS

Particular thanks are due to Kitty Lloyd-Lawrence, Director of the Building Community through Arts programme, Kew Studio, and to

Rosamund Goodliffe, Arts and Education Officer of the Central and Cecil Housing Trust, Kew, for their inspired efforts in this field.

REFERENCES

Ackroyd, J. (1995) A smooth transition. Dissertation, Birkbeck College Library, London.

Bandura, A. (1989) Perceived self-efficacy in the exercise of personal agency. *Psychologist*, **12**(10), 411–24.

Besdine, R.W. (1978) *Treatable Dementia in the Elderly*, Hebrew Rehabilitation Centre, Rosindale, MA, USA.

Bruner, J. (1963) *The Process of Education*, Vintage, New York.

Csikszentmihalyi, M. (1975) *Beyond Boredom and Anxiety*, Jossey-Bass, London.

Csikszentmihalyi, M. (1992) *Flow: the psychology of happiness*, Rider, London.

Ernst, P., Beran, B., Safford, F. and Kleinhauz, M. (1978) Isolation and the symptoms of chronic brain syndrome. *Gerontologist*, **18**, 468–74.

Fromm, E. (1975) *The Art of Loving*, Unwin, London.

Gibson, F. (1992) Computers, life history writing and older people. *Generations Rev.*, **2**(2), 12–15.

Grimley Evans, J. (1991) *An Anatomy of Ageing. The Fifth Bayliss Lecture*, Royal College of Physicians, London.

Hodkinson, H.M. (1972) Evaluation of a mental test score for assessment of mental impairment in the elderly. *Age Ageing*, **1**, 233–8.

Ingvar, D.H. (1976) Functional landscapes of the dominant hemisphere. *Brain Res.*, **107**, 181–97.

Jones, S. (1977) Teaching the elderly, in *The Quality of Life in Residential Homes and Hospital* (ed. F. Glendenning), Beth Johnson Foundation and Department of Adult Education, University of Keele, UK.

Jones, S. (1978) *A Residential College for the Elders*, Residential Care Association, Ossett, near Wakefield, UK.

Jones, S. (1980a) The educational experience in homes and hospitals, in *Outreach Education and the Elders: Theory and Practice* (ed. F. Glendenning), Department of Adult Education, University of Keele, UK.

Jones, S. (1980b) Education for the second half of life, in *Living in the 80s* (ed. N. Dickson), Age Concern, London.

Jones, S. (1983) *Learning and Meta-Learning with Special Reference to Education for the Elders*, PhD thesis, University of London.

Jones, S. (1991) Education and life in the long-stay ward, in *Care of the Long-stay Elderly Patient*, 2nd edn (ed. M. Denham), Chapman & Hall, London.

Kirkham, C. (1981) Poetry at Redhills Hospital. *Involve* (Volunteer Centre), 14, Spring.

Koch, K. (1977) *I Never Told Anybody: teaching poetry-writing in a nursing home*, Random House, New York.

Lowen, A. (1976) *Bioenergetics*, Penguin, Harmondsworth, Middlesex, UK.

Maslow, A.M. (1970) *Motivation and Personality*, Harper and Row, New York.

Maier, S., Watkins, L. and Fleshner, M. (1994) Psychoneuroimmunology: the interface between behaviour, brain and immunity. *Am. Psychol.*, **49**(12), 1004–17.

Mulford, J. (1979) *Hospital Job Creation Programme*, unpublished report, Newton-le-Willows College of Further Education, Lancashire, UK.

Naylor, G.F.K. and Harwood, E. (1973) Action research: music for the elderly. *Proc. Aust. Assoc. Gerontol.*, **2**, 26.

Ornstein, R. and Sobel, D. (1989) *The Healing Brain: a radical new approach to staying well*, Macmillan, London.

Orrell, M. and Sahakian, B. (1995) Education and dementia. *BMJ*, **310**, 951–2.

Ott, A., Breteler, M.M.B., van Harskamp, F. *et al.* (1995) Prevalence of Alzheimer's disease and vascular dementia: association with education. The Rotterdam study. *BMJ*, **310**, 970–3.

Royal College of Physicians (1981) Organic mental impairment in the elderly. Implications for research, education and the provision of services. *J. Coll. Phys. Lond.*, **15**, 141–67.

Routtenberg, A. (1978) The reward system of the brain. *Sci. Am.*, **239**, 121–31.

Schulz, R. (1976) Effects of control and predictability on the physical and psychological well-being of the institutionalised aged. *J. Personality Soc. Psychol.*, **33**, 563–73.

Schulz, R. (1980) Ageing and control, in *Human Helplessness: theory and applications* (eds J. Garber and M.E.P. Seligman), Academic Press, London.

Seligman, M.E.P. (1975) *Helplessness: on depression, development and death*, W.H. Freeman, San Francisco, USA.

Seligman, M.E.P. (1990) *Learned Optimism*, Pocket Books, New York.

Sutherland, S.S. (1976) The psychology of incontinence, in *Incontinence in the Elderly* (ed. F.L. Willington), Academic Press, London.

Valk, M. (1980) Poetry can help: the work of Kenneth Koch. *Br. J. Soc. Work*, **9**, 501–7.

APPENDIX

'OTHER PEOPLE'S PAGES': A MODEL FOR A SIMPLE ART AND COMMUNITY BUILDING PROJECT

For staff in care settings where schedules are tight, it is important to be able to spend some time with clients in purposeful activity: motivating them to respond, to learn, to develop skills, to begin to perceive themselves and their environment as one of possibility, not constraint. Working alongside clients on an art project that draws on the unique experience and originality of all participants enriches client and staff relationships and allows all concerned to experience personal growth and satisfaction.

What follows is a model of such a project with a step-by-step guide for implementation. Participants have repeatedly surprised themselves, colleagues and fellow clients with their artwork, and have been asked to sell their work at exhibitions or in book form! Yet the process is simple, with participants working in pairs to encourage and assist each other. It is possible to work with very confused clients as their partners are able to record the lucid moments as they arise and to keep gently returning the attention to the drawing. As the work is initially, and maybe ultimately, abstract, inexperience in art, mobility and manual dexterity are not problems. Workshop sessions of one to two hours are suggested.

The techniques used are drawn from both Japanese art and western graphic design approaches. In Japan there is a notion that 'less is more'. This principle is seen in the tradition of Sumie, black ink painting on a white ground with its eloquent use of space. Japanese Haiku poems allow their authors only 17 syllables in three lines and yet create profound images. In this project, participants are allowed to use only black ink, simple tools and few words, a restriction which encourages creativity and unexpected effects.

STEP ONE

To overcome initial hesitation, it is important that participants understand the need for mistakes, for imperfection. Perfect is lifeless. In Figure 17.1, the two circles by Seika Kawabe, an artist active in the Japanese avant garde calligraphy movement since the 1950s, illustrate this perfectly. One has little character and is expressionless, while the other is full of vitality and individuality.

STEP TWO

To encourage participants to let go and allow their own individuality to come through, it is also important to understand that creativity requires experimentation and play; it requires a stage of childlike exploration. Some participants may go on to draw from life or imagination using the techniques they have been exploring. Others will prefer to keep their marks abstract. Provide several sheets of cheap, smooth, white photocopying paper, black ink, a variety of brushes, pens, twigs, bits of string to dip and drag, etc. Encourage all participants to cover several sheets with experimental marks before, if wished, going on to draw natural objects (these do not require symmetry and once drawn are easily recognizable).

STEP THREE

The next stage of the process requires an adult, selective, critical approach. Cut L-shaped pieces of card and use these to 'frame' parts of the work. Move the frames around trying different formats, squares, rectangles or the pillar format so much used in Japan. Draw participants' attention to the space left by the marks made, to the weight, direction and balance.

STEP FOUR

Even a small mark, or accidental effect, will be impressive and thought-

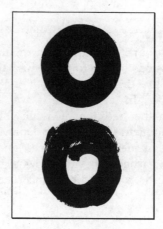

Figure 17.1 'Circles' by Seika Kawabe illustrates the individuality of imperfection.

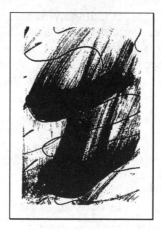

Figure 17.2 'Passing birds' by Margaret Ray: editing experimental marks for a striking image.

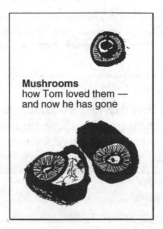

Figure 17.3 A common food and a few words evoking powerful emotions.

provoking when isolated and presented well. Titling work or using phrases and short poems such as Haiku allows a further level of expression and effective communication between partners and later between artist and audience. Figure 17.2 shows a design called 'Passing Birds' taken from the first experiments of a woman who had not drawn for years and who now found her abstract lines suggesting to her birds in flight, while she herself was confined to a wheelchair.

STEP FIVE

It is important to present the work 'professionally'. Use a good word-processor to typeset the words, a restrained, elegant style of typography with plenty of space around the enlarged or reduced images and good white paper to print and publish the final cards or books. Figure 17.3 is an example of this type of work produced by a lady in a residential home for older people.

STEP SIX

Invite everyone: colleagues, staff, family and friends to respond and to celebrate. Mount an exhibition. Throw a party. Present 'Other People's Pages'.

Art education 18

INTRODUCTION

A successful experiment carried out between 1970 and 1975 showed clearly that people of advanced years, even while living in long-term wards in elderly patient departments of hospitals, welcome the opportunity to learn something new. Awakened interest developed and concentration improved, particularly when a suitable room was set aside away from the wards, creating a space for quiet and study for the introduction of the subject.

Whenever people are segregated away because of calendar age, preconceived ideas can be created as to what 'they' want or do not want to do. Many interesting aspects were revealed from the comments of those on the receiving end of the project. The following are some brief details of the history of the research and of its interesting recent developments. Included are ideas for the benefit of staff wishing to extend the interest of their residents in all types of residential care institutions, particularly elderly patient departments of hospitals.

THE PROJECT

HISTORY

In January 1970, the King Edward's Hospital Fund for London gave a grant for the development of a project: 'Art for the Elderly in Hospitals'. This was later also supported by a grant from the Centre for Policy on Ageing (then the National Corporation for the Care of Old People) and the Hayward Foundation. The project lasted for five years and involved the long-term care departments of ten hospitals in the London area, based on the art classes introduced at New Cross Hospital, London in 1966, then part of Guy's Hospital. In order of development, the ten hospitals were:

New Cross, Cheam, Neasden, Hither Green, Lennard, St Charles, St Mary Abbots, New End, Princess Louise and Western. The purpose was to provide opportunities for the serious study of art on an equal footing with that already provided for able-bodied adults in the community. The research emphasized the importance of the following three development areas.

1. *Suitable accommodation* This involved persuading the elderly patient departments of the ten hospitals in the London area to provide a room away from the long-term wards suitable for use as a studio.
2. *From their point of view* Opinions of the older people and of the hospital staff were monitored and valued as each new class was introduced and formed the basis of the development of these ten different studios.
3. *Training courses* These were designed and organized specifically for specialist art tutors interested in extending their teaching to older people living in residential care. Courses now extend to care staff themselves interested in introducing creative interests to their residents.

The students selected for this educational provision were of course the most important people involved. Their average age was 80 years. The students were confined to wheelchairs and the majority could use only one hand. Most of them had been in hospital for at least five years. For these people, formal education finished at an early age, and few had any previous instruction in art.

We were dealing with an age group that we ourselves had not yet reached so it was not easy to imagine with any accuracy what life was really like looking out onto the world through the eyes of an older person living in these wards, trapped physically, yet with a sensible and alert mind. Therefore, their comments were vital throughout the project and formed the guidelines for its development.

Emphasis was placed on the classes being as much for art appreciation as for active participation, bearing in mind that the patients might not necessarily choose to study the subject of art if a wider choice were presented. Once it had been really emphasized that they did not have to paint or draw if they did not want to, opinions and interest came readily within the quiet atmosphere of the studios. Some showed a desire to look at art and other reference books or examine natural objects through a magnifying glass, which later could become the inspiration for practical work.

In 1975, a purpose-built studio was completed, especially for the long-stay older patients at New Cross Hospital where the original art classes began and where the long-stay department of Guy's Hospital was then housed. On completion, a metal plaque was fixed to the outside wall announcing 'ART STUDIO – This art studio provided especially for the use of elderly patients was built with the help of a grant from the King

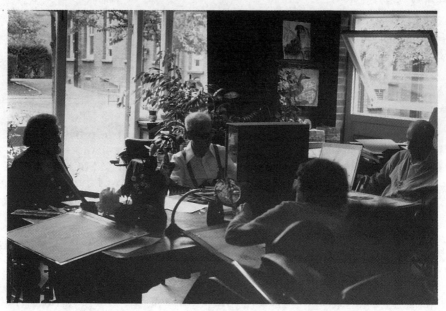

Figure 18.1   Purpose-built art studio leading on to a garden: New Cross Hospital.

Edward's Hospital Fund and opened in October 1975'. The new studio was also financed by Guy's Hospital. The kiln for pottery was financed by the League of Friends.

At one stage, there were four classes a week taking place in the studio at New Cross Hospital covering pottery, still life, plant drawing, print making, calligraphy, painting and drawing. In addition, a class was organized each week for the staff. The studio was built adjacent to the hospital day centre and had french doors leading on to the garden (Figure 18.1).

As well as painting and drawing materials, all the ten studios contained the nucleus of a small library with art and other books for reference, opportunities for examining natural objects, and facilities for film and slide projection. Of the original ten hospitals involved, three were closed as part of the Department of Health and Social Security's spending cuts in 1979. The remaining seven continue to have flourishing studios and to form the pattern for classes elsewhere in the UK.

Each of the new classes, after the first four months, settled down to a steady group of between 10 and 14 students, with a nucleus of approximately six students who developed a sustained interest. All the classes had some people who came regularly for at least two years. All the tutors reported considerable improvement in the skill and understanding of the subject by their older, often very physically disabled, regular students. An increase in their visual observation and ability to concentrate after the first six months was also noted. They were learning. Among the opinions most repeated by a variety of older students as the classes progressed was an appreciation of a room set aside from the wards, especially for the work in hand: 'somewhere quiet where we can concentrate'.

Here, in addition to the often existing bingo and sing-songs, was an activity with a serious element of learning. Nursing staff were often surprised to see their older patients studiously concentrating on a painting or completely absorbed as they looked at colour reproductions in a well-illustrated book on art.

Media and studies included drawing and paintings, fabric printing, calligraphy and in some studios, pottery. Three studios eventually bought their own kilns. Here, the older people had the opportunity to gain first-hand knowledge of pottery (Figure 18.2), and to observe and take part in the exciting process from biscuit firing to glazing of their own pots. In most cases these activities were experienced by the older people for the first time.

As classes progressed, sketching out of doors and visits to galleries were arranged, as well as slide shows within the individual studios. These were all very much appreciated, and as one 82-year-old woman, living in the elderly patient department of a hospital, said: 'I had always wanted to visit a gallery, but my husband was never interested in such things and I

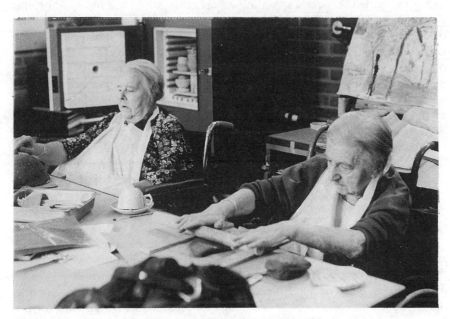

Figure 18.2 An opportunity to gain first-hand knowledge of pottery.

had a big family to bring up. I never thought I would ever have this opportunity'.

Exhibitions of the older students' work took place in all the hospitals concerned. These were generally held in the studios and linked with the annual hospital fêtes. Good mounting and presentation will enhance any art work, and paintings by older students are no exception. Framing and mounting of their pictures for the hospital exhibitions gave added dignity and quality to the exhibits, which delighted the artists and was appreciated by staff and relatives of all generations.

Two major exhibitions representing the work produced in the ten hospital studios took place. One exhibition, in December 1975, was held at County Hall, Westminster, with the support of the then Inner London Education Authority, and the second was held at the Royal Festival Hall, London, with the support of Counsel and Care for the Elderly, in March 1979. The aim of both these exhibitions was to promote the idea of the project, and was an opportunity to show selected works of a high standard produced by older students, not just for the interest in the unique background of the artists who had produced them, but as paintings in their own right, giving pleasure to all generations. Some of the exhibiting artists visited these major exhibitions to see their work in a professional setting.

The tutors were qualified art specialists, trained on a course especially designed for tutors interested in extending their teaching to older people living in residential care. Presenting an art class in the setting of a hospital or residential home is very different from the atmosphere of school or college, to which most of the tutors were accustomed. It was important therefore that they had a prior understanding of the role of hospital and other residential care staff, in order to slot in to this particular environment successfully. An insight into the lives of their prospective students when they were not attending the class, as well as knowledge of particular methods, art materials and approaches, is all of great value to a tutor before embarking on this type of teaching.

The first of these training courses took place in 1972 at the University of London Goldsmith's College and was called 'Teaching Art to 80-Year-Olds'. The course continued in London annually under the title 'Art for the Elderly in Residential Care'. Two further courses for tutors from all parts of the country also took place, one of which was directed by the Department of Education and Science.

The trained tutors were employed by their local education authority and attached to the appropriate adult education centre or institute while taking the classes in the hospital studios.

As well as being trained on the course mentioned, the majority of the tutors often had considerable experience in creating an enthusiasm for art in adults and schoolchildren of all ages and interests. These tutors successfully created a similar enthusiasm in their students within the hospital studios. All the older people selected for the project eventually developed a real interest in the subject, either through art appreciation or through practical experience in one medium or another.

ESTABLISHING AN ART CLASS

The importance in hospitals, in particular, of early meetings between all interested members of staff cannot be over-emphasized when introducing new classes in residential care institutions. This is necessary to gain interest and to make sure everyone is adequately informed beforehand. At these preliminary meetings, the staff must first decide whether there is a nucleus of older people who have already expressed a positive inclination towards new ideas and who may benefit from joining the classes.

Suitable accommodation for the classes is of prime importance. All institutions are short of space, and it is, therefore, essential to discuss these matters right from the beginning. The variety of type of space and accommodation provided by hospitals and residential homes for this type of interest seems to be unlimited in its originality as each new class is established. It is amazing what accommodation can be discovered when it is inspired by the interest and enthusiasm of the staff to get the class going successfully.

Although every situation is different, the following are basic essentials.

1. An internal telephone should be in the room, or very nearby. Tutors are seldom trained in first-aid or other nursing skills, and it is essential that they can reach trained nursing staff in an emergency.
2. Toilet facilities should be within easy reach of the studio.
3. The room should have adequate heating, be reasonably soundproof, and with good light – daylight where possible.
4. A water supply and sink, ideally in the room or close by, is essential. If pottery is envisaged, plenty of shelf space, and a sink especially for this purpose with a built-in sediment tank beneath it within the working area, would be needed.
5. A wall area for the display of students' work and teaching aids.
6. Some sturdy tables high enough for wheelchairs to be pushed under.
7. One or more cupboards for storage, large enough to contain A1 paper (594 mm × 841 mm) as well as other art materials.
8. The room should be large enough to accommodate six to eight people in wheelchairs at a table or tables for painting, clay modelling or pottery, and, in addition, to enable two or three students to sit quietly examining natural objects, reference or art books, or observing the others working.
9. If possible, the room should have access to a garden.

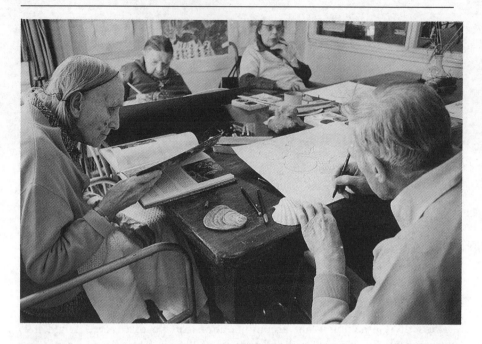

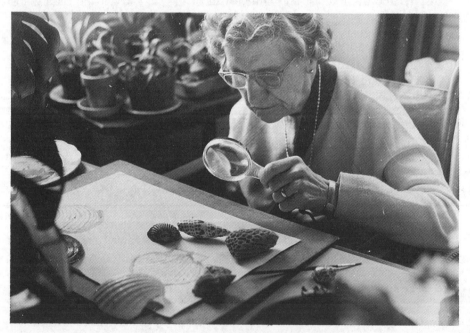

Figure 18.3   'We like somewhere quiet where we can concentrate'

These facilities can be extended as money and other considerations permit.

Every effort should be made for the area or room allocated to be exclusively for the use of the art classes so that it truly becomes 'the studio' in which art paraphernalia can be left, and in which an atmosphere of quiet study can be created (Figure 18.3).

Having provisionally chosen an appropriate room for the classes, a formal meeting can take place. This should include all hospital or residential care heads of departments concerned with the older people who may be involved, as well as representatives from the local education authority if a tutor is to be invited. The meeting would:

1. check again that the proposed room is not planned for other uses, as it is important that both students and tutor feel secure in establishing the classes and building up an atmosphere for learning in a stable situation;
2. make sure that the room really is geographically in a suitable position, for example, unhampered by difficult stairways;
3. choose a suitable day and time for the class;
4. discuss the availability of porters if the class is being introduced in a hospital;
5. ensure that all are adequately informed of the educational nature of the classes, including the art appreciation element, and of the type of older person most likely to benefit from attending the classes;
6. discuss financial matters, for example, cost of materials and payment of students' fees.

On the success of these first meetings rests the establishment of successful smooth-running classes for the next few years. Their importance cannot be too highly emphasized.

MATERIALS

From the allocation of money agreed upon during the first meetings, materials can be ordered for the new classes. The following were used successfully and are suggested as basic requirements. Tempera block paints, 2¼ inches (57 mm) in diameter, arranged in plastic containers, each holding six blocks, were found to be ideal and were provided in the classes in this project (see details of suppliers at the end of the chapter). These six-block containers are heavy and make a steady base for those students with the use of only one arm. The colours can be mixed boldly, adding white for an opaque effect and water for transparencies. The six colours suggested are: red, orange, blue, yellow, black and white – using Ostwald colours or equivalent, where possible, as these are especially designed to be equally balanced in tone for creating new colours. This palette of predominantly primary colours gives wide scope for accurate colour mixing. Opportunities to discover that blue and yellow make green, that red, yellow and blue makes brown, and that red and blue becomes violet are very much enjoyed by those being introduced to the delights of colour mixing for the first time.

Brushes should be of good quality and include both bristle and sable. Suggested sizes are: bristle, sizes 3, 4 and 6; sable, sizes 2, 4 and 6. A selection of both white cartridge and grey sugar paper should be sufficient in the early stages. Water pots should be heavy to avoid spilling by unsteady hands. White china plates are heavier, therefore steadier, than plastic, and are a good substitute for expensive artists' palettes. Charcoal, a variety of felt-tipped pens and other sundry items would be purchased at the discretion of the tutor. If pottery is to be introduced, be sure to use only non-toxic glazes. An extractor fan should be fitted in the room in which the kiln is housed.

It is better to purchase a few good-quality materials than a large amount of substandard equipment. Do not be tempted to accept poor-quality materials for your class because it is 'only for beginners'. Students learning new skills need every encouragement. Good-quality paper is especially important, since it is not likely to disintegrate with water and pressure of the brush.

If money permits, it is well worth while purchasing some art and natural history books containing first-class prints, with the hope that these will form the nucleus of a small library. One or two large magnifying glasses should also be available. Arrangements for the local library to supply books on art and related subjects at regular intervals add variety to the small permanent studio collection. This could be followed by volunteers and others sharing the interest of the books with the prospective students during their general visits and conversations before art classes commence.

Plants can enhance the appearance of the new room. Choose varieties that will not be affected by central heating and can successfully survive the tutor's holiday periods. Tradescantia, small plants and cacti have proved sturdy in this respect, and can form the basis of a larger collection. The art tutor would of course be very much involved in setting the scene of the studio and making the room inviting for that very important first visit of the students. The aim should always be for the room to become a focus – attractive to both staff and patients alike.

In the meantime, staff may wish to talk to the older people about the classes, and must be sure to explain to prospective students that they do not have to paint if they do not want to, emphasizing that the classes are as much for art appreciation as for participation, and explaining that they have a choice and may come to visit the new studio 'only to look' if they wish. Many an item has been bought on the initial understanding that you do not have to buy.

It is important also for the tutor to give as much time as possible before the classes begin to visiting the wards from which students are to be selected. These visits will give the tutor a valuable insight into the environment in which the prospective students are living when they are not attending the art class. Getting to know the staff and hearing their opinion of the patients is also very valuable to the tutor. Chatting informally with the older people themselves in the ward gives both tutor and prospective students a chance to understand each other's point of view before the idea of the art class is delicately explained. The final selection of older people to join the first class should always be the result of a joint agreement between staff, patients and the tutor. The introduction of the classes to the older people should never be hurried, so that they feel always that it is in their time and as they choose. They should always feel free to just visit or participate on a regular basis if they wish.

After the classes have taken place for a few weeks, and are becoming established, further follow-up meetings should be arranged. These should be, as before, with the appropriate heads of departments from the hospital or residential home and representatives of the local education authority. They should be held at regular intervals of approximately three months. The aim of the meetings should be to monitor the progress of the classes to overcome initial problems, or perhaps to organize the first visit to a local gallery (Figure 18.4), sketching out of doors or to plan a future exhibition of work.

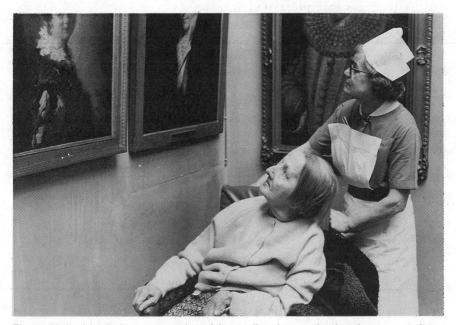

Figure 18.4 'I had always wanted to visit a gallery but my husband was never interested in such things'.

NEW DEVELOPMENTS

Since the project was completed, many hospitals, nursing and residential homes throughout the UK have introduced educational opportunities and creative interests for the benefit of their physically disabled older patients and residents. The basic essentials still apply, that is:

1. the importance of a room suitable for use as a studio;
2. continued enquiry as to the needs of the students, with development guided by their wishes;
3. courses and/or meetings for tutors, volunteers, and care staff to prepare before introducing the classes.

Some consultants may well say that the need is now different and that the older people in elderly patient departments of hospitals today would not benefit from a learning situation as they did in 1968 when initial classes at New Cross Hospital commenced. Yet new classes continue to begin in hospitals and residential homes, where rooms are provided for use as studios, with older people benefiting and appreciating opportunities to study art seriously. An art tutor who has had considerable experience in teaching older people in hospitals and other residential institutions said: 'Through the practice of art they evolve a sense of worth and confidence, and discover that their point of view matters'.

In the elderly patient department of Greenwich District Hospital, London, the older students have begun a new interest as they work in their studio with stained glass. One lady in her 70s, who had been in hospital for at least five years, produced to her own design a crucifix in coloured glass which now hangs in the hospital chapel in a position above the door which she chose herself. Working with glass could be dangerous, particularly for a disabled person, yet this was made possible with the guidance of a trained tutor and suitable working facilities. In this hospital in 1992, an exhibition was held of the older students' work. This exhibition celebrated 21 years of established art classes for the older day hospital patients and older people in short and long-term care. Classes are continuing at this hospital.

NEW TRAINING COURSES

Trained tutors are teaching in all parts of the country, not only to those of advanced years living in hospitals, but in a similar manner in all types of residential care accommodation, including sheltered housing, day centres and clubs. Courses have been extended to advanced levels for the previously trained tutors, and for course organizers, to encourage continuity. For care staff, the general national vocational qualification in health and social care now includes sections on artistic and creative activities in the intermediate and advanced courses.

WHERE A TUTOR IS NOT AVAILABLE

In some areas of the country, it has not always been possible to obtain a tutor. For this reason, various courses in creative interests and educational opportunities as well as the general national vocational qualification have been popular among managers and care staff, and certainly enable them to fulfil a need among the older people concerned. Enthusiasm for a subject by an amateur as well as a professional can interest others around. As a result, rooms have been successfully set aside and educational ideas have been introduced. Subjects have varied from art to wine-making, the history of kings and queens, computer uses and nature studies. As subjects have progressed, more knowledge and study is needed by staff and residents alike. Members of local clubs are being invited to visit and exchange ideas with residents and occasional return vists are arranged. There are now opportunities for serious progressive learning.

Although much success can be achieved by care staff, volunteers and other members of the community, the aim should always be to invite an adult education specialist tutor in the subject to the group whenever possible – maybe for a limited number of sessions – in order to widen the perspective of the chosen interest for everyone. In the UK, tutors are employed by their local education authority. The students concerned, through their appropriate hospital or residential home, pay the old-age pensioners' students' fees in the same way as they would if they could go to an adult education institute. In some areas of the country, these fees are financially assisted further by their local borough.

INTEGRATION NOT SEGREGATION

In one residential home for older people, a resident said: 'It is very nice here and we have beautiful grounds, but we are cut off from the mainstream of life'. In the elderly patient departments of hospitals also, people, because of their age, are segregated from other generations. Where the pursuit of the knowledge of art has led to classes going on visits or other generations being invited in, the stimulated comments from the older students involved show clearly the need for a wider involvement with the outside world. Efforts to enhance mobility and transport for such visits are truly rewarded. Sketching out of doors, including the hospital grounds, brings contact with other generations. Passing members of staff and visitors are enlightened to see what the older long-term patients are doing as well as heightening the overall awareness of the students as they concentrate on their work.

In the Royal Hospital, Chelsea, London, where classes have continued since 1986, the extension of art appreciation has led to a contact with the Courtauld Institute of Art. Now a visit to a gallery is arranged each term. In addition, the students exhibit their own work in an exhibition held annually for the general public. After observing her patients attending the art class and enlightened by their development, an assistant senior nursing officer said: 'There is nothing to compare with seeing a patient blossom into discussion and laughter from a new interest'.

At a residential home for older people, where transport to the adult education art classes was arranged, residents said: 'We like to see the young people and to listen to their conversations, especially at tea break in the canteen when they come down from the other classes in other subjects'.

At Greenwich District Hospital, patients visiting the elderly day hospital attend art classes provided, but when treatment finishes so do the art classes. The art tutors and volunteers have successfully arranged for the older people concerned to travel from the isolation of their own homes to their local adult education art class where they now continue their studies alongside other age groups.

GENERATIONS TOGETHER

In 1968, I conducted an additional project, bringing together children aged between three and five years from a children's home and the long-stay older patients already attending the art class at New Cross Hospital. Here were two groups of people, young children living in a children's home and older people living in long-term care in hospital, who had become deprived of family life through living in institutions.

This project, lasting nine months, was preceded by a visit to the art class by a group of children, in this case with hearing disabilities. They had come to see the paintings produced, especially by the older people, for the hearing aid department of the hospital. It was not practical for the children who had come from the school for the deaf to visit the class regularly. However, the success of the meeting between the generations inspired the further development for research.

For the longer-term project, a children's home in Lewisham, London, was approached. The matron was very interested and co-operative and willing for with a group of her children to take part in a pilot scheme. It was arranged for a group of children aged between 3½ and 5 years, with members of their care staff, to visit the art class at New Cross Hospital one morning a week on a regular basis.

Many notes were produced for this study. The older people concerned were told of the proposal in advance, and their personal opinions sought. It was also explained to the children about the visit beforehand. This paved the way for the first meeting to the studio. Three children were selected for the first visit. On arrival, everyone was introduced by name. The children either spontaneously ran towards a particular older person, or sometimes, more shyly, approached on invitation. Within ten minutes, a close relationship between the generations was established.

After two meetings an adjustment was made. There appeared to be a slight sadness by the older students who, although taking pleasure in seeing the children, did not have a child to be 'responsible' for themselves. It was agreed to increase the number to five or six children on each visit. This proved to be more successful. The paintings produced at this time were sometimes joint efforts, or sometimes individual paintings by the children, with guided instruction from the older person. Although the elderly students beforehand had created a concentration and confidence in their own paintings when alone with their tutor in the studio, it was observed that they had now become more alert while assuming a kind yet definite authoritative manner with the children, of which the children at once took notice.

After approximately six to eight weeks, a second adjustment was made. The older students now expressed the need to have a separate time to concentrate on their own paintings with the tutor as before, emphasizing that 'not for one moment should the children be turned away'. The temporary art studio was conveniently divided by a glass partition so that it was easily arranged for children to paint in one section, and the older students in the other, with both being able to observe through the glass. This proved to be a much happier situation. The children began working separately and then gradually wandered naturally into the room with the older people to show their work for approval and guidance. Towards the end of the morning, the children mingled freely between both rooms. The atmosphere became rather like a normal home with the children running in and out freely.

A third adjustment was made after a few weeks, when the older students asked whether they could, in addition, have a time separate from doing their own paintings to give guidance exclusively to the children. The class was then divided so that approximately half the session during the two-hour meetings was devoted to this purpose. During this period, the children joined the older people with enthusiasm, going almost always to their particular older partner in painting. This time the correct balance of the art class between the generations was achieved.

During these special sessions, a spontaneous learning situation between the two generations quickly emerged. The most popular instruction was guidance in the forming of the letters of the alphabet and numerals. The older people became tutors of their very interested pupils and were thrilled to find the children learning under their tuition. An atmosphere of calm concentration was observed, with interruptions of praise and

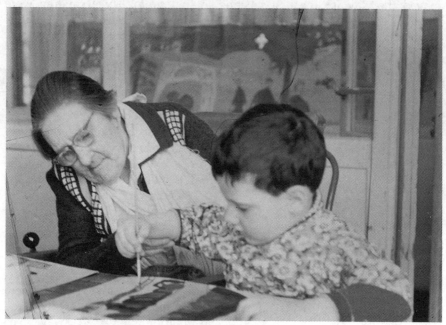

Figure 18.5 'An atmosphere of calm concentration was observed'.

laughter. This final arrangement of working partly in separate rooms and partly together established a successful pattern for the rest of the project.

The elderly people:

- became more alert;
- took on a responsible role with the children;
- developed close relationships with the children;
- showed a personal concern for the children's welfare: 'do they need their hands washed?', 'where is he going?', 'she needs a hanky';
- spoke with a kind yet authoritative voice, took a lot of interest and were delighted when the children progressed under their tuition;
- gave their opinions regularly and with confidence as the weeks progressed;
- showed a balanced attitude towards the children, not sentimental.

As regards the children, the children's care staff said 'we do not have the time to give this sort of personal attention to the children'. They noticed that, by their quiet assurance, the older people gave confidence to the children, and said that the children were definitely quieter with the older people than they were in the children's home. The matron of their home said: 'they are always happier on returning from the art class'.

The above project raises the questions:

- do the children receive something nearer to a grandparent/grandchild relationship?

and

- the older people a purposeful involvement bringing them nearer their rightful place with other generations in society?

In 1968, children living in children's homes stayed in one home until they were 5 years old and were then transferred to another home with older children. Most of the children involved in this project were already five years old or had become five years old as the project progressed, and so were due to be moved. For this reason, the research finished after nine months. As the weeks passed and the normal art class resumed, the older art students commented about the children and often wondered how they were getting on.

Since these early days, a number of studies between generations have been made both in Europe and particularly the University of Pittsburgh, USA. An intergenerational study in the UK to transfer an educational class for able-bodied young adults to the grounds of a residential home is in preparation, giving older physically disabled people in residential care equal educational opportunities in art within their immediate environment, and enabling examination of the benefits of this unique integrated learning situation between the two generations.

CONCLUSION

The provision of educational opportunities in art for older people living in all types of residential care, and in day centres and clubs, has proved successful in the project described. Here, suitable accommodation and trained tutors were provided on a scale equal to facilities offered to adults of all ages attending mainstream classes in local education institutions. Education authorities should heed the early pioneers of adult education and continue to make tutors available to this segregated area of the adult community. Further, planners of the future should not only include a space for quiet study in all buildings where older people are expected to live in residential care or where they spend time in day centres, but also extend their designs to be equally suitable for possible intergenerational adult education classes taking place within the residential care setting.

Each successive generation of older people will have different needs. We must make sure, therefore, that the opinions of older people in the future continue to be considered by successive younger generations with regard to educational opportunities, or for that matter, anything else.

APPENDIX

SUPPLIERS OF ART MATERIALS

Calder Colours (Ashby Ltd) Nottingham Road, Ashby-de-la-Zouch, Leicestershire LE65 1DR, UK (tel: 01530 412885; fax: 01530 417315) stock Tempera block disc paints in Ostwald colours or equivalent in plastic containers, as well as other art materials. They will supply materials locally in the UK and to all parts of the world through local art dealers.

The following firms stock brushes, paper, poster paints in Ostwald colours (not Tempera blocks) as well as a variety of other general art materials:

Daler Rowney Ltd, 10 Percy Street, London W1
(tel: 0171 636 8241): mail order system for UK residents.

Daler Rowney Ltd, PO Box 10, Southern Industrial Estate, Bracknell, Berkshire RG12 8ST (tel: 01344 424621; fax: 01344 486530) will export directly or through local distributors.

Daler Rowney Ltd, 2 Corporate Drive, Cranbury, NJ 08512-9584, USA (tel: 609 655 5252; fax: 609 655 5852).

Plus One Co Ltd, 5-5-20 Minami Tsuknguchicho, Amagasaki City, 661, Japan (tel: 816 426 1337; fax: 816 426 1558).

The Artland Co Ltd, 301-307 Lockhart Road, 3/F Lockhard Centre, Wanchai, Hong Kong (tel: 852 2511 4845; fax: 852 2519 6817).

The Art Friend, BLK 231, Bras Basah Complex, Bain Street, Singapore 0718 (tel: 65 336 3271; fax: 65 3370 743).

Pottery Crafts Ltd, 8–10 Ingate Place, Battersea, London SW8 3NS, UK (tel: 0171 720 0050; fax: 0171 627 8290) stock kilns suitable for use in hospital studios, i.e. FL.50 15 × 12 × 18 inches, Firecraft front-loading, internal volume 1.87 cubic feet. They will supply and despatch the above kilns and other pottery materials, including non-toxic glazes, to all parts of the world.

Dramatherapy 19

WHAT IS DRAMATHERAPY?

Professional dramatherapists are relatively new, having developed in the UK as a body since the early 1960s. They evolved along with the new wave therapies. Peter Slade established the use of dramatic play as essential to child development, and has paved the way for drama in education. Brian Way extended its use into personal development, and Sue Jennings and her colleagues pioneered remedial drama and its progression into the field of therapy. 'Sesame', a branch of the Religious Drama Group, took volunteer actors into institutions to perform and to involve patients in their performance. From these varied sources, a new profession has emerged.

The therapeutic use of drama is, however, as ancient as man. Its roots lie in the rituals, dances and actions of our ancestors which were used to promote the welfare of their communities. Each community had a counsellor, confidant and leader of rituals called the shaman, who in time became particularly associated with the rituals of healing. The fact that he was consulted about both personal and community problems illustrates that the links between social organization and health were recognized long before they were rediscovered in more recent times.

Considering drama, *per se*, will help one to understand dramatherapy and its application. The word 'drama' is derived from the Greek *dran* – a thing done. So it is about action. However, nothing dramatic can be achieved without the vital addition of creativity. Drama is also about imagination, feeling, symbol and metaphor, the latter representing the 'as if' quality of drama. Landy (1986) writes of the interactive meaning of drama for individuals: 'For drama to occur it is necessary for the actor, one who acts in everyday life, to distinguish between either one aspect of the self and another or between self and non-self'.

Drama can be seen as a continuum, the components of which are:

ritual–play–movement–mime–dance–games–role play–theatre. The drama-therapist can use components at all levels of the patient's ability, and the activities suggested below are adaptable to all levels of individual need.

RITUAL

Ritual has already been referred to. There is a tendency to relate it only to primitive societies and magic. However, there are many rituals in the present which we cannot disregard, both personal – those that people create for themselves – and cultural.

Children often have a bedtime ritual of bath, story and to bed with a good-night kiss. Without their ritual, they feel unhappy and fear disaster. Adults have similar rituals of going to bed and getting up in the morning, completing chores, etc. They are often referred to as routines, but can become imbued with a sense of security.

Cultural rituals are accepted as the norm – particularly the religious ones surrounding birth, death and marriage. They may not be highly valued as such in our society, but they have their uses. The rituals around death, for example, allow for expression of sympathy to the mourners, help them to come to terms with bereavement and facilitate the grieving process.

PLAY

Drama is an extension of play. It is accepted that children learn through play, but all can learn from the play element in drama. The 'make-believe' involvement of acting 'as if' it were real allows for a detached objectivity which promotes a sense of security. The action is not real, but once-removed, and therefore safe for experiment.

Play is a part of drama only if it is used to some purpose and deliberately undertaken for dramatic action to take place.

MOVEMENT/DANCE

These elements are all basic to life. Infants move instinctively. Finding a joy in the movement itself, they experiment with more movement. The more active they are the more they discover, thus strengthening muscles, learning co-ordination and balance, and gaining confidence in their bodies. Repeated movement develops rhythm and continuity, and enters the realm of dance.

Adults tend to lose this facility to enjoy movement for its own sake and spontaneous dance. Schooling teaches that there is a 'right way' to do things, and an appropriate time and place. Yet movement as part of dramatherapy can still be a medium for learning or re-learning – for example, balancing skills or co-ordination after a stroke.

Movement is important at all ages, but particularly to older people. If limbs are not exercised regularly, they become stiff and painful and finally cease to be of use at all. Exercises, unless enjoyable, can be a bore. Motivation will then fade and action suffer. Exercise that is built into an enjoyable dramatic context is more liable to be undertaken.

MIME

Mime is a word that can be misleading. Mime artists are highly trained and skilled people with muscular control and expertise beyond the capabilities of the untrained. Perhaps a more useful terms is 'non-verbal communication'. Most professionals are aware of the need to understand and co-ordinate body language and speech as an important component of social skills training.

GAMES

Organized games can be simply a recreation, but, if used with a specific purpose in mind, can form part of a therapeutic programme. Games are basic drama that can be used either creatively on their own, or as a 'warm-up' to other dramatic activities.

ROLE PLAY

Each individual has many roles in society (Moreno, 1946). As people grow older, roles change and often diminish. Practice is often needed to expand present roles, and rehearse new ones. There may be grief and bereavement over lost or diminished roles. Moreno writes: 'Working with the "role" as a point of reference appears to be a methodical advantage as compared with "personality" or "ego"'.

The word 'role' is taken from the name given to the written part an actor played in Greek theatre. It was written on a 'roll'. Modern actors research the role of the characters they are playing, i.e. the feelings and attitudes the characters will have in the situation in which they are depicted.

Real life roles are about a place in society, be it family, professional or social. There is an expectation of accepted behaviour in this role. Role play as therapy often concentrates on behaviour. Dramatherapy pays heed to the theatrical source of role, emphasizing feelings and attitudes as of equal, and sometimes greater, importance than behaviour.

THEATRE

Theatre is the presentation of a story, mime or sequence of events by one person, or a group, to another person or group. It is a good medium for allowing people to become more aware and understanding of experiences so far unknown to them. The audience identifies with characters on stage, and they 'live' the events portrayed 'as if' audience and players were one. As well as being a means of escaping from the reality of every day, this is also an opportunity to view experiences 'once-removed'. This exchange of experiences between audience and actor – be they painful, pleasant, amusing or desired – allows for acceptable access to feelings that are normally hidden. The therapist then has an opportunity to discuss personal issues and feelings with patients either individually or in a group.

Theatre is the communication of experience, and the higher the standard of the actor's performance, the clearer the communication. In all other aspects of drama, the therapy is in the doing, and not in the standard of performance. Involvement in performance is the only time when the patient is concerned with the standard at which he works.

For a patient, the experience of being part of an audience allows:

- involvement in make-believe by 'the willing suspension of disbelief' (Esslin, 1976);
- an opportunity to view life experiences through metaphor;
- a sense of being part of a corporate body with the other members of the audience;
- interaction with other members of the audience;
- an opportunity to escape from reality.

The experience of being a performer can be equally rewarding by:

- encouraging creativity and imagination;
- creating a new social role;
- creating self-confidence and enhancing self-esteem;
- accepting the discipline of theatre by setting boundaries;
- relating to other members of the group in a different way, and learning to work as a team.

THE USE OF DRAMA

Dramatherapists can call on any or all of these components of the continuum to meet the needs of the individual or group with whom they are working. Depending on the needs and abilities of the group, the dramatherapist may either take them through activities in a planned programme of experiences selected from the continuum, or use issues as they arise and select action spontaneously. Either method constitutes a dramatic process in which the flexibility of movement within the continuum is a response to the needs of the participants.

Patients are admitted to hospital because they are sick, and because the ensuing disabilities cannot be accommodated at home. This may be a continuing state or a temporary one. Dramatherapy is rooted in action and creativity, so the dramatherapist, whilst acknowledging disability, works with the preserved ability of the patient towards the goal of rehabilitation (discussed later in this chapter) or healing.

WHY DRAMATHERAPY?

Now that the nature of dramatherapy has been described, it is necessary to consider why it is needed and what it may contribute to the life of someone confined to residence in hospital.

A hospital ward offering extended care is a community of 20 or more residents and, overall, may be as many staff. Those involved, be they residents or staff, will possess very different abilities and will come from very different backgrounds, yet all, in their own way, personal or professional, are trying to come to terms with the challenge of living or working, over long periods of time, with illness or disability.

All patients within themselves, and by the use of the remaining attributes, physical or mental, have to adjust to their disabilities and meet and express their personal needs. Additionally, they have to make social adjustments. These will have commenced at the time when hospital life was foreseen but not implemented, and will continue through transfer to extended care and the subsequent learning about and coping with new patients and staff. Illness notoriously turns us in upon ourselves (consider trying to be sociable with a raging toothache) and enforced social adjustments at this time will be particularly taxing and potentially overwhelming.

The social adjustments are in two directions. Towards fellow patients there may, out of anxiety, be either identification ('I shall get like that') and/or a distancing ('I'm not like these other people'). Anxiety may also be felt towards caring staff, in or out of uniform, who will carry authority to impose strange and uncomfortable clinical procedures. Furthermore, professionals, even if only in the quest for objectivity, will distance themselves in terms of human relations. The closeness of patients to ward orderlies and cleaners, more so than to doctors and nurses, is well known. In a ward, most relationships are short-lived; staff do their jobs and go home. Social mobility, at least for staff, and maybe for patients, is high, with all that that means for lack of social cohesion.

Staff are part of the ward community and also have their own groupings. They have professional standards and import personal values from their home life. They will have to cope with the projected image that patients have about them and get on with each other in a multidisciplinary team. Their needs also bear attention.

It is common experience that the diversity of illness and personality seen on any one ward is enormous, even when attempts at stratification have been made into, say, psychiatric or elderly communities, or into medium and extended care. A stroke may, to a greater or lesser extent, impair physical autonomy; depression may impair drive; or confusion (in either the short or long term) may impair mental autonomy. There are many more variations when the subtleties are considered. Disability may not be total, or multiple disabilities may be present in different combinations, so one patient may be physically active and optimistic (but totally confused) while another is physically dependent but mentally sharp, with a third being depressed in a way that augments physical disability. A naturally anxious person shows more distress than someone who is more phlegmatic. Some will conduct an aggressive search for aid while others will be unnaturally subservient.

Then there may be premorbid personal problems without direct connection with the illness, but still of great relevance to the individual: personal issues such as variations in mental and physical aptitude may influence the presentation of illness, or social issues such as poverty, lack of or problematic family supporters, burdensome family responsibilities, no home, or the necessities and chores of giving up a home.

Finally, in any long-term hospital ward, there is an element of terminal care. Facing death oneself as a patient or in others as a relative or staff member includes coming to terms with both the anxiety of anticipation and the management, afterwards, of bereavement and mourning.

This attempt to understand the minds of disabled patients and the nature of the community in which they live in a broader context illustrates the complexity of the task of those responsible for treatment and life in an extended care hospital ward. A patient will want to feel understood as a person, and the provision of extended care does not stop once strictly professional/technical needs are met. There is a 'well' side to the patient's existence based on a rich individual experience of life, as well as a 'sick' or dependent side. The broader view does not invalidate the need for professionals to diagnose, classify and care for the types of physical and mental disabilities seen, but to stop there is premature. An individual treatment plan in extended care requires that all facets of life are considered.

Some regard permanent hospitalization (or residential care) as the interval between social and physical death. Need it be so? Clinical staff are well trained in making traditional diagnoses or assessments but are not so well trained in looking beyond strictly biomedical/nursing needs (this is discussed later under 'The role of staff in providing quality of life').

Table 19.1 Maslow's motivational goals (after Maslow, 1943)

1. Physiological	Homeostasis for e.g. food, fluids, heat
2. Safety	Particularly in the face of unfamiliarity
3. Love	Affectionate relationships
4. Esteem	For self and from others
5. Self-actualization	Creative self-expression

What is there over the strictly biotechnical horizon? There are many models by which human nature and needs can be classified, but some that seem of particular value in making the task of extended care more meaningful and easier to understand are described below.

MASLOW'S HIERARCHY OF HUMAN NEEDS

Maslow (1943) looked at human motivation by arranging goals in rank order: from those that are primitive and the most demanding, particularly if unsatisfied, to those that are complex and creative but which are also vulnerable in the face of challenge (Table 19.1). There are various cultural paths to each goal.

Maslow described the most primitive and demanding needs as those for physiological stability, e.g. food, warmth and fluids. At this level needs must be met, even in the face of hazard to higher-order needs. This is survival. Next in turn comes safety: protection from threat and physical danger. Safety, once assured, is followed by the social need to belong: to be able to give and receive friendship and love. Then, in turn, there is a need for esteem, autonomy, self-respect, achievement, and the appreciation and respect of others. Finally there is self-fulfilment of a creative kind: self-actualization.

As the most primitive of these needs are the most demanding, it is only when they are met that the individual feels free to indulge needs of a higher order; once biology and safety are assured, then interest can turn to social and creative needs. However, these needs, being tender plants, require nurturing.

The environment of a conventional hospital ward, in Maslow's terms, provides food, warmth, and reasonable safety (but accidents and cross-infections too). A sense of belonging may be actively discouraged if resettlement is the aim: autonomy is often eroded (but need it be excessively so?), respect may come more from professional rather than from individual concern, and the opportunities to create and contribute are minimal. Wards like this don't do very well beyond Maslow's second level. However, there are models of rehabilitation which, if implemented, may help towards a better way of life.

SOCIAL REHABILITATION

The dangers of institutional care are now too well known to require more than brief mention. It is only too easy for the patient to fall into the 'sick role' and accept, enjoy and even exaggerate the dependency that this brings.

Rehabilitation attempts to offset these tendencies by maximizing role performance in individual patients, by making them the principal determinants of, and actors in, their own lives. Physical rehabilitation maximizes accomplishments in a physical world; psychosocial rehabilitation develops role performance in a social world.

The gains from rehabilitation may be large or modest but are appropriate even when small. In any case, the valuation of 'gains' is relative; not everyone aspires to the heights, and in difficult circumstances there can be job satisfaction for the carer even when gains are small. It is important for all staff, whether professionally trained or not, to understand the value of apparently simple daily activities in rehabilitation. Sharing a photograph, or a story from the past, or the physical contact of an arm round a shoulder or a hand held can be important professional as well as human activities and should be appreciated as such. Resettlement, i.e. the placement of a patient outside hospital, may be one aim of rehabilitation, and perhaps in hospital care the ultimate one but it is not the sole aim.

Social rehabilitation is achieved by defining, in collaboration with the patient, appropriate roles as personal targets for growth and change, small or large. Understanding and motivation will need to be conveyed by explanation; patients need to know what is expected of them. Appropriate skills will need to be learned, strengthened, or re-learned, so that the roles may be undertaken. For example, assessment and discussion with a patient may reveal that he wants to make friends with other patients but lacks the necessary social skills. The defining of the task may have motivated him to learn how, say, to find an opening to a conversation, something that has never been easy for him, and is now more difficult because of dysarthria following a stroke. He is then helped to learn the necessary skills and is given sufficient practice to make them acceptably easy and free from anxiety.

Rehabilitation theory (Bennet, 1977) tells us that roles are always multiple and changing, e.g. with age and work status. What roles are available in an extended care ward? Which can we create? The very fact of admission to such a ward suggests that the condition is more than transitional and that some degree of pre-admission role failure (or of role imbalance, because of failure by others to attenuate role demands) has occurred. Confidence in any or every role performance may have been eroded, so keeping roles 'open' is vital to self-esteem. The role of 'patient' may, to some degree, have to be accepted, but not to an excessive or disabling degree, and the patient may need help to strike a balance.

The role of 'decider' should be open to all, although the complexity of the decision may need to be matched to the clinical disability. Some may be very able at financial affairs; others, because of memory or cognitive loss, may be capable of little more than deciding what to eat or wear at that moment in time.

THE ROLE OF STAFF IN PROVIDING QUALITY OF LIFE

What can be achieved in practice? Staff are hard-pressed and oriented towards the professional rather than the expressive side of patient care. Nevertheless, however, even if not competent in some of the broader roles of total patient 'care', they can help to provide an acceptable milieu by involving others, such as dramatherapists, who do have the necessary skills. Patients may reach the outside world by outings, but something of its quality can also be imported into the ward. So a patient may expect more of a doctor than a prescription, more of a nurse than a facility with bathing, and more of a dramatherapist than physical exercise, etc., etc.

Staff time is always precious, and its allocation raises the question of priorities. How is time and effort apportioned between the demands of heavy nursing and the need for quality of life? There is here an opportunity for conflict, which can be either creative or destructive depending on the way that it is handled. The potential for conflict in extended care, and how it may be handled, is well illustrated in a study of residential care of the physically disabled conducted by Miller and Gwynne (1972). It has lessons for all those engaged in long-term care. Initially the authors set out to investigate low staff morale in a residential care home. In the process, they identified two conflicting ideologies of care in staff. On the one hand, there was a traditional, humanitarian strategy in which patients, seen as sick, passive and compliant, were subject to active intervention by others (Table 19.2). This was called the 'warehousing' model. On the other hand, there was a liberal strategy that respected individuality and independence and called for effort and a contribution on the part of the client. Because it emphasized growth, it was called 'horticultural'. This was excellent for those who could cope, but inability to meet expectation led to a sense of failure, scapegoating and exclusion. Balanced decisions were needed: when, in the face of true dependency, to offer care, and when to switch to the 'DIY' growth model, perhaps in the same patient, when the task was within their reach.

Individuals, in real life, present with a mixture of autonomy and dependence. A single strategy aimed at only one, say dependence, will always be inappropriate when autonomy is present, and vice versa. Any one strategy, if used exclusively, will always be wrong some of the time.

Table 19.2 Systems in the care of the physically disabled (after Miller and Gwynne, 1972)

Humanitarian	Liberal
Preserve life	'Really normal'
Offer care	Promote autonomy
Problems	*Problems*
Dependency	Failure/exclusion
'Warehousing'	'Horticultural'

Not either/or but 'Which approach at which time?'

Inappropriate strategies will lead to unnecessary suffering for both the patient and staff. The art is to know when to use which strategy, and that is an art that requires much and constant thought, some experiment and rehearsal and a lot of experience; it is not easy. For this reason, Miller and Gwynne considered that the best way of maintaining a balance was to make 'supervision' available to staff so that problems can be analysed and solutions debated and, if necessary, rehearsed. It does not necessarily involve a line manager. Indeed, there may be disadvantages in exploring some of the complex human reactions to caring within a professional hierarchy. Rather it means an opportunity to share and be helped to understand one's personal and professional reactions with others who are in the same boat. It is a psychotherapeutic or counselling model that should allow the ventilation of personal feelings, and understanding of the feelings and roles of others. It gives an opportunity for problem-solving and, perhaps, rehearsal of responses.

BRINGING IT ALL TOGETHER

Attention has been drawn to the multiple problems that a patient may bring to a long-stay ward. The carer must find a middle path between essential and excessive support for not only the individual but for the group, and tensions may arise in both patients and staff that need to be attended to if the community is to prosper. A case has been made for exploring personal and group issues and for setting realistic goals for both clinical and social rehabilitation in which some of the higher aspects of human expression are given consideration and outlet.

The very words of social rehabilitation form a bridge between clinical practice and drama; there are so many in common: role, performance or role play, rehearsal, which is analogous to repeating rehabilitative tasks under supervision, and dialogue (over conflicts).

Table 19.3 The contribution of dramatherapy to the life of the long-stay ward

For the patient
1. Helps to enrich life and contribute to self-esteem and creative expression.
2. Helps to explore emotional problems of disability and to rehearse coping strategies.
3, Helps to develop personality and skills that may be needed in a new way of life.

For the member of staff
1. Increases job satisfaction from the enriched life of the ward community.
2. Helps in sharing with other professionals and in developing solutions to the problems and conflicts of care.
3. Helps in assessment by seeing the patient in a different social context.
4. Helps in formulating broad treatment plans.

There is also the enriching and sensitizing effect of artistic appreciation or expression, the exploration of self through role play and reversal, and the use of dramatherapy to take the patient out of the sick role, both for assessment and therapy. For staff, although dramatherapy is not the only tool for 'supervision' and exploration of the interaction of professional and personal, it is one such tool which can help to promote understanding and cohesion. These contributions are summarized in Table 19.3.

HOW MAY DRAMATHERAPY BE PRACTISED IN EXTENDED CARE?

Reference has already been made to the value of the play element of drama, and the metaphoric 'as if' quality of its application. This section will demonstrate some specific ways in which dramatherapy can contribute to life and work in a ward offering extended care.

QUALITY OF LIFE

Drama should be enjoyable, and games, play readings and improvised plays can contribute to creating a friendly, relaxed and stimulating environment.

Inviting a theatre group into the ward makes a social occasion, and a trip to the theatre, if that is possible, widens horizons and is an event in itself. Drama used with the overall goal of improving quality of life is therapy in its broadest sense.

SOCIAL ADJUSTMENT

With other patients

The anxiety caused by unfamiliarity can be mitigated in the dramatherapy group. If there is a regular group session, newcomers can be helped to find their own place in the ward community. There is usually a ritual of introducing new patients to the group. It may be simply a formal introduction, or group members may introduce themselves, adding three personal statements they would like the newcomer to know. Some other introductory games are:

1. Throw a ball around the group, each person giving his/her name as they catch it.
2. When people are aware of some names, they can call the name of the person to whom they are throwing.
3. Find three things you have in common with your partner. These may be very obvious things like both having blue eyes or wearing spectacles. It does not matter how simple they are, the sharing will move to a more personal level when the group is ready.
4. Tell your partner about your favourite TV star/actor/sportsman/piece of music/ book/painting.

These simple games can help to ease the anxieties of being 'the new patient'. It makes sense to use the games within the security of a group session, where the content of dramatherapy is explained and accepted. The relationships formed in the group, and the discussion commencing there, will be developed outside it.

With members of staff

Patients usually relate to staff, particularly those in uniform, in a fairly passive manner. The staff are authority figures who will tell the patients what to do, or will minister to them if they are disabled. This attitude fosters dependency, and whilst that may sometimes be necessary, it is important to encourage personal choice and independence as far as possible in order to avoid the negative effects of being in an institution. Some methods of encouraging alternative ways of relating are:

1. Available staff join the dramatherapy group as ordinary members entering into the games and activities with enthusiasm; the shared experience can become a bond which helps to create a different kind of relationship.
2. A ward noticeboard shows photographs of staff and patients, both as they are seen on the ward, and with their families. This may be part of reality orientation, either in specific sessions or informally, and it is available at any time.
3. Trust exercises can be a means of creating a trusting, cohesive group. They can encourage trust in oneself, and also hold a measure of responsibility for others. If staff are prepared to join the dramatherapy

group, it is possible to promote a different quality of trust. Also, if patients find themselves responsible for the wellbeing of a staff member, opportunities for a more reciprocal relationship occur. Some simple trust exercises are: (a) Close your eyes and allow a partner to take your hand. Discuss your feelings. (b) Close your eyes and allow a partner to lead you across the room. It is important to stress that the leader is totally responsible for the other person's welfare, and must avoid bumping into furniture. Discuss your feelings. (c) For the more able: stand in a circle, and, with each supporting the other, by joining arms; stand on one leg. This can also be done in pairs. Discuss your feelings. It is particularly necessary to discuss each trust exercise because some people find them very threatening.

4. Touch is a very important means of communication which can be explored openly in the dramatherapy group. Some people enjoy physical contact, others do not; staff may feel it is not professional to use touch as a means of communication. It is important to be aware of the feelings of each individual, in both the group and ward. An older patient may appear endearing, or perhaps be distressed, and the impulse may be to offer comfort with close physical contact. This may be just what the patient needs and wants, in which case it is appropriate. However, if the individual is one who finds touch difficult, staff should restrain their impulse and consider the needs of the receiver. Indiscriminate use of physical contact can be seen as patronizing.

It is not only important to consider touch while socializing. It is easy, when under pressure in a busy ward, to communicate stress to patients by the manner of touching them whilst carrying out routine procedures, thus communicating staff problems to patients.

REHABILITATION

PHYSICAL REHABILITATION

The need for movement after illness or surgery needs no emphasis. Older people who have pain or difficulty in moving are at risk of further permanent disability if they do not exercise. Encouragement and motivation are often necessary to get people on their feet. Physiotherapists may visit regularly, but their work can be complemented in dramatherapy groups. It is essential to consult the physiotherapist in selecting the group members and finding suitable exercises, to avoid undoing the good work done by them. Here are a few suggestions for keeping patients mobile.

- Throwing and catching a soft ball whilst sitting in a circle.
- Kicking the ball across the circle, still seated.
- Playing 'balloon football'. The group face each other in two lines. The

aim is to keep the balloon(s) in the air. If a balloon reaches the floor behind a team, then the team sitting opposite, who have patted the balloon, score a point.

- Walking in time to music, especially marches, helps a rhythmical step, co-ordination and balance. Try singing 'Onward Christian Soldiers' as the group walk around the room.
- Swing arms to a waltz tune. If possible, waltz with the more able.
- Those who are more mobile hold hands in a circle for support, and then gently rise onto tip-toe.

WHEELCHAIRS

Most games and exercises can be modified for people confined to wheel-chairs. Given sufficient helpers, the group can create 'wheelchair dances'; these are fun, giving a sense of movement and skill to people with limited mobility.

Adapting to being confined to a wheelchair is a process that is not always given much attention. In fact, the chair can become part of the body image. The time needed to get from one place to another is different. Work around personal perceptions of the chair as part of the body image: how big is it? how long does it take to do things? This is particularly useful for people in self-propelled chairs. Here are some ideas of the kind of games one can invent:

- Place obstacles around the room and see if people can complete the course without bumping into things.
- Guess how long it will take each individual to complete the course. Then check it out.
- Place furniture with varying gaps. Speculate on whether a wheelchair will pass between without touching. Check it out.
- Ask the patient 'What would you like to say to your wheelchair?' Then, 'if the wheelchair could talk, what do you think it would say?' This is a useful way of helping people express their feelings about their lack of mobility.

SOCIAL REHABILITATION

Rehabilitation, at its best, aids patients to return to their usual way of life. For most of the patients in continuing-care wards, this is unrealistic, and rehabilitation has to be about making the best possible use of the abilities left to the patient after illness. In the social sense, this may mean learning to live with relatives, in a residential home, or permanently in hospital. For people who have lived alone or with only a partner for several years, this adjustment can be difficult. Dramatherapy can be valuable in learning to adapt to role changes and learning (or re-learning) social skills.

Social skills training

- Games which encourage eye contact, such as ball games, name games, and games of exchanging chairs with others.
- Pass an object around the circle, feeling its texture and sharing reactions.
- Tell your partner about a book you've read, or a TV programme you've enjoyed.
- Describe a place you know well to a partner.
- Describe an outfit that would be suitable for your partner to wear to a wedding/trip to the seaside/visit to the theatre etc.

Role exploration and training

- See how many roles you have in common with a partner.
- Mime an action associated with a favourite working/social role. This should promote considerable discussion and sharing.
- Tell a story of some interesting event in which you played a leading role.
- If a patient is to move into other accommodation, it would be possible to set up a simulated situation to 'try out' in fantasy, experimenting with different approaches.
- If a difficult interview (perhaps with a relative or prospective residential home staff) is pending, rehearsal in a role simulation can be helpful.

EMOTIONAL REHABILITATION

It is important to remember that a variety of strong and possibly conflicting feelings will have been aroused by admission to hospital. Unless these emotions are acknowledged and allowed expression, the patient will have difficulty coming to terms with the new situation. There is an administrative ritual for admission to hospital, taking details of next of kin, personal property and a medical/social history, but there is no accepted ritual to ease the transition for the patient.

There may well be a sense of bereavement if a patient has to give up independent living. Actual bereavement, the death of a carer, may be the reason for admission. Loss of roles may be felt acutely, with a feeling of having 'come to the end of the road'. There may be mourning over lost social life and a feeling of social death. Patients may be facing up to the prospect of physical deterioration and death. There may be anger towards the family who have allowed hospitalization, or towards the illness or disability itself. Frustration at restricted mobility is common. There may also be a feeling of relief at being cared for, and for no longer being responsible for day-to-day chores. All or any of these feelings may exist at the same time, leaving the patient disturbed and confused.

Dramatherapy is an excellent medium for exploring feelings and coming to terms with life events. If people are not aware of their individual feelings, but are tense and upset, it is possible to work metaphorically, perhaps starting with appropriate stories and myths. Working on a fantasy level allows people to enter into situations that engender the same feelings being experienced in real life. This 'once-removed' method of looking at emotions creates a secure environment, and encourages objective appraisal. Some ideas for encouraging expression of feelings are:

- Find an individual body posture showing how people are feeling this moment. Discuss similarities in the group.
- An individual chooses objects (cushions, buttons, pieces of cloth etc.) to represent feelings, noting the size, weight and colour (sculpting). The patient can then debate the importance of each feeling and differentiate between them.
- Patients draw a picture of themselves depicting their emotional state. It doesn't have to be a work of art – pin-men/women can be very expressive.
- Individuals write a 'secret' fear or anxiety on pieces of paper that are then shuffled and distributed at random. Each person is then asked to speak about the subject on their new paper, as if it were their own fear or anxiety. Anonymity breaks through shyness and fear of being exposed.

Patients often feel that they are alone in their emotional response. Opening up subjects for dicussion allows people to share their feelings. It is a great comfort to discover that one is not alone, particularly with 'bad' feelings.

RELATIVES

Patients are not alone with their mixed feelings. Relatives may have the same sense of loss and separation, fear disability and death, be angry with the patient for being ill and at the same time relieved to hand over the caring to professionals, yet feel guilty as well.

Dramatherapy support groups for relatives could help them to express and cope with these feelings. This would ultimately benefit the patient by improved and hopefully more honest relationships. Techniques similar to those suggested for patient groups could be used.

Many people suffering from dementia are admitted to extended care wards. Visiting friends and relatives are often at a loss for means of communication. They can be encouraged to join the 'enrichment' groups.

A shared experience, even if it is a simple game or sing-song, can be a means of communication.

STAFF

SUPPORT

Hospital staff are frequently under pressure. Most disciplines are under-staffed, and individuals feel they are working at full capacity. There is often a failure to realize the emotional strain put upon them. Apart from feeling overburdened, staff have to come to terms with their own feelings aroused by contact with patients.

Working with older, often terminally ill patients is, for staff, a constant reminder of their own ageing and mortality. Inevitably, staff grow fond of people in long-term care, and the death of a patient can be a source of bereavement. Equally, staff can dislike patients, particularly if the patient is disagreeable or difficult. There is a widely held view that staff should like all their patients, so feelings of guilt may arise.

Lack of opportunity to express and share feelings creates yet another burden, and increases the risk of 'burn-out'. Dramatherapy staff support groups could help to resolve the problems of individual members of staff. Similar techniques to those suggested for patients can be used, along with role play and role reversal.

SUPERVISION

It has already been noted that Miller and Gwynne recommend staff super-vision to look at group processes within teams. 'Process' supervision is not about management, but about psychodynamics. The team sets aside a regular time for meeting with an external supervisor to look at what is happening in the relationship between staff and patients, and the interper-sonal relationships within the staff team. This method of analysing interac-tion is accepted in the field of psychotherapy, and is becoming more common in the helping professions in general. Sculpting, role play, role reversal, projective techniques and many other elements of dramatherapy are invaluable in supervision groups.

SUMMARY

Dramatherapy is a process of artistic involvement with a therapeutic intent. It can be applied to improve the quality of life of people in conti-nuing care. More specifically, it can enable patients, relatives and staff to express and explore emotions and come to some resolution of conflict. Given some training and stimulation of ideas, most staff members could work at the 'quality of life' level. Further training is necessary to work psychotherapeutically. As most staff are already working to their full capacity, a dramatherapist included as a member of the team would be invaluable.

REFERENCES

Bailey, C.H. (1981) Drama in health education. *J. Br. Assoc. Dramather.*, **5**, 1–9.
Bennet, D.H. (1977) Psychiatric rehabilitation, in *Rehabilitation Today* (ed. S. Mattingly), Update Books, London.
Esslin, M. (1976) *Anatomy of Drama*, Abacus, London.
Fairclough, J. et al. (1977) Drama for the blind. *J. Br. Assoc. Dramather.*, **1**, 14–16.
Grainger, R. (1987) Evaluation in dramatherapy. *J. Br. Assoc. Dramather.*, **10**, 17–22.
Jones, L. (1984) Dramatherapy and research work. *J. Br. Assoc. Dramather.*, **8**, 11–18.
Landy, J. (1986) *Drama Therapy*, Charles C. Thomas, Springfield, Illinois, USA.
Langley, D.M. (1981) Dramatherapy in the training of psychiatric nurses. *J. Br. Assoc. Dramather.*, **5**, 19–20.
Langley, G.E. (1983) Dramatherapy with the elderly. *J. Br. Assoc. Dramather.*, **7**, 13–19.
McLuskie, M. (1983) Dramatherapy in a psychiatric hospital. *J. Br. Assoc. Dramather.*, **6**, 20–5.
Maslow, A.H. (1943) A theory of human motivation. *Psychol. Rev.*, **50** 370–96.
Miller, E.J. and Gwynne, G.V. (1972) *A Life Apart*, Tavistock Publications, London.
Moreno. J.L. (1946) *Psychodrama* (first volume), Beacon House, Beacon, New York, USA; 5th edn, 1976.

FURTHER READING

Langley, D.M. (1987) Dramatherapy with elderly people, in *Dramatherapy, Theory and Practice* (ed. S. Jennings), Croom Helm, London.
Langley, G.E. (1982) Quality of life in extended care, in *Conference Report: Quality of Life in Extended Care*, Royal College of Psychiatrists, London.
Langley, G.E. and Kershaw, B. (1982) Reminiscence Theatre, Theatre Paper No. 6, Dartington College, Totnes, Devon.
Langley, D.M. and Langley, G.E. (1983) *Dramatherapy in Psychiatry*, Croom Helm, London.

APPENDIX 1

PHYSICAL REQUIREMENTS FOR THE PRACTICE OF DRAMATHERAPY

1. A pleasant, uncluttered, well-lit room with a carpeted or smooth wooden floor, depending on the activities to be undertaken.
2. Assured freedom from interruption, for a defined period, from phones, catering trolleys, and 'Oh I'm sorry I didn't know!'
3. Preferably freedom from uninvolved observers; join in by all means, or stay away.

4. Record/tape reproduction.
5. Props such as: balls, photographs of old haunts or recent activities, things to hold, touch, reminisce or talk about, percussion instruments, objects such as cushions to represent feelings in projective games, simple drawing materials, lengths of fabric.
6. Reasonable access to toilets.
7. Appropriate seating for all.
8. Comfortable casual clothes for all.
9. Extra lights, such as coloured or spot-lights, are not essential, but can be a useful adjunct.

REPORTS OF APPLICATIONS AND EVALUATION

'Dramatherapy', the Journal of the British Association for Dramatherapists (from the Association address as listed), contains many articles on work in progress. Evaluation to date is mostly at the descriptive level but this is not inappropriate (Langley, 1983). A 'cross-over' trial of dramatherapy with patients suffering from schizophrenia sets a model for a more rigorous approach (Grainger, 1987), while others have used dramatherapy techniques as a research tool (Jones, 1984), in training nurses (Langley, 1981) or as a health education tool (Bailey, 1981). It has also been used with the blind (Fairclough *et al.*, 1977) and in psychiatric hospitals (e.g. MuLuskie, 1983).

APPEXDIX 2

FOR ADVICE/INFORMATION

The British Association for Dramatherapists (41 Broomhouse Lane, Hurlingham Park, London SW6 3DP, tel: 0171 731 0160) publishes a membership list of names and addresses.

DRAMATHERAPY TRAINING COURSES RECOGNIZED BY THE BRITISH ASSOCIATION FOR DRAMATHERAPISTS

The Central/Sesame Course in Drama and Movement in Therapy
The Central School of Speech and Drama
Embassy Theatre, Eton Avenue
London NW3 3HY. Tel: 0171 722 8183–6

Post-Graduate Diploma Dramatherapy Course
University College of Ripon and York St John
Lord Mayor's Walk
York YO3 7EX. Tel: 01904 656771

Post-Graduate Diploma Dramatherapy Course
University of Hertfordshire
College Lane
Hatfield
Hertfordshire AL10 9AB. Tel: 01707 285 300

Graduate Diploma in Dramatherapy Course
The Institute of Dramatherapy at Roehampton
Roehampton Institute
Digby Stuart College
Roehampton Lane
London SW15 5PU. Tel: 0181 392 3215/3063

Post-Graduate Diploma in Dramatherapy Course
South Devon College
Newton Road, Torquay
South Devon TQ2 5BY. Tel: 01803 386384

Dramatherapy Diploma Department of Counselling
City College
The Arden Centre
Sale Road
Northende
Manchester M23 0DD. Tel: 0161 957 1500

Music therapy and the functions of music with older mentally ill people in a continuing care setting

INTRODUCTION

Music has occupied a place in the world of healing and health since historical records began. I propose to concentrate on discussions and descriptions of music therapy and related approaches with people over 65 with predominantly emotional, psychological and physical problems relating to old age, rather than go into extensive detail about the qualities of music itself. The latter are well covered in the literature elsewhere (Storr, 1992; Bunt, 1994; Sloboda, 1995). What is essential here is to understand the essence of why music as used in music therapy is important with this population. As Juliette Alvin wrote in the chapter about music therapy in the first edition of this book 'The evocative power of music is immense. It can bring to our imagination stories, places, people – in the past and present'. In the early days of music therapy, there was emphasis on activity-based work with older people using music as a stimulating medium leading to enjoyment and revitalization, and less emphasis on the psychotherapeutic approach in music therapy. Recently, the latter approach has become more prevalent in the UK. There are many obvious valid uses of music in music therapy, and there are also many unanswered questions about exactly why music is therapeutic. However, it is well recognized that music can help social interaction, help people explore memories and associations, develop a sense of achievement, facilitate self-expression and stimulate movement. As Bunt (1994) writes 'Music helps us to feel the essence of emotions; it is about feelings. We can all laugh with pleasure, for example, but perhaps music brings us closer to appreciating the essence of pleasure'. This statement could be equally true of dealing with sadness, tears, perhaps of grief for a partner who had died, or in preparation for our own death. Music therapy has an important function because of the innate qualities of music in addressing many issues of old age, including the onset of confusion related to dementia so often seen in continuing care.

DEFINITIONS OF MUSIC THERAPY

There are many definitions, and I quote just a few. The Association of Professional Music Therapists (1995) defines music therapy as: 'a framework in which a mutual relationship is set up between client and therapist. The growing relationship enables changes to occur, both in the condition of the client and in the form that the therapy takes. . . By using music creatively in a clinical setting, the therapist seeks to establish an interaction, a shared musical experience leading to the pursuit of thera-peutic goals.' This definition reflects the British emphasis on improvisa-tion, but recently Towse (1995) has described an approach with older people with functional illnesses emphasizing the importance of receptive music in music therapy. She describes clinical reasons why this is important:

> For elderly people there are several advantages in using receptive music, the most important of which is that the technique is drawing upon the person's abilities, rather than highlighting disability. This is particularly important when dealing with someone who has suffered a stroke as the ability to play may be affected by perceptual distortion as well as the obvious physical handicap. The capacity to listen to and enjoy music, however, appears to remain intact. Using receptive music that is familiar evokes memories and associations of people, places and events in one's life. Preoccupation with the past carries with it obvious dangers, but for elderly people who are aware of becoming increasingly dependent on others, descriptions of past events provide reassurance that they enjoyed the same independence as the (inevitably) younger therapist. The skills of the therapist should enable the conversation to move from the past to the present.

I take a different view, arising out of the fact that most of my work has been with people who are in advanced stages of dealing with dementia, and for whom interacting through music is often the only means of contact with the outside world (Odell-Miller, 1995). I believe that all approaches are valid and the music therapist's role is to decide which musical approach is necessary, and when. Whether music is improvised or listened to within the music therapy context, the music cannot be predeter-mined, just as changes in the relationship between the therapist and patient cannot, and this is one factor that highlights the difference between music therapy and music for entertainment or educational purposes.

Another short but practical definition that I often use is found in 'Music Therapy and Mental Health' (Scott *et al.*, 1986): 'Music therapy in the field of mental illness concentrates on the use of music as a means of communication and interaction'. As described by O'Connor *et al.* (1993) such therapy can achieve:

• a reduction in the levels of anxiety;
• increased quality of attention;
• increased span of attention;
• increased interest in communication;
• increased capacity to communicate self-states with others – verbally, musically and through action;
• an increased capacity to experience a range of emotions;
• an increased capacity both to exercise and develop the functions of mental organizations [moods, feelings].

REVIEWS OF MUSIC THERAPY

Much has been written about music therapy in various parts of the world although the literature covering its use with older mentally ill people is not as prolific as in other fields, e.g. learning difficulties. In the hope of encouraging readers to explore the literature, some useful publications are mentioned here.

Detailed reviews of music therapy, specifically with older people and also those with mental health problems, may be found in a recent music therapy textbook (Wigram *et al.*, 1995). In this book, chapters by Towse, Hanser and Clair, and Odell-Miller cover between them existing research and literature in this field, which until recently was not prevalent. As already mentioned, Towse writes about the use of receptive music in music therapy, and discusses issues raised in such an approach, i.e. a psychotherapy approach with listening to music as part of the process. Hanser and Clair discuss family work, where family members and/or caregivers bring favourite tapes to family sessions with a client with Alzheimer's disease to aid working together to understand difficulties and help the suffering person. Research is mentioned, and evaluation shows that music therapy is effective in encouraging participation, capturing attention and cutting down confusion during the sessions. A full account of research carried out in the 1980s is included (Odell-Miller, 1995). This research showed that:

1. music therapy is associated with high levels of engagement among participants than reminiscence therapy, although this difference is not a significant one;

2. patients who have received music therapy show higher levels of engagement half an hour after they have received music therapy than they show at the same time on a different day, although this difference is not a significant one;
3. patients show a significantly higher level of engagement during music therapy sessions when involved in this therapy regularly (weekly) than they do when involved intermittently.

Music therapists, such as Towse, Hanser and Clair, were stimulated to carry out research because the existing information is sparse. For example, since its inception in 1969 the *British Journal of Music Therapy* had only published four articles before 1986 specifically about music therapy with older people, e.g. Allen (1975). These recent chapters indicate a changing trend.

An Australian music therapist, Bright (1972), published a book specifically outlining her work with older people, and more recently has described grief work with older adults (Bright, 1995). Thus we see a changing trend in the literature, where music therapy with the older population is covered more fully than in previous years.

MUSIC THERAPY AS A SPECIFIC TREATMENT

It is becoming more accepted that older people, particularly those who are confused, can benefit from an approach which takes into account unconscious process, understanding meaning, symbolic representation and interpretation. Here, Towse (1995) is interesting reading, and she concentrates on listening to music as a form of psychotherapy and its potency. Much less is written about a live improvised approach which also may incorporate listening as and when necessary. This section will describe the latter music therapy approach and summarize some casework.

A description of our local music therapy service (Odell-Miller, 1992) provides an introduction to music therapy in a psychiatric setting. Music therapy is available both in small closed groups, open groups, and in individual settings. There are several models of therapy, and the framework used most widely here is a psychodynamic model. 'Music therapy for elderly people with dementia attempts to alleviate the disruptive symptoms that are brought about by cognitive disfunction, working also with the emotional disorders, anxieties and losses that come with the ageing process. There is a potential for change through the patient experiencing and being held in the facilitating environment of the therapy. The non-verbal nature of this type of communication is an important alternative way of interacting with clients.

The following list of possible benefits may be helpful in understanding the nature of how music therapy can help: increased motivation and decision-making; improved quality and level of engagement; developed awareness of the self and others; increased socialisation and developed relationships; opportunity for expression of [an] individual's emotional state; physical stimulation; relaxation; improved self-image; intellectual stimulation; an opportunity for reminiscence and a sharing of experiences; improved reality orientation.' Within this, what is being offered is defined in terms of the client, and the agent or person referring them.

In a day centre for older mentally ill people, group sessions have catered for:

1. cognitively impaired, confused clients, aiming at enhancing remaining social skills, sensory stimulation and personal expression, and
2. functionally impaired clients, who are not currently psychotic, clinically depressed or confused, aiming at developing, reinforcing and generalizing relaxation techniques, using music, imagery and touch massage.

In individual sessions, aims differ according to referred clients' needs and diagnosis, and utilize song material known to the clients to facilitate expression of feelings within a verbal psychodynamic approach. Doyle, an Australian-trained music therapist and manager of the day centre, uses a specific approach including pre-composed song material, and touch massage, which she has additional training in (Doyle, 1992).

The reader may be wondering what place psychoanalysis has within this field, and it has indeed become an important resource for informing the work of music therapists during the last two decades. Although it may not be appropriate to share interpretations with clients who are confused, it is important to understand at times symbolic representation, and who we may represent for the client therapeutically as a music therapist colleague writes 'Music and the playing of instruments may evoke feelings of sadness or resistance' (Davies, personal communication). It may be important in order to help the client further, to understand something of why this might be. This will be speculative and perhaps we can never properly 'know'.

Understanding the transference and counter-transference phenomenon and having regular clinical supervision can help music therapists work with disturbed people in a long-term setting where change may be little and infrequent. Indeed, there may be no motivation for change for continuing care residents, who may have resigned themselves to never being discharged to community life. Depression may be enormous, and this, coupled with the confused or psychotic expression of some patients, requires staying power by the therapist.

During my 17 years of experience as a music therapist in psychiatric residential settings, an overwhelming factor has often been hopelessness and despair on the part of patients/clients and staff alike. It is not uncommon, as a defence against this, to find hostile attitudes, conflict and forgetfulness developing in staff teams. The conflict can be between those who believe in something hopeful for the patient (which is sometimes only possible after acknowledging their own negative feelings about caring for these people), and those who have lost all sense of hope for the people in their care. It is important for a music therapist to understand these phenomena in order to work in a multidisciplinary setting, and to know that there may be unconscious feelings amongst staff arising from looking after confused people all day, which, if not understood, could get in the way of the music therapy process. Regular liaison is essential for things to work for the benefit of the residents. It helps to understand that perhaps staff forget to bring the patient to her music therapy sessions, although she has been coming for 20 weeks at the same time on the same day each week, as a result of becoming unconsciously forgetful or confused like the residents.

Music therapy is practised and understood on many different levels, as we have seen, ranging from an outcome-based research project, to a psychoanalytically informed way of understanding the therapy. A constant feature within this, is the musical skill and improvisational nature of the work, providing a special dimension often difficult to explain in words. It is perhaps pertinent to mention that training of a music therapist is intensive and more details about training courses can be obtained from The Association of Professional Music Therapists. Musical skill, maturity, sensitivity and an open but strong therapeutic 'attitude' are fundamental qualities needed before embarking on training, which is all at postgraduate level in the UK. Music therapists have developed referral and assessment procedures that are imperative to enable services to function within a multidisciplinary setting. Information contained for example in the Psychiatric Services for the Elderly booklet (O'Connor et al., 1993), Arts Therapies brochure (John et al., 1994) and leaflets produced by Darnley-Smith and O'Connor (available from the author) enables both hospital- and community-based carers and professionals to make use of the service. Only then can referrals be made. Table 20.1 shows some summarized cases referred to the music therapy service between 1990 and 1995. To enable the reader to gain a fuller understanding of what actually happens in music therapy, some clinical material is now described.

EXAMPLE OF GROUP WORK IN A RESIDENTIAL SETTING

Connie was an 88-year-old lady with Alzheimer's disease in advanced stages. She had little recognizable speech, but her personality seemed to reveal itself through vocalization and gesture on the continuing care ward. She had no family or relatives close to her, having lost her husband ten years previously. During her earlier life, she had been a teacher and raised three children. She wandered aimlessly around the ward when not engaged in any specific activity, and was referred for group music therapy

Table 20.1 Summarized cases referred to the music therapy service between 1990 and 1995

Year of birth	Reason for referral	Period of therapy	Nature of problems/ diagnosis	Outcome/summary
1920	Manic depressive psychosis Dementia	2 years	Severe isolation – little or no language used	Ongoing patient – now speaks occasionally about himself and his feelings
1909	To maintain social skills and interests Used to play brass instruments	3 years	Severe depression in response to dementing illness – manic tendencies	At times able to experience recognition and insight into himself. Linking up with others through improvisation
1913	Individual assessment and support	1½ years	Long-term institutionalization, diagnosis of schizophrenia	Ongoing support – less withdrawn at times
1924	Recently bereaved. Severe aphasia. No way of communicating	2 years – in progress	Music therapist asked to assess as well as providing a therapeutic and accessible setting	Patient used instruments and sound to communicate. Shared musical relationship has helped her accept her 'state'
1910	Very confused, angry and disorientated. Unaccepting of situation	3 years	Angry – unaccepting response to situation. Several memory problems – confusion, loneliness	Used music to release some of the confused angry feelings. Helped her relate to others
1912	To improve stimulation and improve his level of communication	2 years	Gradual deterioration due to dementia. Initially his insight led to depression	Music was the only medium to connect with his emotional life

by the consultant psychiatrist 'to provide a place for her to interact with others through a non-verbal medium, and to provide a place for her to express herself in a secure setting'.

After an initial four-week assessment period showing that music therapy could be of benefit, she attended the weekly music therapy group for four years. During this time, she deteriorated physically, but seemed to maintain a sense of self, and a will to socialize and interact. These phenomena were particularly prevalent during music therapy sessions. On the ward, she often shouted at others, seemingly in anger and frustration, and occasionally hit out at others.

Music therapy sessions

There is no such thing as a typical session, but instruments and space within the room are available for clients to use with the therapist. Group sessions here last for 45 minutes, and instruments used are tuned and untuned percussion, including gongs, drums, tambours, cymbal, maracas, metallophone, kalimba, bass xylophone, recorder, guitar and voice. How much or little the therapist structures a session musically or otherwise depends on the clients' needs and the therapist's assessment of these.

During the first part of the session, I usually allow space for each person to acknowledge their presence. This may involve a verbal greeting, shaking hands or a musical interaction. Connie always seemed excited on arrival at the sessions, and recognized everyone as if saying hello, through her disjointed vocalizing. She used this as a chance to express her individuality by using an instrument (usually metallophone or maracas – her choice) whilst vocalizing. I would improvise with her, singing in a style that supported her often agitated jerky rhythms, sometimes using her name, or vocalizing on other sounds, e.g. ha ha, etc. Gradually a rapport built up through this interaction, and each person was greeted in a way particular to them. Connie developed a way of 'following me' around the group, by gesturing or pointing rhythmically or even by walking around. She would often greet others, and each person would have the chance, in these early moments of the session, to introduce themselves, musically, with my musical support on instruments during improvised sections. Occasionally in this section, if the atmosphere was chaotic or members seemed unsettled, I would play a pre-composed or improvised piece for listening, in order to help members focus on themselves and the group in a more settled way. Connie often seemed to relax during these moments, and her agitation seemed to subside, helping her feel more at peace with herself and the group.

The middle time in the group was centered around building improvisations between the whole group or in threes or pairs, where interaction and expression seemed more intense and perhaps allowed more in-depth feelings to be shared verbally and musically. For example, Connie would sometimes hum or beat in a particular way, and I would develop this musically. This could lead to others joining in, or remain as a dialogue between two members.

Connie developed a preference for the bass metallophone, and would share this with another member, Mary. They were increasingly interested in making music together, using the 'white note' scale, with a feeling of interaction and dialogue. I would support from the piano or with the recorder, if it seemed important to be close to them. I would describe this as the therapist taking a containing role, within which other members of the group could join. Sometimes I would play firm harmonic rhythmic chords in the bass whilst another member improvised in a free way, perhaps aggressively drumming at irregular intervals.

During Connie's therapy, I identified that she needed to express herself loudly at times and that this would often be followed by a quieter period of reflection, when she would sometimes be tearful. This was seen as useful for her, and I would try to show support and understanding by reflecting to her musically or verbally how she might be feeling. She, and others, seemed to find this useful, after a group improvisation.

In the final part of the session, it is important to enable things to close in a way that helps members sense an ending, to prepare them for going back out of the therapy session. In work with people who are not confused, more responsibility for this would be given to group members. However, it was important with this group to aid this process by sensing the atmosphere, and Connie particularly responded to this approach. She seemed to become more aware of the ending during her years in therapy, and would often settle and sit as if contemplating saying goodbye. Occasionally song material was improvised around a theme of ending and goodbye, perhaps putting Connie and others in touch with their own experiences of endings, grief and death. However, with Connie, it was not possible to be certain, only to sense that she often seemed to want to express profound emotion, developing into hugging, kissing and clinging onto Mary, her neighbour, or a helper in the group. She would then be able to settle again, and leave peacefully as if the group had 'contained' these feelings. I would be aware of a need to slow down, or speed up the musical and rhythmic pulse according to the mood of the group, and sometimes each member would be involved in a separate goodbye with me, sharing an instrument, or improvising on their own chosen instrument with harmonic or melodic support from me on piano, violin, voice or recorder.

Connie, whilst physically deteriorating through the effects of Alzheimer's disease, was able to experience an emotionally expressive place within which she could be contained in her final years, most importantly on a non-verbal level. She related to others in an excited and exuberant way, and seemed to value the consistent relationship with others provided by the group. I could understand perhaps something of what she was experiencing, and often felt she was 'clinging' to a familiar nurturing relationship reminiscent of other relationships she may have experienced.

She moved wards three times in four years, and, as she had no family visiting her, she had generally a bereft, isolated existence. The group provided a stable space within which she could be herself, and deal with these last years of her life. She remained involved and engaged until shortly before her death, despite her physical frailty.

EXAMPLE OF INDIVIDUAL WORK IN THE COMMUNITY

So far we have considered music therapy taking place in a hospital setting. However, music therapy services are now increasingly provided outside the hospital setting, for example in state and privately run homes and in day centres.

The function of the multidisciplinary team has been of primary importance for Norman, a musician in his mid-50s. He suffers from a complex form of dementia, simultanagnosia, resulting in severe perceptual problems. His life has been spent specifically as a pianist, and in teaching improvisation and composition. His ability to improvise is still not very much impaired although he can no longer read music.

He was first referred by the psychiatrist, who had a clearly defined area of music therapy in mind: 'we wondered whether it would be possible for you to assess Norman and see if it would be possible to help him work through some of the emotional implications of his diagnosis' (from the referral letter). In later letters, once the therapy had been under way for several months, the psychiatrist wrote 'Although he has considerable difficulty expressing himself, he did explain to me that he found weekly music therapy visits very helpful, and his wife has commented that he seems brighter after these sessions'. This is an ideal investment of music therapy, as all those in the team including his wife believe in the importance of therapy. Two other key people are the community psychiatric nurse, who visits weekly to help with practical coping strategies and provides support to Norman and his wife, and the psychologist, who has aimed at 'trying to help the couple understand his neuropsychological strengths and weaknesses'.

After one year of music therapy, he is now more cognitively impaired, and occasionally confused over his wife's identity: 'She's not my wife, she looks after me'. He has a good relationship with her and is affectionate but has occasionally been aggressive recently as a result of frustration. He recognizes me, and often refers immediately to the fact that we will play music. I represent for him carer, fellow musician, pupil (he was a lecturer in music) and transferentially I feel that I also symbolize partner, child, pupil and nurturer at different times. He is developing more of a rapport with me musically and often says 'I feel this is so good for me – it's just there, music is here – you touch it and you get it'. He also has recently begun to improvise on his own between sessions, something which he had no inclination to do when we first met because he was afraid of the piano: 'It comes up to hit me'. It seems that this fear has subsided, the more our work develops, and that, through improvising, he has recognized a way of expressing himself in an area in which he feels expert and confident. During the first year of therapy, he has become more disoriented, often needing me to point him towards the piano or into the therapy room as if he cannot orient himself to the situation. However, his interactions through improvisations, with me using voice, violin and piano are still developing. The role of the other team members has freed him up to have music therapy for himself and his wife has always respected the privacy of this, and enabled proper boundaries to exist although the work takes place in his home.

The work cannot be fully understood without actually hearing the tapes of sessions in both this case and the previous one, but I hope that these case studies have at least given some insight and understanding into music therapy processes and possible interventions.

MUSIC WITHIN A CONTEXT OF THERAPEUTIC ACTIVITY

In the first section of this chapter, we looked at the many general therapeutic qualities of music. This section will describe these more general functions of music, and activities that are therapeutic but different from the specific treatment of music therapy. For older people who are looked after in continuing care settings, or by carers in homes or in their own homes, various activities such as concerts, sing-songs, music projects and tea dances are organized by a variety of organizations. 'Live Music Now' and The Council for Music in Hospitals are two such organizations, and Arts Councils often give grants to enable people to gain access to music and musicians who may otherwise not have it. Others in the caring field also involve themselves in such work, including doctors, nurses, other therapists, psychologists and social workers who have an interest or skill in music. Where a music therapy service exists, music therapists may also encourage such events, and be involved as part of a local project or activity, but this would be separate to and in addition to their specific music therapy work. Towse (1995) writes about her post as a music therapist: 'A significant feature of the post is that a distinction exists between music as therapy, and as entertainment. The latter is important, but is not organised by the music therapist'. In my opinion, in surveying music therapists working with the older population around the country, this distinction is in operation, but music therapists may jointly organize and advise about such events together with other agencies and professionals. In our own service, several such projects have been extremely beneficial, particularly to older people living on continuing care wards. The entire BBC Philharmonic Orchestra rehearsed in the main hall of the hospital during a project set up jointly by the local Arts Council, and education authority. People who had not been in the presence of a whole orchestra ever, or for some years, were able to wander in and out and experience the orchestra in rehearsal. Many older people were shocked by the volume of the orchestra, and were able to express strong opinions about this and some of the 20th century music played which they were not perhaps familiar with. This was a real experience, one of exhilarating excitement, and of activity too, when people could touch and explore some of the instruments. A particularly memorable moment was when one older resident, who has suffered from manic depression for many years, was able to get onto the orchestra lorry and have her photo taken with members of the orchestra. Her father had long ago been part of the management team of a large orchestra, and she is still talking about this special experience three years later. Another occasion was a percussion workshop organized by local agencies, and planned very carefully with music therapists. A professional percussion player worked with groups of older clients, giving them a one-off experience of playing the instruments, talking about his role, and creating a piece of music. In this activity, the music was more of an end in itself, which was appropriate only for people who felt they could cope with this, i.e. they were expected to 'get it right'. This was certainly therapeutic for some in raising self-esteem and encouraging feelings of achievement and fulfilled a different, more educational, function than music therapy treatment.

In our service, within the multidisciplinary team, we have felt it important to develop strong multidisciplinary links. This has enabled a positive supportive environment to exist which has in turn helped the multidisciplinary team cope with some of the disturbing phenomena often found in continuing care 'institutions'. The tea dance, for example, acts as a support for staff and clients alike. It is organized by the occupational therapist assistant, together with advice and involvement from arts therapists, dramatherapists and music therapists. Visiting musicians provide music, as well as music therapists at times. It is an event as much like 'normal' life as possible, where there is entertainment, socializing, dancing, visual aspects (flowers and table decorations) and tea. People can participate as much or as little as they choose. It is not a formal therapy, takes place fortnightly, and is a special occasion. Apart from the obvious benefits gained by older residents and relatives, the event is important in helping the team deal with the 'darker' side of this difficult caring work, and has helped improve relationships between therapists and nursing staff. The latter welcome attending with clients, and the particular milieu and environment created by a mixture of music, tea, dancing and conversation make this an important community event. It should be emphasized that many people participating in these events are able to orient themselves within such settings, and that those referred for specific music therapy treatment are often those who are not able to benefit from such events, and need more individual help.

CONCLUSION

This chapter has aimed to give an overview of music therapy and the therapeutic use of music with older people. To find out more about any aspect of music therapy, the Association of Professional Music Therapists and the British Society for Music Therapy will be able to help, particularly in the area of training, further training and literature:

- Association of Professional Music Therapists, 38 Pierce Lane/Fulbourn, Cambridgeshire, CB1 5DL
- British Society for Music Therapy, 25 Rosslyn Avenue, East Barnet, Hertfordshire, EN4 8 DH.

REFERENCES

Allen, D. (1975) Music therapy and geriatric patients. *Br. J. Music Ther.*, **8**(3), 2–6.
Association of Professional Music Therapists (1995) *A Career in Music Therapy*, APMT, Cambridge, UK.
Bright, R. (1972) *Music in Geriatric Care*, Agnus and Robertson Ltd, New South Wales, Australia.
Bright, R. (1995) Music therapy as a facilitator in grief counselling, in *The Art and Science of Music Therapy – A Handbook* (eds A. Wigram, B. Saperston and R. West), Harwood Academic Publishers, Switzerland.
Bunt, L. (1994) *Music Therapy: An Art Beyond Words*, Routledge, London.
Doyle, S. (1992) *Annual Report of Music Therapy Service*, Mental Health Service, Addenbrokes NHS Trust, Cambridge, UK.
Hanser, S. and Clair, A. (1995) Retrieving the losses of Alzheimer's disease for patients and care-givers with the aid of music, in *The Art and Science of Music Therapy – A Handbook* (eds A. Wigram, B. Saperston and R. West), Harwood Academic Publishers, Switzerland.
John, D., Appolinari, C., Odell-Miller H. *et al.* (1994) *Arts Therapies in The Mental Health Services*, Addenbrookes Publications, Cambridge, UK.
O'Connor, C. *et al.* (1993) *PSE (Psychiatric Services for the Elderly) Booklet*, Addenbrookes NHS Trust, Cambridge, UK.
Odell-Miller, H. (1992) *Changing Models of Music Therapy within a Mental Health Service*, BSMT Publications, London.
Odell-Miller, H. (1995) Approaches to music therapy in psychiatry with specific emphasis upon a research project with the elderly mentally ill, in *The Art and Science of Music Therapy – A Handbook* (eds A. Wigram, B. Saperston and R. West), Harwood Academic Publishers, Switzerland.
Scott, M., Odell H. and John, D. (1995) *Music Therapy and Mental Health*, revised edn, Association of Professional Music Therapists, Cambridge, UK.
Sloboda, J. (1995) *The Musical Mind*, Oxford University Press, Oxford, UK.
Storr, A. (1992) *Music and the Mind*, Harper Collins, London.
Towse, E. (1995) Listening and accepting in *The Art and Science of Music Therapy – A Handbook* (eds A. Wigram, B. Saperston and R. West), Harwood Academic Publishers, Switzerland.
Wigram, A., Saperston B. and West, R. (1995) *The Art and Science of Music Therapy – A Handbook*, Harwood Academic Publishers, Switzerland.

PART THREE
Improving quality of life: case studies

Having set the scene in the previous two sections of the book, this section aims to show how ideas and concepts can be put into practice within specific homes in the public and private sectors. The final two chapters give an overview of what has been achieved in the voluntary and private sectors.

The Nightingale Centre 21

INTRODUCTION

Until comparatively recently, in-patient services for people suffering from dementia have been largely illness-focused, directed towards symptom control and overlooking the patient's residual abilities and past interests. In the face of competition for finite resources, the high physical care demands of this very dependent client group invariably took precedence over the need for therapeutic social activities.

Despite token homage paid to the concept of holistic care, close examination rarely supported any evidence that this was, in fact, being delivered, and many patients spent long periods of time sitting on wards with little, if anything, to occupy them. Where there were attempts to provide activities at ward level, these were very much on an *ad hoc* basis and tended to be unstructured and lacking individuality. Usually there was an inverse relationship between patients' levels of incapacity and the recreational input they received.

THE EARLY YEARS

The creation of the Nightingale Centre, opened at Graylingwell Hospital, Chichester, in 1989, represented one unit's attempt to redress the balance and consider the social and psychological needs of patients with a dementing illness.

A redundant ground-floor Nightingale-style ward was identified to house the centre, and the Friends of Chichester Hospitals agreed to fund the project. Since the centre was to be sited within the old Victorian institution, the amount of structural alteration would necessarily be limited, but the intention was to provide a quiet non-clinical environment within which patients could participate in meaningful activity away from the ward setting.

To contain costs, the majority of the work was completed in-house by the hospital estates department. False walls were strategically deployed to create smaller, more intimate areas, and some fine old pieces of furniture were retrieved from storage and restored. Soft furnishings were carefully chosen to reinforce the domestic ambience. The design of the centre incorporated wheelchair access to all areas and, where appropriate, adaptations to assist with mobility, while at the same time attempting to retain a homely, rather than a hospital, effect.

On its completion in 1989, the centre included a craft room, a fully equipped kitchen, in which patients could prepare simple meals under supervision, and areas for more passive pursuits, such as music appreciation and television/video viewing. The large day room (Figure 21.1) could be subdivided by screens to provide areas in which small groups could function. There was also an enclosed garden, accessed via a ramp, with a greenhouse, a raised fish pond, (Figure 21.2), a paved patio with seating and a barbecue area, and a lawn.

Staff recruitment attracted considerable interest from applicants from a wide variety of educational and professional backgrounds, and the interview panel could afford to be rigorously selective. No previous experience in working with older mentally ill people was required and candidates were appointed on the basis of their creativity and ability to

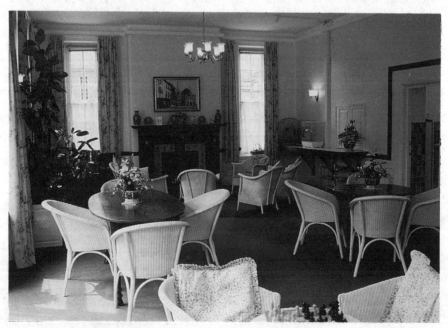

Figure 21.1   The large day room.

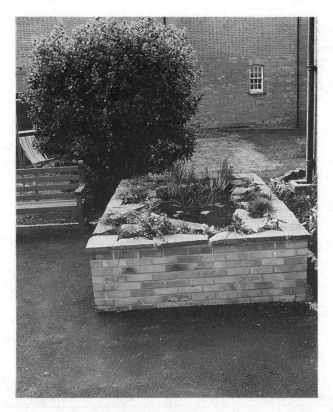

Figure 21.2   The garden with raised fish pond.

communicate. The degree of autonomy with which they would be expected to work was reflected in the Whitley nursing grade B allocated to the post. For its first four years, the centre was managed by an unqualified but experienced nursing assistant who had been closely involved throughout the development phase.

The initial focus of the centre was primarily to provide therapeutic activities for patients from the five single-sex continuing care wards and the mixed-sex admission/assessment ward which at that time comprised the Department of Mental Health Services for the Elderly. The patient population represented a broad spectrum of abilities, and, while most patients were suffering from dementing illnesses (albeit at different stages of the disease process), a sizeable minority had a diagnosis of functional mental illness. The latter group had mostly been transferred from the rehabilitation unit after many years of hospitalization as their physical dependency increased, but their level of cognitive functioning remained relatively intact. The varying needs of this disparate care group were matched by the range of activities offered by the centre, generating considerable interest from other organizations and attracting praise for its innovative practice at that time.

A CHANGE IN FOCUS

Subsequent developments, outlined below, have led to a change in the structure and function of the centre. Following the manager's retirement, which coincided with the acquisition of trust status and associated restructuring, it was decided that the needs of the client group had changed to such an extent that professional supervision was required. A head occupational therapist, based in the unit's day hospital, assumed managerial responsibility.

A recently appointed activities co-ordinator (occupational therapy technician 2), working under the direction of the occupational therapist, is responsible for the operational management of the centre. She is currently supported by three full-time and two part-time unqualified activities assistants. They continue to be paid as B grades under the Whitley nursing pay scale.

The activity co-ordinator has developed, and continues to develop, the role of volunteers within the centre. There is an active recruitment campaign, via advertisements in the local press. Respondents are sent job descriptions and application forms. References are taken up and prospective candidates are interviewed to establish hobbies, interests, skills, experience and personality. Those who are accepted work the hours they are able, whenever they can. There is no upper age limit for volunteers, and, indeed, many from the older generation are particularly well able to establish a rapport with the patients they help to care for. Basic instruction in the procedure to follow in the event of fire and in handling wheelchairs is given. There are plans to expand the training programme for volunteers in the future.

In the last two years, introduction of the Community Care Act has resulted in a change in the patient profile and a significant increase in average dependency. Many of the activities that were successful in the early days of the centre are no longer appropriate and the majority of the therapeutic programmes offered are now focused towards the more profoundly handicapped patients.

CURRENT FUNCTION

The philosophy of the centre is founded on the principle that each individual, no matter how impaired, retains the capacity to enjoy and participate in social interaction. For many people, the connotations of dementia are totally negative, with memory loss and declining intellect presenting an unrelieved picture of dwindling faculties and increasing failure. The sufferer's potential for sociability, often retained late into the illness, is frequently ignored. Depression, a common feature of dementia, may result in poor motivation, while inactivity appears to accelerate the progress of the illness, a vicious circle that the services provided by the centre aim to check by introducing pleasurable experiences into the patient's life.

Within the centre, activities focus on residual abilities and provide the opportunities to succeed that are lacking in so many other areas of the patient's existence. The wide range of activities available encompass social, domestic, physical and cognitive factors and are all designed to take account of the patient's skills, interests and individuality. Each patient is individually assessed, previous interests established, remaining skills identified and programmes developed. A programme is sent to all wards, detailing the events planned for the week, both on a group and on an individual basis. Forthcoming social events and attractions are advertised on a large noticeboard mounted outside the wards.

Activities are carried out in group settings, both small and large, and on an individual basis. The emphasis is on adapting each activity to the individual's functional ability, if necessary breaking it down into small steps and ensuring it is free of the risk of failure as far as possible.

Practical pursuits, such as art, cookery and gardening, are often planned on a one-to-one level to allow close supervision. Large groups are organized regularly, and dancing, music, parties and outside entertainment are popular. Boules and croquet are played on the lawn.

A minibus, equipped to take wheelchairs, is available weekly for individual or group outings to places of interest or of special meaning to patients. Excursions may include cricket matches, picnics, pub lunches or a day at the races. There are currently two drivers, both qualified nurses, within the Department of Mental Health Services for the Elderly, who had been tested and approved by a local driving school to drive the minibus. One of the centre staff is planning to take the course in the near future.

Staff from the centre accompany patients wishing to attend the fortnightly interdenominational services in the chapel. The hospital chaplain, an accomplished guitarist, visits the centre on alternate weeks to lead singing sessions. The songs, secular and pastoral, are much enjoyed by all participants. Red Cross volunteers also visit every two weeks and provide hand care and hand massage, a service that is available to relatives as well.

Every fortnight, staff assist a small group of patients in the planning and preparation of a special meal to which their relatives or friends are invited. Numbers are deliberately restricted to three to six, plus guests, to promote an atmosphere of intimacy. Wine is served and table settings are reminiscent of a high-class restaurant. The occasion is always a great success: patients, both male and female, enjoy the opportunity to potter in the kitchen and derive great satisfaction from preparing a meal for others under supervision.

Many patients appreciate spending time in the shop and reminiscence room. Both of these are furnished and equipped in period style, encouraging recollection of earlier times and exploiting the relatively intact long-term memory. Items of memorabilia can be removed from either of these areas to encourage group discussion.

While the centre retains a dedicated establishment of its own, its staff also work in close liaison with other disciplines. In conjunction with physiotherapy staff they run a weekly physical exercise group, which includes activities such as skittles, armchair hockey, walks, dancing and exercise to music, in all of which people confined to wheelchairs are able to participate.

Nursing staff from the wards also attend the centre with their patients and have become increasingly involved in suggesting, planning and implementing activities. This has enabled staff, whose chief priority is meeting physical needs, to look at another dimension of care, equally important to the patient's quality of life. Many have seen responses not encountered on the wards, enabling them to make a more objective assessment of their patients' capabilities and limitations. In the interests of safety, one ward moved all its patients and staff to the centre for the day to allow essential structural work to be carried out unimpeded. This proved such a success that, although the refurbishment is complete, they have continued to repeat the exercise.

THE ROLE OF RELATIVES

Relatives are always actively involved in the assessment process and are welcome to attend sessions with patients. Their participation is particularly useful in providing support and encouragement and they, in turn, appreciate the opportunity to contribute to the programme of care and to gain positive feedback at first hand.

The centre also provides a comfortable and relaxing venue for the monthly relatives' support group. The activity co-ordinator attends, canvassing their views on, and ideas for, the activities offered.

ORGANIZATION

The day is divided into morning and afternoon sessions, although more than one activity will be taking place at any one time to take account of the limited attention span and range of abilities and interests of the client group. The activity co-ordinator maintains a register to monitor attendance, which is totally flexible depending on individual need, varying from one to seven sessions per week.

Patients attending the centre originate from the admission/assessment ward and from the remaining three continuing care wards within the unit. While patients from the latter are never excluded from attendance other than for physical illness or extremely disruptive behaviour, occasionally patients from the former, who are still insecure in the hospital environment, require a little time to settle into the ward.

The Nightingale Centre initially operated from 8.30 a.m. to 4.30 p.m., Monday to Friday, with some flexibility to allow for evening activities, such as barbecues. The service has now been extended to seven days a week. Although it is unmanned outside the original opening hours, the keys are available for any relatives or staff from the wards to use at other times. Relatives, in particular, often use it as a quiet retreat away from the ward where it can be difficult to ensure privacy.

EXPANDING THE SERVICE

Whereas in the past the centre itself formed the focus for all activities, the emphasis has since shifted towards providing a service on the wards. The old system of providing activities exclusively within the centre contained a number of inherent disadvantages. The logistics of transporting patients, the majority of whom were wheelchair-bound, presented a problem, requiring considerable resources in terms of manpower and time. The service was sometimes viewed as elitist by ward staff since patients with more challenging behaviour were difficult to contain within the centre and hence tended to be excluded. The practice of separating care into components of social care, taking place in the Nightingale Centre, and physical care, carried out on the wards, risked reinforcing the fragmented and biased view of the individual that the centre had been designed to overcome.

The Nightingale staff now spend a proportion of their time working on wards with staff and patients, developing ward-based expertise in providing meaningful occupation for patients. This also gives them an opportunity to get to know patients away from the centre and to share information and ideas. Every activity assistant has a particular ward to which they act as link person, and they attend the ward handover at least once a week, contributing details about patients' social performance at the centre.

Many patients within the unit are now profoundly disoriented and physically frail and their ability to engage in participative activity is extremely limited. In an attempt to remedy the deficit in the service to this client group, *Snoezelen* therapy has been introduced. This was initially developed in the Netherlands for people with learning disabilities but its use has since been found to be effective with patients with dementia. The word '*Snoezelen*' is derived from the amalgamation of two Dutch words, meaning sniffing and dozing. *Snoezelen* therapy relies on sensory stimulation within a controlled environment, using a unique combination of light, music, vibration and aromatherapy to induce relaxation through the tactile, auditory, olfactory and visual sensations that the patient experiences.

A room on one of the wards has been used to house the *Snoezelen* equipment and can be used at any time by staff or relatives. *Snoezelen* therapy has proved very useful for restless and/or agitated patients, who usually respond very quickly to this soothing assault on the senses. The experience is obviously pleasurable to patients, many of whom are reluctant to leave the room. Its 24 hour availability means it can be used to take account of diurnal variations in behaviour, such as evening wandering, and the equipment can be transported for use with bedbound patients.

CONCLUSION

Within the next two years, the Department of Mental Health Services for the Elderly will be moving to community-based units in which social activity will be an integral part of individual treatment programmes. The Nightingale Centre has been instrumental in paving the way forwards, promoting a more balanced and sensitive response to the needs of the older people who use the psychiatric services in Chichester. It has demonstrated that people with dementia still retain the capacity to enjoy life, to gain pleasure from personal achievement and social interaction, and to appreciate the opportunity to explore new creative outlets.

The Bolingbroke
Hospital long-term care
project

22

INTRODUCTION

The Bolingbroke Hospital long-term care project provides nine multiply handicapped older people with the highest standards of personalized accommodation. The project provides a personalized home within a hospital. To achieve this the furniture and furnishing were specifically designed. The rooms are decorated with fabric-covered panels that hang from a specially designed picture rail, so each person can choose their colour scheme. The bedside lockers, wardrobe and chest of drawers also hang from a rail, so that the floor is clear and to facilitate personalization.

Using this method, personalization becomes easy. The basic research for the project took three years. The underlying hypothesis concerned the impact of personal belongings (Millard and Smith, 1981). Although it was opened in 1987, it still attracts visitors from home and abroad. Then few people in the UK accepted that single-room accommodation for long-stay patients should be the norm. Now few doubt that long-term care of older people should be provided in single rooms, and the next step is to get universal training for all who work in long-term care.

Writing about the spread of civilization, Lord Raglan used the analogy of a fish touching the top of the pond to illustrate the spread of ideas as ripples. Using that analogy, the Bolingbroke Project is like a koy carp; visitors ask 'How much did it cost?', but we do not know the design cost. Its design represented the combined efforts of innumerable people from different walks of life, all of whom shared a common vision of providing a better world for long-stay patients.

Major co-operating agencies were the staff of the department of geriatric medicine attached to St George's Hospital Medical School in Tooting, the Bolingbroke Hospital nursing, therapy, administration, domestic, works and catering departments, the Hotel and Catering Division of the University of Surrey, the London College of Furniture, the Department of Health and Social Security Architects' Department, Charles Den Roche of Simple Systems, whose company designed the method of wall hanging, and a host of others, including carpet and equipment manufacturers, visitors, patients and relatives.

If you want to undertake a similar project, do not mention the cost. This is important, for until you know what you can do, you do not know how much it will cost. The most important thing is to decide what you want to do, then when you know what you want, raise the money to do it. Eventually our project cost us £15 000 more than a simple upgrade.

If having read about the project you wish to visit, then visits are arranged, with the permission of the patients, on Wednesday afternoons, between 2.00 and 4.00 p.m. Prior booking is essential: write to the Ward Sister, Charles Ryall Ward, Bolingbroke Hospital, Wandsworth Common, London SW11. You will see a standard of living that an affluent society can easily afford.

This brief chapter gives no more than a flavour of the project. It concludes with an update and photographs of the ward that give a glimpse of its splendour.

SOCIAL POLICY SIGNIFICANCE

A false premise is that the care provided out of institutional settings is superior to that provided within. Support for this misconception is widespread among professionals and the population at large. Consequently, hospital long-term care is seen as second best and incapable of meeting the needs of those for whom it provides. Therefore, care in the community is fostered because it is thought to improve choice. Few people, however, would choose to be sick, to be disabled, to have no money, to live in a poor house, to have no family and friends. It is not the poor who choose, it is the community in which they live that makes the choice.

Negative attitudes relating to institutions are deep-rooted. On one level, the institution is seen as a place of punishment or confinement. In his book *Erehwon*, Samuel Butler used the analogy of punishment for ill-health and treatment for crime. The crime of the aged long-stay patient is to not be rehabilitable, to be difficult to treat, to be a widow(er), and to have no children or friends.

The use of wards in isolated long-stay psychiatric hospitals for older people enhances the view of punishment for sickness. Similarly, the open wards of our long-stay hospitals punish people for being sick: stripped of their possessions, dressed in other peoples' clothes, addressed by their first names, long-stay patients wait for death.

The concept that long-term care is punishment is enhanced by the fact that many departments of geriatric medicine have allocated beds in old workhouses. Older people remember the workhouse for what it was: a place of confinement and punishment for those who had not learnt the benefit of the work ethic. The image is dependency: the stigma is uselessness. Couple inherent environmental defects with the lack of staff training, and it is hardly surprising that 'care in the community' is perceived as the answer to all problems. Yet hospitals are part of the community, and, irrespective of how good the care provided at home is, some older people will still need to be tended within institutions (Millard, 1994). Consequently, for older people with complex problems, long-stay hospital care is the right choice.

THE DANISH PERSPECTIVE

The roots of the Bolingbroke Hospital long-term care project lie in a visit to Denmark sponsored by the King Edward's Hospital Fund of London. The intention of the visit was to see the lack of physician-led rehabilitation. That was seen to be correct, but the overwhelming impression of the care of older people in Denmark that the group came away with was the quality of the accommodation in nursing and residential homes. All residents had single rooms: private lavatories were the norm and residents were encouraged to furnish their rooms with their own possessions.

Denmark chooses to tend its sick older people in a way that respects older people's contribution to their society. The Danes are aware that their society will, if the worst comes to the worst, tend them in their old age. In so doing, Denmark shows how it values its old people, as it does not throw them in the dustbins of their affluent society. Yet all is not perfect, for the lack of rehabilitation, coupled with the absence of a geriatric medical service, forces too many into care. In 1979, extra beds were to be found in the bathrooms and corridors of acute hospitals, and old wards were still being used for people waiting for places in nursing homes.

After the visit, we were convinced that the British long-term care system required Danish standards of accommodation, while the Danish healthcare system required British concepts of rehabilitation. People visiting Denmark without knowledge of rehabilitation may leave with the wrong impression. It is important to recognize that the quality of long-stay care shows how a society values the older people whom it cannot rehabilitate. It does not demonstrate that community care, based on rehabilitation, is not the best option for the majority. Personal belongings, single rooms, fabric-covered walls, etc, ice the cake of our department of geriatric medicine, but the project is not the cake. The cake is an effective dedicated medical department committed to diagnosing, treating, rehabilitating and supporting older people and their carers.

REHABILITATION IN PERSPECTIVE

The NHS, rehabilitation and operational planning are three healthcare legacies of World War II (Timm, 1967). The concept of a national health service was rooted in the depression (Pater, 1981); the split of responsibility between social service departments and hospitals for long-term care came about because of a combination of complaints concerning the aftercare of discharged chronic sick patients and the movement of the population that took place because of the bombing of London during World War II (Means and Smith, 1983). The complaints about aftercare led to an inquiry that recognized that the chronic sick were suffering from lack of medical leadership, teamwork, rehabilitation; the bombing of cities showed that frail older people could manage in seaside hotels. Thus, at the start of the NHS, responsibility for the chronic sick was placed on the hospital service while responsibility for frail older people remained with local government.

THE ROOTS OF THE PROJECT

Defined medical responsibility for long-term care is the key to quality control (Millard, 1993). To cope with this responsibility, the St George's

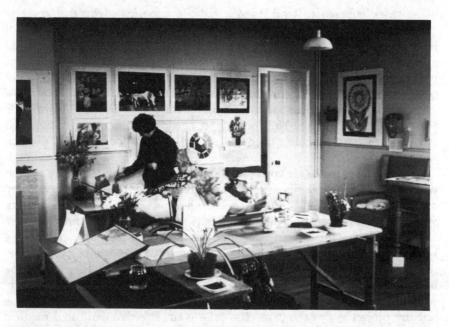

Figure 22.1 Art at Cheam, 1973: the art teacher, Mrs Audrey Huntley, and two artists.

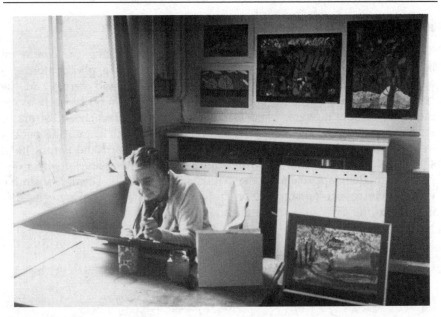

Figure 22.2 An artist at work.

department of geriatric medicine provides a no waiting list, active, therapeutic, needs-related service with combined acute rehabilitation wards and
long-stay wards. The department has been developing since 1968. Our
new way of looking at long-term care started in 1972 when an art teacher,
Mrs Audrey Huntley, came to an isolated long-stay hospital. Within a
year, she had taught long-stay patients to paint. Soon visitors were
coming to the hospital, not out of pity for the older residents, but to
admire their work (Figures 22.1 and 22.2).

The next major influence was the film 'Away from the Workhouse'
made in Professor Hall's department in Southampton. This film developed
the concept of patient committees. To see for ourselves, we took a coach-
load of staff and one patient from Cheam Hospital to meet the staff and
residents of Ashford Hospital. Thereafter we introduced a patient
committee. This simple action resulted, among other things, in a ward
Christmas party, a cheese and wine evening, a summer barbecue and an
evening bonfire and fireworks. At that stage, proud of our achievements,
Roger Burton, the department's social worker, and Professor Millard,
visited Denmark. There we saw in-patients surrounded by possessions.
The effect was striking. We felt like burglars in their rooms.

Soon after, Chris Smith, a psychologist doing an MSc course at St
George's, helped to test the hypothesis that personal belongings have a
positive effect.

PERSONAL BELONGINGS: THEIR POSITIVE EFFECT

The test was simple. Second-year medical students taking the course on ageing were divided into two groups: one group saw a photograph of a patient surrounded by family photographs, flowers and cards; and the other group saw the same patient in bare surroundings. In each room, individual students were asked to complete an adjective check list and a semantic differential test in which subjects were asked to rate the patient in the photograph on a bipolar scale. The results (Millard and Smith, 1981) showed a trend for the students who saw the possessions to be more positive in their approach to the patient. Thereafter, it seemed a simple matter to introduce personal belongings into long-stay care. However, that is far from the case. Impediments abound.

IMPEDIMENTS TO PERSONALIZATION

ASSET STRIPPING

Long-stay patients undergo social asset stripping. The path to a long-term care ward is not an easy one; few come directly from their own home. Most have passed through other places first. A child's home or a residential home often intervene, and personal belongings are discarded at each stage. Consequently, for many long-stay patients, even the simple goal of two photographs is impossible to fulfil, let alone retrieving their cherished possessions.

INSTITUTIONAL RULES

Institutionalized staff resist change. Staff ask questions such as 'Why put photographs behind her bed when she is blind?' 'Who is to be responsible if they are broken or stolen?' 'What about fire, dust, clutter, infection?' At each turn, the inertia of the institution has to be overcome.

UNSUITABILITY OF THE ENVIRONMENT

At Cheam Hospital in Sutton the long-stay patients were housed in four 18-bedded Nightingale wards designed for infectious diseases. You can't put pictures on curtains. Beds were often under the windows. Equipment attached to the walls got in the way. Many reasons intervened. We therefore compromised with patient identity boards and a wall-mounted board on which to pin photographs. Despite the compromise, by 1983, less than a third of the patients had a few personal mementos.

BELONGINGS DAMAGE WALLS

Picture nails damage the walls. Long-stay patients stay for a long time, but they are still transient. Others follow. Wards are expensive to decorate. Wilful damage must be avoided. The first principle taught in schools of hotel and catering is care of the environment. If you want to run a nice hospital or residential home, make sure that notices are not stuck up with Sellotape, as sticky tape damages the walls and leaves unsightly marks.

AN OPPORTUNITY TO EXPERIMENT

In 1979, on his appointment as Professor of Geriatric Medicine, Professor Millard gave up working in the London Borough of Merton and moved to run the geriatric medical services for part of the London Borough of Wandsworth. Wandsworth had no geriatric beds in the district general hospital at that time. All the beds were in long-stay hospitals. Although much good work was being done, the hospitals were inadequate for modern diagnosis and treatment, so, in 1980, the decision was made to transfer the patients from St Benedict's Hospital to the Bolingbroke Hospital. Thus, in 1981, the Bolingbroke Hospital, a 100-bedded acute hospital, received 96 long-stay patients on transfer from St Benedict's Hospital. To capitalize on the forced marriage of acute and long-stay hospitals, it was decided that all wards should become acute; within one year, five had succeeded. The failure of one ward to succeed was the opportunity we needed.

THE BOLINGBROKE PROJECT

Bolingbroke Hospital had five Nightingale wards, each containing between 15 to 21 beds, and one ward, the Charles Ryall ward, previously used as the private patients' ward, with six single rooms, two twin rooms and a three-bedded bay at the far end of the ward. However, it was badly in need of redecorating, replumbing and rewiring. The staff in the single-room ward had developed a first-class rehabilitative environment. Their reward was the transfer of the long-stay patients from the ward that had failed to become acute.

KEYS TO SUCCESS

APPOINT A PROJECT CO-ORDINATOR

Key to the success of any innovative project is the employment of an individual who shares the dream. The salary of a technician's post in the medical school was supplemented by the St George's Hospital endowment funds to employ Ms Rosemary Horsfall as a research assistant. Trained as a nurse, she had for several years been casework co-ordinator with the charity Counsel and Care for the Elderly. She brought knowledge of statutory and voluntary-sector residential and nursing homes and shared our desire to develop a model unit. Her contribution ensured our success.

SELECT THE WARD-BASED STAFF

Choice of the correct nursing staff comes next. All the nurses, trained and untrained, on day and night duty, working in the Charles Ryall ward were interviewed individually by the project co-ordinator, Professor Millard and the senior nurse manager. All wanted to move – so all stayed.

People who visit now would be surprised to find that many of the nurses they see who run the ward so well were in the original group. The reason for their desire to move is retrospectively clear. People dislike change. In the case of the staff of the project ward, they had already had one major upheaval. In addition, they had succeeded in the primary task of developing a rehabilitative environment and their success was to be punished from the glamour of acute and rehabilitation to become long-stay.

Freedom of choice is a myth. People talk of the rights of staff and patients to choose. In reality, there is little choice. Managers choose what happens to wards and the staff and patients accept. If a managerial team decides to change the operational policy, they must sell that policy to the staff whom they employ. Rosenthal and Jacobson in *Pygmalion in the Classroom* showed that 'If children are failing at school, you should look at the teachers and not the taught'. Similarly, if patients are mismanaged, one should blame the managers not the staff they employ.

BUILD THE TEAM

An inherent problem in teamwork is conflict. It is tempting to try at any cost to avoid the traumas associated with the building of a team. Yet without teams nothing can be achieved. Even if the knowledge required to develop a new style of patient management is contained in one individual, that individual can do nothing on their own.

INVOLVE THE PATIENTS

The patient must be part of the team. Changing the world of long-stay patients involves them more intimately than it involves us. Staff may not like the idea of change, but older people recognize that if life is to advance, change must occur. Regular meetings with patients are essential to success. At our meetings, the patients were made aware of the reasoning behind the project and the objects that we wanted to achieve. Some could not understand, but we did not exclude them. Our motto for the project was 'The best for the worst'. If this is the philosophy, nothing is gained by exclusion. Some of our patients did not live to see the finished project, but both they and their relatives willingly accepted that to achieve our final goal they had to be inconvenienced. How much, neither they, nor we, realized. The contractors had to knock down part of the wall in the ward in which they were housed. We then had ten patients in a ward designed for six, and the patients and staff were overcrowded, cramped and uncomfortable. Yet no-one complained as they were willing participators in the dream.

INVOLVE THE ANCILLARY STAFF

Ancillary staff must also be involved. Involve the porters, the cleaners, the domestics and the works staff. Get them together and tell them what you are doing and why you are doing it. They have ideas and experience and their contribution is essential to the success of the whole; they take pride in their work and have justifiable pride in the achievement. That our project succeeded was to a large extent due to their willingness to help. Without them we would have achieved nothing; ignore them and you will achieve nothing. You can design the finest environment but unless your staff look after it you achieve nothing. Overlook ancillary staff training and involvement and you overlook the most important cornerstone in the building of your new ward.

INVOLVE THE PROFESSIONALS ALLIED TO MEDICINE

A third essential group are the therapists, social workers, dietitians and nurses. They had much of the expertise that we required; as such they needed to be consulted and involved throughout the project. Without them, we could not have developed the idea, formulated and discussed the principles, and developed the teaching.

Each profession has its own skills. Do not expect a ward sister to be an expert in colour co-ordination, nor a therapist to design a bathroom. Each profession has its own knowledge base. You need to involve representatives of the hospital administration, the hospital engineers and the works department. Professional skills need to be complemented by others. Hospital works departments have considerable expertise in upgrading hospitals but they have little skills in designing hotels. If you are to design a hotel within the hospital, turn outwards and involve others.

DEVELOP A DEMONSTRATION ROOM

We started our project by decorating one room. The cost involved was minimal. We wallpapered it, put up picture rails, attached a few pictures and carpeted the floor. This illustrated what we wanted to achieve. We involved one patient and her family in the selection of the colour scheme. Sadly she died three weeks after the room was completed so the next patient entered an already decorated room. However, she and her son ensured our success.

The principle we wanted to demonstrate was that hospital patients could have rooms with their possessions and that visitors and staff could only enter with the resident's permission. The willingness of our first resident, and subsequently of other residents, to allow strangers into their rooms has ensured that the ideas behind our concept spread.

Retrospectively, it seems surprising that all the visitors came to see was a wallpapered and carpeted room. But from that room the whole project grew, and there we identified the basic principles of care.

UNDERSTANDING THE BASIC PRINCIPLES OF CARE

Public and private space

Soon after we began, we realized that we had to separate the public and the private space. We did this because visitors were entering the patients' room space without permission. As the day room was at the far end of the ward, the solution was to move it to the other end. Now the day room is the first space that visitors enter. To separate the unit from the general hustle and bustle of the hospital, the front door has a knocker. The principle is that the day room is public space, while the bedrooms are private space. Separating public and private space identifies territory and has the advantage that it restricts access and prevents casual theft of personal belongings. Our working rule is that no visitors can enter private space without the patient's permission.

Personalized accommodation

The room is the patient's. As it is their room, their name must be on the door. They should choose the colour scheme. Their belonging and their pictures should be on the walls. Personalization damages the walls. In our demonstration room, we learnt that wallpaper gets torn adjusting the bed; wheelchairs knock the walls. Picture nails mark the walls and pictures leave fade marks. In addition, when a patient dies, it is difficult to justify re-wallpapering a room that has only recently been decorated. Redecoration takes time, and time is limited. Hospital beds must be kept in use. Eventually we solved the problem by hanging reversible decorative fabric panels from a specially designed rail.

HELPFUL CONCEPTS

MONEY IS NOT THE PROBLEM

Share the dream. Speak to the League of Friends. Talk to pensioner's groups. Mention it in public lectures. Welcome visitors. We were fortunate. The League of Friends paid for the first room to be upgraded. The King Edward's Hospital Fund for London gave £25 000. The Hotel and Catering Division of the University of Surrey advised us on the room arrangement. The London College of Furniture staff and students designed the new style of furniture and furnishing. The DHSS Architects' Department redesigned the layout. The works aspect of our project eventually cost £250 000, yet the contribution of others was without price.

BUILD A MODEL

Our dream nearly failed because we did not build a model. Architects can understand lines on plans: staff cannot. Our demonstration room showed what we wanted to do. There we learnt the principles of care but we were not knowledgeable enough to develop a comprehensive plan. Fortunately, the late Mr Brian Hitchcox of the DHSS Architects' Department was. He shared our dream of single-room accommodation, then built a model to show that rooms need supporting facilities.

That model, which still hangs from the wall in the education centre, is silent witness to our mistakes. We had totally overlooked the necessity of redesigning the bathrooms and sluices. We had failed to make proper use of the balcony. We had failed to make a proper bridge between the project ward and the next-door ward, and we had failed to even consider the design of the six-bedded bay in an adjacent ward. The model showed we were out of our depth. Now we recommend that all projects should have mock-up rooms and model layouts as these are an essential prerequisite of planning.

RECOGNIZE YOUR OWN LIMITATIONS

The Bolingbroke Project stands as witness to the skills of others. The day it was completed, the Bolingbroke staff realized that we could never even have begun to design the finished project. Our training skills were medical, nursing, therapy and administration. We understood the basic principles of running a department of geriatric medicine. We knew nothing about the manufacture and design of furniture, the way to lay out a hotel room, to plan a hospital ward, to colour co-ordinate or a host of other tasks. The knowledge is vast and our ignorance was extensive. The research into personal belongings established the concept, but the fulfilment of the dream rested on the creation of an environment in which others could bring their professional skills to play.

BUILD ON THE PEOPLE THAT YOU HAVE

Your dreams will never materialize if you denigrate the material with which you have to work. Start where you are, with the staff, the patients and the buildings that you have. Take an inventory of the good things that you have. Recognize what people can do, don't harp on what they cannot. Take pride in providing the best service for the most severely handicapped people for they truly require your professional skills.

If you want to institute change you must broaden your horizons, visit other wards and departments, even in your own hospital. Have an open day on your own ward. Ask others to visit you. Apply for grants to travel elsewhere. Arrange a visit by staff of your hospital to another hospital, and make it an annual event (we do). Then you will see that, although you do some things better than others, others do some things better than you.

UPDATE ON THE PROJECT

The long-term care ward in Bolingbroke Hospital is continuing to provide an excellent standard of accommodation and care for nine multiply handicapped older people. Separation of public and private space and personalized accommodation remain firmly established as the pivotal principles of the project. The corridor walls and carpets have been changed but the decorative panels are still the same. In some cases, however, it proves difficult to obtain personal belongings from relatives.

A recent SWOT analysis (strengths, weaknesses, opportunities, threats) confirmed the many strengths of the project: individual choice for patients, autonomy, homely environment, availability of acute care when needed, a high degree of hygiene and cleanliness, a team spirit amongst nursing staff, and compassion towards patients, especially in terminal care. Amongst the weaknesses were the heavy workload for nurses and the fact that the patients actually get spoiled!

The main threat at the moment seems to be the possible relocation to St George's Hospital, Tooting. Other threats mentioned are cuts as well as changes in nursing staff. Application of the CARE scheme (derived from 'High-quality long-term care', RCP, 1992) as a tool for auditing long-term care, revealed excellent performance on the key indicators of:

- preserving autonomy
- promoting faecal continence
- optimizing drug use
- managing falls and accidents
- preventing pressure sores
- optimizing the environments, equipment and aids

- the medical role in long-term care: specific standards for doctors to adhere to.

CONCLUSION

The Bolingbroke Project stands silent witness to the way that a civilized society could choose to tend its sick and frail dependants. The decorative standards seem to many visitors to be too high. Time has shown that the design solution of hanging furniture and fabric panels from the walls is the correct one. Achieving universal usage requires inventions to be marketed and sold. That requires the skills of others. However, what is certain is that the care of long-stay older patients in the UK will never be the same again.

Figures 22.3 to 22.6 show a view of the front door with its knocker, the dayroom, and the decorative design of two rooms. The chosen pictures do not illustrate the carpets on the floors, the names on the doors, or the blue and pink bathrooms which contain special baths and equipment necessary for the staff to do their work. Hopefully, however, they may give some insight into the project, and perhaps encourage others to try to build a better world where they are.

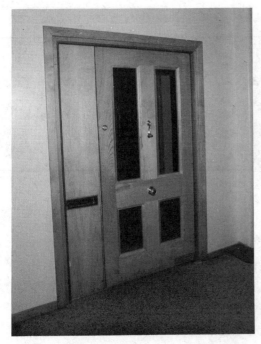

Figure 22.3 Front door and knocker.

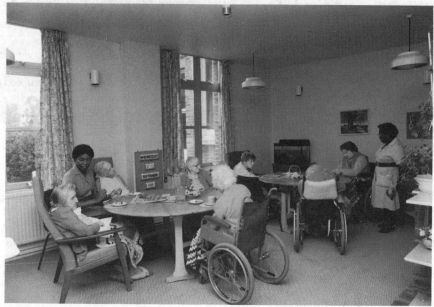

Figure 22.4 Public space.

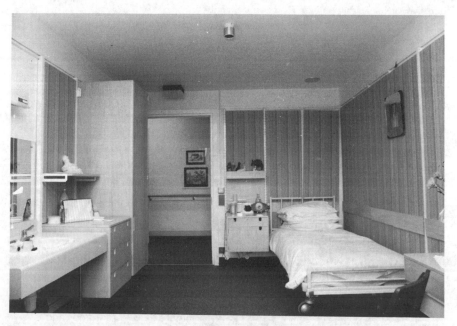

Figure 22.5 The hanging furniture and decorative panels.

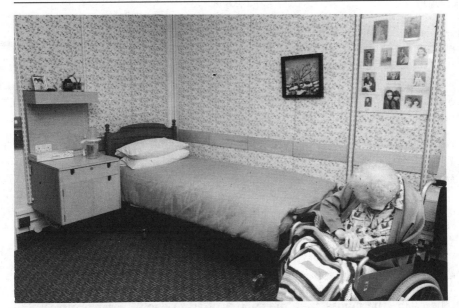

Figure 22.6   A patient in her room.

ACKNOWLEDGEMENTS

We thank Mrs Elizabeth Mosby for preparing the manuscript, the multi-disciplinary laboratory staff at St George's Hospital Medical School for taking the photographs, Ms Charlotte Walden for an early draft of this article, and Dr Paul Higgs for his assistance. In addition, we acknowledge with gratitude the debt we owe to countless people, both living and dead, for the assistance they gave in making a dream reality.

REFERENCES

Means, R. and Smith, R. (1983) From public assistance institutions to 'sunshine hotels': changing state perceptions about residential care for older people 1939–1948. *Ageing Soc.*, **3**, 157–81.

Millard, P.H. and Smith, C.S. (1981) Personal belongings – a positive effect? *Gerontologist*, **21**, 85–90.

Millard, P.H. (1993) The seven principles of planning geriatric medical services. *Health and Hygiene*, **14**, 95–8.

Millard, P.H. (1994) Meeting the needs of an ageing population. *Proc. R. Coll. Physicians Edinb.*, **24**, 187–96.

Pater, J.E. (1981) *The Makings of the National Health Service*, King Edward's Hospital Fund for London, London.

Royal College of Physicians (1992) *High-quality long-term care for elderly people: guidelines and audit measures*, Royal College of Physicians, London.

Timm, O.K. (1967) Rehabilitation; to what? *J. Am. Geriatr. Soc.*, **15**, 709–16.

Jubilee House

23

INTRODUCTION

Jubilee House was one of three experimental homes that were set up to test the feasibility of providing nursing home care for older people within the NHS. The homes were the subject of an in-depth research project, the main aim of which was to make comparisons with existing long-stay wards. Political changes have reduced the number of long-stay care beds within the NHS but the findings are still important to organizers of long-stay care whatever the setting. Valuable information has been gained both from the official report and from the comments of the staff and residents who worked under the research spotlight.

EVALUATION OF THE NHS NURSING HOME PROJECT

The main component of the research was a randomized control trial that aimed to compare residents in the experimental homes with patients in associated long-stay wards. The objective of this was to compare clinical effectiveness, patient satisfaction, staff satisfaction and the cost of the two modes of care (Bond, 1984).

CLINICAL EFFECTIVENESS

No significant differences in clinical care were demonstrated. The nursing home provided nurse-led care with input as needed from a general practitioner. This was compared with the consultant-led care of the traditional hospital wards. The research found that the home care was clinically as effective as hospital care. Before concluding that nurse-led care is generally as effective as medical care, two points must be noted. The first is that referrals to the project could only be made by a consultant geriatrician. This meant that residents and controls had been carefully assessed and any medical conditions controlled as far as possible. Secondly, the homes were led by nurses who were experienced in long-term care and had been specially trained for their role.

COST

The cost of the NHS homes proved, perhaps surprisingly, to be less than for long-stay hospital wards. The researchers considered this to be because the nursing homes had greater flexibility in staff roles. There was no need to stick to rigid shift patterns or rigid boundaries between roles. Their self-contained situations also allowed more control over financial resources. The research team concluded that it should be possible to provide 'good quality NHS nursing home care at a cost that is no greater than hospital care' (Donaldson and Bond, 1991).

PATIENT SATISFACTION

Consumer views were significantly more positive in all three homes than in hospital wards (Donaldson and Bond, 1991). Residents in the NHS nursing homes were less likely to express negative views about staff. They were more likely to state that they had sufficient privacy to see visitors and more likely to have seen sufficient visitors. Those in the long-stay wards were more likely to wake and rise early and to describe their reasons for rising as staff-orientated (Bond et al., 1989).

Residents in nursing homes were found to be significantly more likely to be engaged in meaningful activity during the morning and afternoon and in verbal interaction over lunch time (Bond and Bond, 1990). There can be no definitive measure of quality of life but it seems reasonable to assume that, in frail older people, higher levels of mental engagement and activity do equate with greater happiness. The increase in engagement in the homes was as much due to organizational factors as to structured entertainment. Seating arrangements, particularly during meal times, were designed to encourage residents to speak to each other. The length of meal times allowed them to be social as well as functional. The commitment to resident choice meant that frequent discussions were needed between staff and residents. The researchers point out that enforced activities in the form of 'entertainment' can result in lower levels of engagement than where there is no formal programme (Bond and Bond, 1990).

STAFF SATISFACTION

Several important differences were found in the staff's background and perception of their role (Bond and Bond, 1992). Staff in NHS nursing homes:

- had more education and training related to the care of older people, but had worked in the field for less time than hospital staff;
- perceived their patients differently as having more social needs with greater individuality;
- regarded their work differently, less as 'just basic care' and more as skilled work oriented to the needs of the resident rather than the organization;
- indicated more satisfaction with their job and specifically with variety in their work, use of skills and abilities, sense of achievement and in-service training.

Clearly staff in the NHS homes had a more positive view of their role.

Traditionally, work in long-stay care has been seen as of lower status than other forms of health care. These findings suggest that instilling a sense of pride and recognizing expertise can significantly improve quality of life for residents. The researchers recommend that staff have the opportunity to share ideals of care and work out methods of putting them into practice. Management practices should encourage maximum autonomy for all grades of staff including nursing assistants. If staff are not given a high degree of trust and autonomy, they will not give trust and autonomy to their residents.

The findings have implications for the future training of staff in any long-stay environments. The researchers go on to make several suggestions.

- All staff, irrespective of grade, joining an organization providing long-term care should receive appropriate induction training and ongoing in-service education that reflects the special needs of frail older people. Both staff and residents should be involved in the identification of training needs.
- A mechanism needs to be found whereby health professionals in their initial educational preparation may gain positive experience of long-term settings.
- An element of social gerontology and social aspects of caregiving should be included in the education of all health professionals who are involved in providing care to older people.

ENVIRONMENT

Jubilee House had 21 single and two twin rooms with a large sitting room, two dining areas and various other communal areas. The bedrooms were furnished, but residents could bring their own furniture if they wished. Each resident had a domestic-style commode that could be left in the room without giving a clinical appearance. Most residents used a commode at night and some preferred to use them during the day. The saving in staff time of having these facilities always available easily justified the expense of their purchase. All rooms had a TV aerial point and some residents had private telephone lines installed. Once settled in a room, the resident was encouraged to think of it as their own. They could arrange the furniture as they liked, bring as many of their own possessions as they liked and even decorate it to their own taste. No changes were made without the resident's agreement.

An anticipated disadvantage of single rooms was that residents would be reluctant to use the communal areas and risk becoming isolated. Contrary to expectations, the main sitting room was the place where residents chose to spend the major part of their day. This seems partly because it was the main entry point to the home. Residents sitting here were able to keep an eye on all comings and goings. Although some residents preferred to eat in their rooms, the dining rooms were well used. Both were furnished with round tables seating four people. The height of two of these tables was raised, as the optimum table top position varies from person to person. Finding the correct level can be critical for those who are struggling to eat independently despite disabilities. A pleasant ambience to the dining rooms was seen as a priority. Meal times should be a pleasure, something to be looked forward to rather than a task to be completed as quickly as possible. A measure of success was that staff chose to eat with the residents rather than using their own dining room.

When first opened, Jubilee House was furnished with chairs that were colour co-ordinated with the general decor. It was soon apparent that this was too restrictive. Disabled people who spend much of their day sitting in an armchair must be able to choose one that exactly suits their needs. What is needed is variety in the shape of the back and wings, in height and depth of the seat, and in design of the arms. The enormous advances in continence care products meant that chairs could be selected from domestic ranges without being restricted to wipe-clean fabrics.

Residents at Jubilee House were all physically disabled so they all used pressure-relief cushions and mattresses. This was initially expensive but the cost benefits of saving in staff time and the near eradication of pressure sores should prove persuasive to any financial manager. Similarly, the initial outlay on a good selection of sturdy hoists saves time and reduces the chance of injury.

PHILOSOPHY

The underlying philosophy of Jubilee House was that residents should run their own lives as far as possible. The home's written philosophy was prominently displayed. It was regularly reviewed by staff and residents and could be amended, by general agreement, at any time. This means that it remained a live statement and a yardstick by which all decisions could be measured. The basic philosophy has remained unchanged since Jubilee House opened:

> The rights of the resident to independence, individuality and dignity will be respected at all times as will their right to exercise choice and make decisions. Residents will be consulted, either directly or, if this is not feasible, through a friendly 'other', in all matters affecting their health and welfare. They will have control over their daily life, including times of awakening and taking meals, with recognition of their need for privacy, fellowship and entertainment at appropriate times.

Over the years, only one addition has been made. That is that other people's safety must not be compromised. This has been made explicit because otherwise the philosophy would be invalidated by occasionally making exceptions to it. Two circumstances brought about the need for this addition. Mr Cole continually dropped his lighted cigarettes as could be seen by innumerable small burn holes in the carpet around his favourite seat. Because of the risk of a serious fire, we had to take charge of his matches and insist that he should only smoke when a member of staff could sit with him. So that this didn't take on a punitive feeling, we also told staff that they could have a cigarette if they were sitting with him. (Mr Cole's cigarette consumption went up!) The clause has also been invoked when a resident's increasing disability made the use of a mechanical hoist the only safe way to get her into bed. She had been using her own bed that was not suitable for our mobile hoists. Exhaustive enquiries failed to find a practical alternative so, rather than risk injury to staff, the bed had to be changed.

It is important that all staff are aware of the ideals of the home because the nature of long-stay care means that different needs may conflict. Health requirements and personal choice are often at odds. Optimum mobility, for instance, was encouraged but never demanded. That may be the principal aim of a rehabilitation ward but our goals were different. A resident may have been advised to stop smoking or to rest on his bed for part of the day but the decision was theirs no matter what the medical implications.

PATTERN OF LIFE

Routine was not discouraged provided it was structured by the individual resident and not the institution. Cleaning schedules were arranged to suit the residents so that they did not feel pressure to be up at a certain time. Baths could be taken at any time and as frequently or infrequently as the resident chose. Cooked breakfasts were prepared on demand between 8 and 9 a.m. but cereal, toast and tea or coffee were available all morning. The advantage of the flexible breakfast was that residents could eat when they were up and ready. They were more relaxed and more able to help themselves. There was no pressure for individuals to tailor their morning routine to the needs of the institution. Residents were able to take their time, chat to their companions and linger over a second cup of tea. Those who thought this system would prove expensive on staff time were proved wrong. Time needed to individually prepare tea and toast was balanced by not having to wake residents to prepare them for breakfast.

A variety of diversional and social events were organized but there was no compulsion to attend. Regular sessions were arranged for the differing needs of residents. As the residents change, so does the popularity of different forms of entertainment. Activities proving most popular were often the simple ones such as a group of residents meeting once a week in the office for coffee and a chat with the clerical officer.

Recognition of the importance of personal territory was one of the original reasons for testing the nursing-home style as an alternative to the long-stay ward. Nobody entered a resident's room without knocking and waiting for a reply where possible, or allowing a reasonable pause if mental state or dysphasia made it impossible for the resident to respond. Staff had no right of entry. Most residents liked the security of occasional visits from staff during the night, but those who preferred to remain undisturbed had the right to do so.

All residents had a lockable drawer to which staff had no access. This could be used for valuables, drugs for those few residents who were physically and mentally capable of administering their own medicines, or simply for private belongings. On one occasion, a resident forcibly demonstrated his right to refuse treatment by locking away his speech therapy exercises and refusing to relinquish the key.

Many residents extended their desire for personal territory beyond the confines of their own room. There was a pattern of people claiming their own spot in the sitting room and their own place in a dining room.

Keeping in touch with their local community was an important part of the concept. To this end, the League of Friends provided a small car converted to take one wheelchair. A major advantage of this over a larger minibus is that the ease of loading and driving meant that it could be used by relatives with minimal instruction. Residents could tour the local town and sea front or visit friends rather than waiting for larger excursions that are complicated to organize and not to everybody's taste. Contributions to the cost of petrol were voluntary but most residents preferred to pay their expenses. The car became so popular that a booking system had to be established. Emphasis on smaller outings did not preclude the more organized trips for which a minibus could be hired.

A survey of residents' opinions showed close family relationships to be their highest priority. Staff training emphasized the need to make visitors welcome and to facilitate whatever role they wished to take. Where communication with residents was difficult, regular visitors told us that they found it easier to have other things to do within the home. The husband of one resident looked after the home's budgie and several relatives adopted their own flower bed. Relationships seemed more natural when periods of conversation were broken up by other activities.

Tea bars gave visitors the opportunity to make themselves a drink. A spare bedroom was available for overnight accommodation and friends could join residents for a meal (a small charge was made for these facilities). A well-stocked toy corner and a slide in the garden made Jubilee House popular with younger visitors.

OPPORTUNITIES FOR CONTROL BY RESIDENTS

Many of the innovations at Jubilee House have involved 'pushing back the boundaries' to see how far residents could and would wish to be involved in the running of their home.

The residents' committee was a major influence in shaping home management. Our hope that it would function with no staff input proved unrealistic, but the care assistant who convened meetings was nominated and elected by residents. The few necessary communal structures to daily life were decided by the residents' committee. Lunch and supper times were changed more than once according to their instruction.

As residents realized that the committee gave them a genuine role in the management of the home, they became more vocal, more likely to express any dissatisfactions, and more likely to raise matters unprompted by staff (Miller, 1986). One grievance raised by residents was that they did not like the way that death was handled in the home. We had been devoting our energies to comforting the relatives and the body was removed with a minimum of fuss to avoid upsetting the other residents. The residents felt excluded. They wanted to take a much larger part in the process. At the instigation of the committee, regular bulletins were given to all residents if anybody was ill and a garden of remembrance was created. Far from wanting death to be handled discreetly, residents wanted to discuss their grief for the death of a friend and their wishes and fears concerning their own death.

A more recent development was the involvement of residents in the employment of new staff. This had the dual advantage of giving residents control over a vital part of their lives and of demonstrating to new staff that the opinions of residents are highly valued. Being part of a panel interviewing prospective employees proved too tiring even for the most mentally alert of the residents. A compromise was to ask candidates to wait for their interview with a group of residents. The views of these residents were sought before a final decision was made.

NURSING CARE

The fundamental structure of the nursing process involves a continual cycle of assessment, planning, implementation and evaluation of care. The logic of this cycle is hard to dispute but the application of the process has seen a plethora of documents that are, in the main, more appropriate for use in acute than in long-stay areas. The result has been that many long-stay nurses have shied away from using the process. At Jubilee House, the nursing process was accepted enthusiastically. The structure was adapted to meet the needs of an area where changes are slow but time is always in short supply and where the majority of staff were unqualified care assistants and worked part-time. The written plans were unconventional but they were tailor-made to help the qualified nurses collect information, organize their ideas and communicate their decisions simply and quickly to the rest of the team (Sander, 1987).

With a care staff consisting predominantly of unqualified assistants, it was important that the expertise and skill of the trained nurses were used to their best advantage. Staff nurse and care assistant worked side by side meeting the residents' needs, but the plans for care were drawn up by qualified staff working as primary nurses. These primary nurses had up to six residents for whom they were responsible. Any task they performed for the resident was an opportunity to make an assessment of their needs: was the integrity of their skin threatened; were they taking sufficient fluid; was their pain control adequate?

Individuality of care is increased by primary nursing. With only one trained nurse on duty at a time, it was impossible for primary nurses to give all the care needed by the residents. However, they could use their specialized knowledge and skills to assess, plan and evaluate the care given. Part-time staff were primary nurse to fewer residents but the relationships they developed proved very beneficial.

So successful was the primary nurse scheme that we extended it to encourage special relationships between care assistants and residents. These care assistants were responsible for helping residents to arrange domestic affairs. This might include looking after their clothes or helping them to buy birthday presents for their family. The help in buying presents was particularly appreciated by many residents because it gave them the chance to maintain an active role as loving parent or spouse.

As there were more care assistants, they were linked with fewer residents and even closer relationships are possible. One resident had no visitors because her family were distressed by the personality disintegration that was part of her dementing process. Her care assistant made contact by letter when she requested information about the resident's past lifestyle. It was not suggested that they should visit, but such a rapport was built up that the daughters felt that they wanted to see their mother when 'their' care assistant was there to support them.

It had been the custom for primary nurses and care assistants to volunteer for their special relationships with residents. As we gained confidence with the system, this was reversed so that, where feasible, residents choose staff. A resident whose care assistant left demonstrated her feeling of control over the situation by expressing the change as 'I've taken on Rosie as my new care assistant'. This system could be threatening to staff as they might be exposed as unpopular with residents. It is to their credit both that they willingly accepted the scheme and that no member of the staff has ever been shunned by residents.

The trained nurses have skills and knowledge that they should share with their residents rather than impose on them. Their expertise is needed to prevent complications arising from underlying disabilities. Staff at a Jubilee House study day were asked why they need trained staff when there were no dressings and no catheters. The answer was, of course, that there were no dressings and no catheters because it employed trained nurses.

CONCLUSION

The evaluation of different modes of care concluded that nursing-home-type care is preferable to traditional wards. This is not just a matter of environment. Staff attitudes, self-esteem and training were also significantly different between the two types of care. The role of the nurse is not to control and order the lives of residents but rather to offer a wealth of expertise that can help them to make the most of the years remaining to them. No matter how political changes influence the care of older people, this project has demonstrated that, with the right attitudes, the right education, and the right environment, long-stay care can be a dignified and enjoyable end to a long life.

REFERENCES

Bond, J. (1984) Evaluation of long stay accommodation for elderly people in *Gerontology: Social and Behavioural Perspectives* (ed. D.B. Bromley), Croom Helm, London.
Bond, S. and Bond, J. (1990) Outcomes of care within a multiple-case study in the evaluation of the experimental National Health Service nursing homes. *Age Ageing*, **19**, 11–18.
Bond, J. and Bond, S. (1992) *Evaluation of Continuing-Care Accommodation for Elderly*

People. Overview of a Survey of Nursing Staff, Report No. 60, Centre for Health Services Research, Newcastle upon Tyne.

Bond, J. Gregson, B.A. and Atkinson, A. (1989) Measurement of outcomes within a multicentred randomized controlled trial in the evaluation of the experimental NHS nursing homes. *Age Ageing*, **18**, 292–302.

Donaldson, C. and Bond, J. (1991) Cost of continuing-care facilities in the evaluation of experimental National Health Service nursing homes. *Age Ageing*, **20**, 160–8.

Miller, L. (1986) The making of a home. *Nursing Times*, **82**(24), 40–1.

Sander, R. (1987) The nursing process in long stay care. *Geriatr. Nurs. Home Care*, **7**(2), 20–2.

Balmoral: a long-stay ward without nurses

24

INTRODUCTION

The impetus for the project came in 1987 when a team of people, all newly appointed to provide services for older people in South-West Hertford-shire, decided to set aside time to develop a philosophy for in-patient services. The group, guided by an external facilitator, had very little diffi-culty in agreeing a philosophy, but implementing the standards was to prove far more challenging and indeed set us on a route that was to question the most basic assumptions with regard to a conventional model of long-stay or continuing NHS care.

BACKGROUND

Abbots Langley Hospital consisted of a set of 'Nissen' huts built in 1945 to care for the returning Canadian troops after World War II. The hospital was sited in the grounds of a large mental institution. In 1987, there were five wards providing long-stay care. These Nightingale wards each had 21 beds, a dayroom and a toilet. The single-sex wards were conventionally nursed by a sister, staff nurses, enrolled nurses and auxiliaries. The 'medical' model of care meant fixed times for everything: drug rounds, meals, toileting, bathing, visiting and going to bed. Choices were minimized as it was believed that the patients were no longer able to make them and that anyway the caring staff generally knew best. This model meant that people were beautifully cared for physically but their psychological needs were often overlooked.

Beyond the hospital the attitude to long-stay care was 'hostile'. Restric-tions in finance and manpower, across the region and indeed the country, resulted in service rationalization and subsequent closures of long-stay beds with patients transferred to private or cheaper options elsewhere. We were not immune and were facing serious difficulties in recruiting and retaining nursing staff to work in an isolated setting of relatively low status.

PHILOSOPHY

The NHS has a statutory responsibility to older people who are physically frail such that they cannot be cared for elsewhere and require long-term residential hospital accommodation which becomes their home. The philosophy that we agreed was:

- continuing care provided for life;
- dignity for the individual;
- flexibility of approach, interpretation and style of care;
- freedom to make choices, e.g. when to go to bed;
- very careful selection of patients for continuing care;
- respite care to be provided within the continuing care facility.

MANAGING THE CHANGE

IMPLEMENTING THE PHILOSOPHY

The introduction of the philosophy included a presentation to every member of staff at the hospital and discussions with ward sisters about changes necessary to implement the philosophy. Some changes involved new structures such as the introduction of a multidisciplinary panel to consider selection (Golding *et al.*, 1987) and the creation of an activities and recreation department headed by a senior nurse. Although staff had for many years provided entertainment and outings, such events were limited by staff availability, whereas the new vision was of a range of daily activities that patients could choose to attend. This change was not only an immediate quality service improvement but an educational tool that would allow staff to see the range of activities that long-stay patients could enjoy and in which staff could become involved.

By 1989, the multidisciplinary panel was meeting fortnightly, backed by a system that allowed potential patients and/or their families to visit prior to admission and to go on to choose their preferred ward. The activities and recreation department had blossomed, and with the help of an array of volunteers and relatives offered a range of activities in a newly opened centre – a closed ward renovated through the charity of a local building company and including a hairdresser, shop, tea bar, bar, activity room and general lounge area. Although much had been achieved, life on the wards remained largely unchanged, i.e. institution not customer-led.

Despite efforts by the team which produced short-term changes, real changes that were dependent on attitude shifts were failing. Choices continued to be made for not by patients, for example patients were selected and 'sent' to activities. Regimens based on nursing shift patterns and efficient institutional functioning proved resistant to intervention. Not only had the 'medical' model largely survived unchanged, but in places attitudes had hardened as staff felt implicit criticism in attempts to change long-established patterns of care. They were antagonistic to the activities department which they saw as involved in the light and enjoyable work of continuing care with the hard slog of physical care left to ward staff.

Based on their experience over two years, the team began to focus precisely on the factors supporting and inhibiting progress. A major impediment appeared to be a tendency to keep patients 'safe'. This is not to suggest that the team wanted to expose patients to dangers but rather to extend personal choice and help patients to maximize their enjoyment of life. Whereas relatives and volunteers were enthusiastic and involved in delivering such experience possibilities, the qualified nursing staff had real problems recognizing opportunities for patient freedom of choice. This led the service manager (himself a nurse) to question the appropriateness of nurses as main caregivers in the holistic care of long-stay patients. That thought, coupled with nursing recruitment difficulties, led to a series of considerations and investigations.

- A survey indicated that qualified staff were spending 14.7% of their time on tasks that might require nursing qualifications.
- Some elderly people with similar levels of disability and stability but different personal circumstances to those in the hospital continued to live at home supported by their families who acted as carers. Such carers, although learning certain skills such as catheter care, were not required to become qualified nurses.
- In such circumstances, who provided those services defined as possibly requiring a qualified nurse? The answer was that some tasks were completed by the patient or carer (e.g. self- or assisted drug administration), some by carers (e.g. catheter care) and some by the district nurse with occasional patient contact with a general practitioner if the patient's condition changed.

It seemed that a major reason for nurses' involvement in continuing care was the tradition of providing continuing care in a hospital setting, and hospitals are staffed by nurses. Once acknowledgement was given to the notion that the medical hospital model was not appropriate, it followed that care need not, even should not given care requirements and the shortage of qualified nurses to meet acute needs, be delivered by nurses.

A NEW CONCEPT TO MAKE THE PHILOSOPHY OPERATIONAL

From the conclusions above was born the idea of running a pilot unit staffed by carers rather than nurses. Medical care would be provided by a general practice and overseen by a consultant geriatrician. The unit would be supported by a nurse advisor (modelled on a district nurse) with no managerial control on the unit but with full control over all nursing issues relating to patients.

Before problems of implementation could be tackled, it was necessary to gain backing and support not only from senior hospital management but from professional colleagues, professional staff organizations, relatives and patients. Consultation discussion started with the broad concept and progress of the project required the unit general manager, district management board, health authority, and chief nurse advisor to support the idea of a hospital ward staffed without nurses. Some of the major issues debated included:

- the perception that the driving force for using unqualified staff was relative costs, i.e. the venture was a cost-cutting exercise. However, this was not the case and the budget was set to be exactly the same as the other wards;
- the legal and ethical position of unqualified staff giving out drugs: a complex issue with final agreement that unqualified staff could give out drugs under specific conditions defined in an operational policy;
- the division between nursing and non-nursing tasks: the composition of the project team with three qualified nurses allowed an informed debate to lead to a protocol for nurse involvement on the unit.

At meetings with relatives of patients on the existing Balmoral ward, the proposed pilot unit, the proposal was discussed in depth. This was of great importance as the vision of care on the new unit allowed much more input from relatives in day-to-day care. With the relatives' support, the proposal was made known to patients. Two particular reassurances were given. Firstly, if monitoring revealed that care standards fell below satisfactory standards, the pilot would end and traditional staffing would be reintroduced. Secondly, any patient wishing to continue to be cared for on a traditionally staffed ward could be transferred to one of the other five wards staffed by nurses prior to the project or at any time during the project. In the event, no patients were transferred.

Other staff in the hospital expressed concerns that patients would not be properly cared for and that Balmoral's unqualified staff would constantly seek their help. The latter concern with lack of knowledge was reflected also in the general practitioner's concern that he would be called out frequently and inappropriately and bombarded with telephone calls. A further underlying fear of nursing staff was that this could be the beginning of the end – they would become redundant. With the benefit of hindsight, the project team acknowledges that, of the many issues and concerns with which they had to deal, the fear of job losses by the nursing staff was the one that they failed to recognize sufficiently and deal with effectively.

STAFFING THE NEW BALMORAL UNIT

All of the hospital ran with separate day and night staffing and the pilot initially excluded night staff. The day team to be recruited were a manager, deputy, two senior carers and six carers. In salary terms, this roughly translated to equivalent nursing grades: manager, grade F; deputy, grade E; senior carer, grade C; carers, grade B. The manager and deputy were appointed and took up their posts two months before the opening to recruit the rest of the team, devise the operational policy, prepare an induction programme, address their own immediate training needs, and prepare for the handover. The manager appointed had been in the post of voluntary services organizer at the hospital for a year and prior to that had worked for ten years in management with Marks & Spencer and held a psychology degree. The deputy had worked in psychiatric care and had an army background. The senior carers and carers came from a variety of backgrounds: some had worked at the hospital as nursing auxiliaries, some came from the private healthcare sector, some from completely different backgrounds such as shop work. All existing staff on Balmoral ward were invited to apply to work on the new unit (with protection of salaries and terms of employment) or were redeployed to vacancies on other wards.

No formal qualifications were required for any of the posts on Balmoral unit, although the unit manager and deputy were required to have previous management experience, and, like the senior carers, to have worked with older people. However, the major consideration in the recruitment of all the staff was attitude: respect, awareness, compassion, understanding, the ability to form relationships and to work in a team. If staff came to the project with these attributes, then it was believed that they could be taught the necessary skills. For the first year, it was agreed that one of the senior nurses on the project team would act as nurse advisor. After that time, the nurse advisor post would be reconsidered and possibly filled by a district or practice nurse.

The new Balmoral team underwent a two-week induction period which included visits to other homes, teaching on skin care, bowel and bladder care, measuring temperature, pulse and blood pressure, and experience sessions were set up to learn how it feels to be in a hoist, pushed at speed in a wheelchair or to be fed. Staff had to pass a competency assessment devised and examined jointly by the nurse advisor and pharmacist before they could distribute any drugs. The manager introduced a keyworker system designed not only to underpin individual care but to give carers real responsibilities within a team structure and to avoid the hierarchical structure traditional on wards.

THE NEW UNIT

Given that the intention was a change in the delivery of care, the new staff could not work alongside the old staff. Nor could the old staff simply go off duty one day and the new staff appear the next. The solution proposed by the manager for elderly care was the re-opening of a closed ward just down the corridor, with patients transferring over a period of days and the old Balmoral ward then closing. The new manager took a controversial initiative and had a (donated) carpet installed – no other ward had a carpet or considered it practicable. This was the first indication of a series of actions by Balmoral unit staff that not only made the unit perceptibly different, but were to challenge the traditional powers of the central hospital management. The staffing rota was arranged to ensure that the appropriate keyworkers were on duty for the arrival of the patients. The keyworkers were allocated simply on the basis of the unit manager's knowledge of each and of the report on each patient prepared by the sister seconded to manage the closure of the old Balmoral ward. Each carer was keyworker for up to a maximum of three residents (depending on carer experience), senior carers were keyworkers for two residents each, and the deputy and manager were initially free to trouble-shoot as necessary and steer the keyworker process.

The unit took its first seven residents on the Monday of the third week in March 1990. Accompanied wherever possible by their relatives, the patients were wheeled down the corridor in a house move involving a two-minute journey and a change of status from 'patient' to 'resident'. On Tuesday, seven more residents arrived and the final seven on Wednesday. From Monday, the unit had on duty its full shift quota, i.e. five on the early shift and three on the late, and in addition the nurse advisor remained on the unit from 9.am. to 5.pm. for the first two weeks.

THE FIRST MONTH

The first month was a frightening and awful experience for Balmoral staff, a very real test of the commitment of the project team and relatives to the project and a time of frustration and confusion for a number of residents!

Day 1 was fine with a full staffing compliment and seven residents. Even day 2 seemed to follow the guideline operational plan with those seven residents invited to indicate when they wanted to get up or wanted to do something and seven more moving in during that day. From day 3, however, and a 'full house' of 21 residents, the staff were in trouble. The night staff were working to the usual routine so the new 'day staff' arrived at 7 a.m. to find that the lights had been on for some time, all residents had been wakened, a 'back round' had been done, and all residents informed that they must wait until after breakfast to get up. As the new unit's manager had no management responsibility for the night staff, attempts were made to negotiate new ways of working which were dependent on which individual was on duty and their degree of support/ hostility towards the concept.

Carers keen to do a good job in meeting residents' requests worked with one resident at a time, allowing choice of clothes, and discovering the needs and abilities of each resident. They were intent on carrying out unfamiliar tasks well and worked slowly at the resident's pace, so slowly that by lunchtime some residents were still in bed (against their expressed preferences), some had missed the activity session that they had requested to attend, and other difficulties were emerging. One afternoon in the latter part of the week, a member of the recreation staff arrived to act as advocate for a resident attending a film session. The resident had confided that it was many hours since she had been to the lavatory and she was very uncomfortable. The question asked was why this resident's toilet needs were being ignored. This resident was continent and able to speak. Although it had been explained that any time she wanted anything she just had to ask, she 'didn't like to', felt inhibited and was used to a system in which everyone was 'toileted' at the same time on commodes at set hours. Suddenly to have no routines was uncomfortable.

Relatives and patients were encouraged to purchase personal clothing for residents (there had previously been a common pool). These were carefully labelled before being sent to the laundry – but they rarely came back, angering relatives and patients who not unnaturally held the staff responsible. The unit manager had yet more problems. A lack of kitchen security meant the unit's crockery was stolen. A lack of awareness of the need to order provisions (she had assumed a central distribution system) meant that the unit ran out of basics like tea and coffee. Other items used by the night staff but not the day staff (e.g. plastic aprons) ran out to the annoyance of the night staff who were increasingly concerned by the chaos of Balmoral (which was constantly untidy) and exceedingly antagonized by the day staff not having everyone in bed by the time they came on duty. The day staff at that time actually would have been physically incapable of achieving that feat but in fact this was a reflection of the philosophy: residents were not being put to bed at an allocated hour, they were invited to indicate when they would like to go, and several liked to stay up beyond nine o'clock watching television or having a nightcap.

In terms of residents' health, the nurse advisor continued to be prominent on the unit. Although staff quickly got to know the residents and therefore knew when something was different, the judgement about the importance of that difference was slower to come as it depended on experience. The nurse advisor carried a bleep and was bleeped unrelentingly the moment she went off the unit. Always fearing that there might be something really wrong, she assiduously responded quickly, only sounding rather tense on one occasion when bleeped off the M25 for a tiny skin tear!

THE BALMORAL UNIT AT TWELVE MONTHS

A year after opening, the chaos had long been replaced by a service that was attracting a local waiting list and national acclaim through the award of a prize for outstanding service quality improvements.

Residents

Residents had control over their day to the extent of:

- choosing when they would go to bed and get up and choosing from a full wardrobe of clothes what they would wear each day: no clothes, including night-clothes, were communal;
- choosing from a menu what they would eat at lunchtime and in the evening and where, either at attractively set and properly served tables or on a tray, in or by their beds;
- choosing to have a cooked breakfast (served at a set time because delivered from the central kitchens) or if they were happy with cereal, toast and tea, carers would get this when required;
- being free to request a bath any day or a hairdressing appointment;
- having visitors in and going out with visitors at any time and having access to their pension (or having it administered on their behalf);
- being told when a resident was ill (some chose to enter a rota which ensured that a dying resident was not alone), being told when a resident had died and offered the opportunity to pay last respects and to attend the funeral;
- being able to call on the help of a particular friend, the keyworker, for personal help such as reading or writing a letter, help with the telephone or with buying a present for a family member;
- being free to make an appointment with the general practitioner at his surgery (held in an office on the unit) and to see him on their own if they wished;
- being encouraged to choose their own activities. To end the chaos, routines for all aspects and activities were re-introduced after four weeks by the unit manager;
- being encouraged to form a group to make known common concerns and requirements, particularly aspects of life that those of us outside institutions take for granted such as personal underwear and clothing,

which, to maintain ownership, was washed by staff on the unit using laundry machine and dryer provided by relatives; residents went on to ask for proper crockery, lighter cutlery and more outings;
- volunteering for particular duties e.g. folding the laundry, helping new admissions.

Relatives

- Many visited daily and some gave direct care if this was comfortable to the resident.
- Helped in the design of an information pack for the relatives of new admissions.
- Helped on outings.
- Joined staff and residents in a Christmas lunch held in a local restaurant.
- Made contributions constantly to improve the comfort of the unit, e.g. washing machine and tumble dryer.
- Were loud in their praise of the unit and keen for it to continue.

Staff

- The Balmoral team had increased to 15 and taken over night duties. This ensured continuity of care and a single approach.
- Keyworkers and residents had formed close relationships, e.g. one resident acted as a witness at her carer's wedding.
- The nurse advisor spent approximately two hours a week on the unit – the most usual task being deep dressings for newly admitted residents.
- The general practitioner had become one of the unit's strongest supporters on the basis that care on the unit was superior in preventive terms. The initial arrangement of an early morning visit was changed in favour of two set 'surgeries' a week and a 'hotline' phone service, resulting in few call outs.
- The consultant geriatrician visited the unit every two weeks and reviewed one or two residents.
- The general practioner, consultant and unit manager met at regular intervals to consider progress, address concerns or queries.
- A full-scale training programme was written and adopted. Although 'home-grown', the course closely resembled national vocational qualification requirements.
- The two other senior carers not involved in designing the training programme also had special responsibilities, for example arranging general outings and helping as necessary with individual requests.
- Staff sickness levels were low and many staff openly claimed to never have been as happy at work before, feeling valued and self-fulfilled.

The unit itself

- Although the unit was no longer chaotic, it remained 'homely' at best, untidy at worst. The neatness of uniformity was removed when residents brought in their own bedspreads, easy chairs and anything else we could fit in the unit.
- Balmoral was constantly full and frequently people were waiting for admission, while other wards had empty beds.
- Although pockets of resentment remained, generally relationships between Balmoral staff and those from other wards improved. Practices such as keyworking and personal laundry were adopted throughout the hospital.
- Because communal toileting on commodes was abandoned, the pressures on the one 'patients' toilet were intolerable and the second toilet, i.e. the 'staff' toilet, was converted to enable use by residents or staff. This caused some controversy off the unit in areas where facilities for staff and patients were kept completely separate.

Management

Management of the hospital during the first year was not easy but increasingly there were signs of harmonious working between the wards and the unit. However, new challenges were developing from increasing demands for autonomy and rights for residents and staff on the Balmoral unit.

1. The unit manager wished to hold the unit's budget. Clear that the unit was now running more cheaply than a conventionally staffed ward – because of 24-hour rotation on the unit – staff wanted the 'saving' put back into the unit not the hospital.
2. Early in its life, the staff and residents of the Balmoral unit came up with an idea to refurbish the ward to create rooms, albeit communal. Initially resisted, the question was later re-opened.
3. Carers were able to give drugs following assessment, but not controlled drugs. This was a cause of distress on the unit, particularly when patients in pain had to wait for a qualified nurse from a ward to be available to administer a controlled drug.
4. Well aware of the benefits of activities, Balmoral staff were increasingly keen to arrange more of these and different trips – this brought them into conflict with the activities and recreation department.

EVALUATION

Any new venture draws its comments; informally Balmoral was enjoying a great deal of positive feedback from residents, their relatives and friends and also from professionals and professional organizations. However, an important aspect of the project was a planned formal evaluation with a particular emphasis on quality, and clinical psychologists, external to the project, were commissioned to carry this out. They compared two conventional long-stay wards with the new unit (Benjamin and Spector, 1990, 1992). Their findings are summarized below.

- The three settings did not differ much physically and there was a lack of space and privacy, particularly one toilet shared among up to 21 residents.
- The policy dimensions measured showed that the Balmoral unit allowed their residents more options than ward 1 to choose their individual daily living patterns, and were better at communicating to the residents the behaviour expected of them than for either of the ward settings.
- A keyworker system is in operation on Balmoral unit and staff work significantly longer hours on average than staff on the two wards.
- The Balmoral unit is also the only setting to hold regular formal staff meetings, and also has a support group that meets once a week so that problems can be aired.
- The lack of trained nursing staff on the Balmoral unit did not increase the dependence of the unit on other health services within the hospital compared to the ward settings.
- Residents on the Balmoral unit were among the oldest, but had greater cognitive functioning than residents of comparable ages on ward 1 and were similar in cognitive functioning to younger residents on ward 2.
- Measures of life satisfaction and morale did not differ between the settings.
- Residents on the Balmoral unit were found to be significantly more involved in higher activities taking place outside the hospital and did score higher on involvement in self-initiated activities and in involvement in social recreational activities available in the hospital, although not significantly so.
- The Balmoral unit did not experience stressful events more or less frequently than the two wards.

In 1991/1992, the Balmoral project was entered for the Hewlett-Packard Health Care Quality Award. Entries were judged by members of the NHS Management Executive, the King's Fund and leading professional bodies. The project was runner-up and Duncan Nichol (then Chief Executive of the NHS) was so impressed by the Balmoral project that he created a special runner-up award of £5000.

EPILOGUE

In April 1994, Abbots Langley Hospital closed. The site was sold for redevelopment. The patients/residents were transferred to beautiful bungalows built within the district and financed by the NHS. Clinicians and architects had worked together on a design to reflect in bricks and mortar the philosophy of care towards which the whole organization had been striving. However, the purchasers, following an agenda of political correctness and encouraging new market entry after tender, awarded the management contract to a private company. The conventional nursing home model was reinstated overnight in line with Department of Health regulations, and the Balmoral unit ceased to be. For the professionals, carers and relatives who were privileged to be associated with the magic of the reality, the dream will never fade and the opportunity to recreate it would ever be welcomed.

ACKNOWLEDGEMENTS

We would like to acknowledge the contributions of the staff and the project team members Ms Grace Bartholomew, Dr Alan Jackson and Mrs Maura Murray. We would also like to thank the carers on the Balmoral unit, and our supporters throughout, those who taught us to think and check assumptions, those who had the courage to allow us to try, and those who felt able to acknowledge and congratulate the success.

REFERENCES

Benjamin, L. and Spector, J. (1990), The relationship of staff, residents and environmental characteristics to stress experienced by staff caring for the demented. *Int. J. Geriatr. Psychiatry*, **5**, 25–31.
Benjamin, L. and Spector, J. (1992), Geriatric care on a ward without nurses. *Int. J. Geriatr. Psychiatry*, **7**, 743–50.
Golding, R. Lugon, M. Hodkinson, H.M. (1987) Confirming long stay status. *Age Ageing*, **16**, 10–18.

The Retreat experience: continuity and change in the care of older mentally ill people

25

INTRODUCTION

The chapter describes the experience of a concerted programme to improve the quality of life of long-stay, mentally ill residents in a hospital in the voluntary sector. The first part of the chapter outlines the driving forces behind the programme, the changes put in hand, and an emerging philosophy of care; the second tries to assess the effect of these initiatives on the quality of life of residents.

The interim conclusion is that market pressures and a concern to improve the quality of life can be mutually supportive; demand has increased and quality of life has improved. However, the latter judgement remains too focused on quality of care, rather than results for residents. The experience also points to a useful residual role for small 'institutions' in the provision of long-term care.

THE RETREAT

The Retreat is a not-for-profit hospital in the independent sector. It is a registered charity and its governors (trustees) are members of the Society of Friends (Quakers). It has 163 beds for acute and long-stay residents (of whom 86% are over 70) and provides out-patient and counselling services.

It was established in 1796 by a Quaker, William Tuke. The hospital quickly developed an international reputation for 'moral treatment', which, without rejecting medical remedies, emphasized 'occupational therapy, talking, diet, fresh air and exercise' (Stewart, 1992, p. 70) in a very comfortable environment. Another element was the emphasis on community and family. It has also been described as 'a negative phenomenon, an attempt to provide an alternative to the chains and other restraints of the traditional madhouses. The watchword of the new approach was restraint without chains . . . eliminated because the patient would be taught to restrain himself' (Harrington, quoted in Stewart, 1992, p. 51).

THE CHANGE PROGRAMME

DRIVING FORCES

A major re-appraisal of the Retreat's role began in the mid-1980s. A group of Friends, appointed by the representative meeting for British Quakers (1986), noted 'testimony to the quality of care' but acknowledged that 'they were troubled'. One factor was their inability to 'discern anything especially Quaker about the buildings or its social life' (Society of Friends, 1988). More specifically, they felt that:

- the style of work relationships did not reflect the communicating, inter-dependence of responsibility that Quakers expect;
- participation in decision-making was not encouraged;
- there was too little stimulation for patients.

There were also comments on the absence of some mental health professional groups (for example psychologists) among the staff of the Retreat.

A reappraisal of the Retreat's role in the care of older mentally ill people was also necessitated by a significant change in market conditions. The growth in the number of nursing homes with lower charges, led to a fall of such residents by a third between 1985 and 1990. The governors, recognizing 'that to rest content with the status quo would be to place the Retreat's future in jeopardy' (July 1990) initiated a programme of renewal.

THE RESPONSE: A PROGRAMME OF RENEWAL

Management arrangements

One element was the now very familiar management changes: the appointment of a chief executive officer, development of directorates, more structured reviews of performance, business planning, and investment in marketing. However, more important was the attempt to change the management style of the Retreat, to reduce the emphasis on differences in status, defined by hierarchical position, and introduce common conditions of service with fewer, simpler pay grades. Precious distinctions between grades and professions, embedded in Whitley Council arrangements, were held to be inconsistent with Quaker notions of interdependency, based on equality of esteem. Responsibility has also been progressively decentralized, most evidently in delegation of budgets and setting quality standards and targets: team working is developing.

A second element was a review of what the Retreat was trying to achieve, based on the 'contemporary reformulation of Tuke's concept of moral treatment' (The Retreat, 1990a). The 'starting point', from the perspective of one senior manager, was a good standard of basic care, but with significant shortcomings, including no real assessments of older residents, cosseting, very restricted choices and poorly met psychological needs. Many residents had lost their identity and self-esteem.

The thrust of the changes has been in line with current thinking, seeking to encourage choice and independence and changing working practices (e.g. meal times) to reflect these choices. The aim has been to develop a service that meets specified criteria: a 'degree of excellence, the degree to which they [services] embody a sense of obligation, their openness, their financial viability and the presence of participative management' (The Retreat, 1990a).

A major investment in training and education

A second thrust of the change programme was increasing investment in education and training, maintained even when the hospital was making trading losses. In the period 1992–1994, among registered nurses:

- 17.24% second-level nurses converted to first-level;
- 13% commenced/completed degrees or diplomas;
- 11% completed other further education courses;
- 39% completed English National Board courses;
- 58.5% completed in-house courses.

Additionally, 28% of untrained nursing staff commenced work for national vocational qualifications for which 22 staff undertook assessors' courses. Also, a greater commitment to provision of placements for Project 2000 nurses led to an increase in the number of wards approved for training in 1993.

Education had been maintained at a modest level after the nurse training school had closed in the 1970s. Responsibility for training (including supervision of students on placement as part of the general registration course) and continuing professional education was allocated to the deputy director of nursing who had many other duties. Things began to change with the appointment of a part-time tutor in 1989, replaced by a full-time nurse educationalist in 1992. The impact was graphically described by a staff nurse in a study of the educational programme of 1992–1994: 'He [the new manager] did arrive and he started saying what do you know about the nursing process, primary nursing and all that sort of thing? I had absolutely no idea what he was talking about, I just thought he had come off another planet . . .' (Flay, 1994).

The approach to adult learning (Knowles, 1973) also suited the transition to more independent methods of working, a feature of the management changes. The approach presumed a readiness to learn; self-directed learning; the need to apply learning; and that a learner's expanding 'reservoir of experience causes him or her to become an increasingly rich resource', (The Retreat, 1993, pp. 22–23). A learning resource centre was accordingly established in 1993, from which 50% of the nursing staff have borrowed books and computers in the resource centre are now used regularly.

An updated philosophy of care

An updated explicit statement of purpose and values has been developed to underpin the changes. It tries to encompass best professional practice, the tradition of the hospital and Quaker concerns. Much of the content is replicated in comparable documents of other institutions. There is, however, an emphasis on equality. Quakers have a view of the worth of all individuals that makes them uneasy with status differentiations: they have no ministers and historically refused to show deference to rulers, judges and sovereigns:

> The Retreat is a community of people who are essentially equal at a level which goes deeper than their status as patients or staff members with graded responsibilities. Services will reflect this perception of equality which makes true relationship and good working practice possible.

The statement provided the starting point for the subsequent quality initiative.

The process of reaching agreement was intentionally inclusive of as many staff as possible, intended to exemplify values of frankness, equality and openness. The 1986 report described management as centralized, non-participative and non-communicative, with insufficient interdependency.

A draft statement on purposes was considered by a cross-section of staff in a series of five workshops, each attended by up to 20 people and lasting some 2¼ hours. About 35% of the staff (78 in total) and about half of the governors were involved. An external facilitator prepared the definitive statement. Weaknesses in management were highlighted, as well as more general problems of communication, areas where staff needed help and aspects of the Retreat which they valued. The facilitator's report also noted staff doubts about whether the points made would really be carried forward.

The values part of the statement, concerning the conduct of the Retreat's affairs, was the product of a similar subsequent process involving 35% of different staff. Some individual departments also developed their own statements.

The quality initiative

The statement on equality was one of four highlighted in inaugural meetings for the quality programme, which began in 1992. The intention was to be open, non-hierarchical and collaborative: the theme was 'continuous improvement'. Each ward or department was asked to develop two simple standards for itself, using the very familiar Donabedian format (1969): structure, process and outcome. The standards were required to result in an improvement on current practice and complement the Retreat's business plan.

It was (and is) a bottom-up process with guidance and support as necessary from the deputy director of nursing. Senior personnel are updated on developments and thinking in a programme of 'spotlight' meetings for each department and ward in the course of the year.

Principles of care for older mentally ill people

Another, contemporaneous, stimulus to renewal was a fundamental examination of 'the care needs of patients on all the psychogeriatric wards and foreseeable demands in this area'. Undertaken by a working party of medical and nursing staff and two governors (both NHS professionals), it produced a statement of principles and philosophy of care for current residents and any newcomers. The principles were presented as 'subjective statements of need and can be imagined as coming from the individual or from an independent advocate speaking on her/his behalf'. They were that older people:

- have the same human value as other members of society, irrespective of their degree of disability or dependence;
- have the same varied needs as other members of the community;
- have the same moral and legal rights as other citizens;
- have the right to forms of support which do not isolate them from family and friends;
- have a spiritual life that requires nurture and expression;
- are unique individuals with a distinctive pattern of capabilities and needs (The Retreat, 1990b).

The report went on to specify implications of each principle for attitudes and everyday practice. A speedy practical outcome was early closure of a ward where the environment precluded an acceptable quality of life: the 'bed accommodation' was held to be 'manifestly incompatible with daily living space, which becomes noisy and overcrowded, and is at times far from the therapeutic and aesthetic surroundings desirable in treating agitation, confusional states, and various other mental disorders of the elderly' (The Retreat, 1990b).

IMPROVEMENTS IN THE QUALITY OF LIFE?

We used two well-established methodologies to ascertain whether these changes have produced commensurate benefits for residents. One is a measure of disability; the other is O'Brien's notion of 'accomplishments' – what service providers should try to achieve for users (quoted in Emerson, 1989). While neither allow us to begin to answer the central question – 'do users feel their life is richer and more satisfying?' – the material offers occasional (tantalizing) glimpses of user preferences and information on capacity and opportunities to enjoy life.

LESSENING DISABILITIES?

A rating scale (BRS) developed by Clifton Hospital, York was used to chart changes in the behaviour of 24 older patients (average age 67) admitted in April 1994 from a NHS psychiatric hospital. The BRS, derived from the Stockton Geriatric rating scale (Meer and Baker, 1966), covers four areas of disability: physical disability, apathy, communication difficulties and social disturbance. The outcome is a score giving an overall assessment of the individual's disability, which can be compared with a five-point grading system. Grade A represents independence in daily living; grade E represents maximum dependency (Pattie and Gilleard, 1979).

One aim of obtaining the information was to reassure the Retreat and purchasers of the quality of life of patients after transfer from an institution where most had lived for a long time (on average about 25 years). The three-monthly repetition of the test also provided some indication on the effect of a programme, focusing initially on improving communication and lessening apathy, to improve quality. There was some expectation of a temporary deterioration in assessments because of the move, and a slow reduction in lower levels of disability.

Table 25.1 summarizes the overall assessments of the individual's disability, each carried out by the resident's named nurse for five quarters from admission in 1994 to April 1995. The table highlights the high levels of disability of residents on admission: 22 of the 24 fell into the medium- or high-dependency classifications. Levels of disability generally diminished in the first 9 months, reverting to the status quo in month 12, although with variations for individuals. Lower social disturbance scores were offset by higher scores for apathy.

Table 25.1 Assessment of levels of disability: older residents, 1994–1995

Date	Dependency level (number of residents)				
	A	B	C	D	E
April 1994	0	2	9	8	5
July 1994	0	1	11	9	3
October 1994	0	1	11	8	4
January 1995	0	3	13	4	4
April 1995	0	1	9	8	6

One interpretation of the data is that the quality programme prevented the increase in disability expected as a result of the move. However, the data are also a useful reminder that improvements in process do not automatically produce commensurate improvements in outcome.

MORE ACCOMPLISHMENTS FOR USERS?

The second chosen indicator of the changes in quality of life is the development of 'accomplishments' of residents. Information is gleaned mainly from audits, conducted by the ward or department setting the quality standards.

Accomplishment (i): ensuring that service users are present in the community

Most residents have easy access to public facilities for shopping or recreation (cinema, sightseeing, swimming). Of 115 older residents, 10% are considered able to go into town unaccompanied, and 60% accompanied. Of these, the majority shop or join in a recreational visit at least twice per month. For the former, more physically able group, social events are integrated into resident's care plans.

The opportunities and range of community interactions have recently increased: events to which the public have been invited to attend, notably an annual gala, started in 1991; and interaction with families and with professional communities has improved, for example some residents have taken responsibility for making appointments with general practitioners.

The transfer of residents from the NHS psychiatric hospital prompted a sustained effort, wherever possible initiated by residents, to contact their next of kin, by letter or telephone. Contact is being maintained by cards being sent by residents at significant times, such as birthdays and

Christmas. The effect has been an increased number of visits by next of kin and an increased number of home visits by residents.

Accomplishment (ii): ensuring that service users are supported in making choices about their lives

One aspect of the quality programme was increased efforts to improve choice and quality of food. A new menu has been developed based on resident and staff comments during a programme of ward visits by catering staff (of all grades). The choice of vegetables is based on the explicit wishes of patients. Meal times have also been changed and extended, and further improvements are planned.

The extent of the changes is very evident in comparisons of menus for main meals. For example, the choice of main course dishes and vegetables increased from four and two in the mid-1980s to five and five in 1990 and six and five in 1995. In 1995, the choice of vegetarian dishes has also increased to four. There are more fresh vegetables and sandwich alternatives have been introduced. Finally, in a ward where the quality target was a 'pleasant (eating) environment . . . conducive to conversation and relaxation at all times', patient views on the size and shape of tables assisted in the purchase of new ones.

Residents now also determine the choice of decoration for their rooms (single and communal). Paint cards and decorating books are provided by the technical staff to assist residents' choices, often supported by family members or advocates.

Accomplishment (iii): developing the competence of service users by developing skills and attributes which significantly decrease dependency and develop characteristics which other people value

Developing competencies, practical and psychological, is a priority for clinical teams. One example is encouragement of residents to prepare their own food and beverages, a crucial element in self-respect for many.

Examples of competencies that have featured in jointly agreed care plans include improving communication skills, functioning at a 'higher' level, and developing characteristics that others value. Another example is plans to improve budgeting skills for recent residents, one focusing on spending on tobacco. It has prompted a policy of 'responsible' smoking; education and support have helped a number of residents to reduce their dependence on nicotine, releasing funds for spending on other items. Another example concerned personal toiletries. By the end of 1992, 70% of the dependent and 90% of the less dependent residents budgeted and supplied their own toiletries.

Accomplishment (iv): enhancing the respect afforded to service users by . . . ensuring that the choice of activities, locations, forms of dress and use of language promote a positive view of users

One effect of all the initiatives outlined above should be a more positive view of residents by staff. Arrangements for the development of care plans reflects this: they are now expected to be the product of agreement between equally respected parties, rather than between 'parent' and 'child'.

Increasing resident participation in decision-making is consistent with a feeling of being valued. Reference has already been made to encouragement of self-catering for some, and comments and suggestions for menus. Consequent changes (for example providing a range of vegetarian meals) have underlined the residents' influence and competencies in this important area of life. A registration officer noted that in one ward 'puréed fruit (is) a favourite, along with cake and biscuits': in another, staff and patients brought in fish and chip suppers.

The appearance of residents is also something that has featured in the programme to enhance respect and in audits, of which the personal toiletries example is but one aspect. The audit of the latter initiative refers to comments on the improved appearance of the residents by staff from other wards. Also, for some particularly deprived, newly arrived residents, additional personal clothing is being purchased: an explicit, minimum standard for items of personal clothing has also been developed by a specially convened working party.

Accomplishment (v): ensuring users participate in the life of the community

There are numerous examples of residents participating in the life of the community but few have actual membership of organizations. There is active participation in community facilities: for example, extra efforts in 1994 led to increased use of the local swimming pool, and a doubling of monthly sessions from two to four. Two residents also attend courses at the local technical college. Another link, the product of conscious effort, is the increase in the number of events in which the public (not just relatives) participate.

EXTERNAL ASSESSMENTS

External assessments of the Retreat also point to improvements in the quality of care and quality of life. Registration officers had rightly been critical of some aspects of the Retreat's arrangements (for example in pharmacy and dormitory provision). While attention focuses on the acceptability of inputs (staff, facilities) and processes (record keeping, nursing practices etc), a recent thorough report (November 1994), says that the overall assessment is 'encouraging'. There are welcoming references to 'the initiatives being developed throughout the hospital' and in reports on four wards from different registration offices there is specific recognition of improvements and high standards. Another indicator is the increased number of wards approved for training for student nurses in 1993, to which we referred earlier. In one case, this was after approval had been earlier withdrawn.

CONCLUSIONS

The information on the effects of the change programme on the quality of the life of long-term older mentally ill residents is inevitably subjective and patchy. Information is also lacking on perhaps the most crucial aspect of quality: the residents' perspective. However, within this limitation, there are clear indications that the programme has produced real improvements in the daily lives of elderly residents. There are more choices and opportunities, competencies have been increased or at least maintained; and discussions between staff and residents are more equal, and in the case of food, sometimes robust. There is some validation of the internal 'interested' perspective by the actions and comments of purchasers, regulators and training agencies.

Encouragement also comes from the content of the programme. There was nothing particularly novel about it, except perhaps for its uncomplicated nature. Practical, observable improvements flowed from a simple, bottom-up approach to quality; the more elaborate, computer-based systems producing more information were consciously eschewed. There was also determination to see it through: investment in training increased and delegation of budgets went ahead despite falling income.

The approach was also intended to announce a change in management style and relationships. The starting point was Quaker views of relationships between people; equal, based on respect for that of God in all. These were very pertinent in 1796, when the mentally ill were not accorded that respect. They are not irrelevant today. One facet of equality is acceptance of differences and personal choice: an uncomfortable bedfellow for the paternalism implicit in the common application of 'existing societal norms and commonly held expectations and standards' (Barry et al., 1993) to assess quality of life. The changes in the 1990s have tried to apply that belief in equality to modern conditions. There have been efforts to develop different, more equal relationships within the ranks of staff (some successful, some not) and between them and residents. In this context, the new pay and conditions are important, signalling fewer differences between professions and grades.

These changes have not been achieved without questioning and difficulties: there have been changes in senior positions but the period has not been marked by increased staff turnover or sickness, frequently taken as measures of discontent.

Finally, the mini-success also raises issues about the place of 'institutions' in providing long-stay services. The prevailing theories had led the Retreat to a *partial* withdrawal from the 'private' long-stay market: the reasons were price, the national catchment, and the 'inappropriateness' of 'hospitals' for nursing home care. Provision also ran counter to the accepted wisdom, enshrined in government policy, that the community/ nursing homes are the 'best' locations for long-term care. The relevance of community provision for long-term, severely ill people is not yet beyond dispute. Holloway (1994) has also pointed out in a review of the re-provision of a mental hospital in three health districts that 'longer term follow up of the community provision is required to determine how well the new pattern of services manages its residents as they grow old and develop age-specific problems'.

The recent experience of the Retreat suggests that, in the shorter term, it has a role in caring for a residue of 'graduates' of NHS mental hospitals. In the longer term, it remains to be seen whether the alternatives do produce greater improvements in the quality of life for older people that still seem possible within the Retreat.

REFERENCES

Barry, M.M., Crosby, C. and Bogg, J. (1993) Methodological issues in evaluating the quality of life of long stay psychiatric patients. *J. Mental Health*, **2**, 43–56.

Donabedian, A. (1969) Some issues in evaluating the quality of nursing care. *Am. J. Public Health*, **59**, 1833–6.

Emerson, E. (1989) What is normalisation?, in *Normalisation. A Reader for the Nineties* (eds H. Brown and H. Smith), Tavistock/Routledge, London.

Flay, S. (1994) The Effects of Increasing the Educational Opportunities for Nurses Working in the Independent Sector, Dissertation, University of Huddersfield, UK.

Holloway, F. (1994) The RDP Cane Hill closure research project: an overview. *J. Mental Health*, **3**, 401–11.

Knowles, M. (1973) *The Adult Learner. A Neglected Species*. Gulf Publishing.

Meer, B. and Baker, S.A. (1966), The Stockton Geriatric Rating Scale. *J. Gerontol.*, **21**, 393–403.

Pattie, A.H. and Gilleard, C.J. (1979) *Clifton Assessment Procedures for the Elderly (CAPE)*, York NHS Trust, York, UK.

The Retreat, (1990a) *Minute on the Future Development of The Retreat*, The Retreat, York.

The Retreat (1990b) *Policy Group Report. Tube Ward/Care of the Elderly Psychiatric Patient*, The Retreat, York.

The Retreat (1993) *Annual Report for 1992*, The Retreat, York.
Society of Friends (1988) *Report of the Group Appointed by Meeting for Sufferings to Meet with Governors of The Retreat*, Society of Friends.
Stewart, K.A. (1992) *The York Retreat*, William Sessions Limited, York, UK.

Voluntary homes 26

Why should this book have a separate chapter on voluntary homes? Are they significantly different from homes in the private or public sector? If so, in what ways are they different and what have they got to contribute?

Firstly, voluntary homes are differently funded. Not only are they relatively well able to raise capital from appeals and trusts, their revenue needs are also supported by voluntary contributions from corporate bodies or from individuals, including bequests, and they often have charitable status.

One of the voluntary sector's largest activities, and historically one of its most important, has been residential care for older people. In the latest edition of Laing & Buisson's Directory of Major Providers of Long Term Care for Elderly and Physically Handicapped People (1995), there were 81 not-for-profit organizations that ran residential and nursing homes. Of these, the ones with the largest numbers of homes mainly for older people were: Anchor Housing (77), Abbeyfields (62), Church of Scotland Board of Social Responsibilities (43), Methodist Homes for the Aged (39) and Salvation Army Social Services (29). Most (78%) of the voluntary homes are residential homes, but a number of charities have now expanded into dual-registration (9%) and nursing homes (15%) (Laing & Buisson, 1994).

In 1993, voluntary residential homes contributed 51 000 places to the care of older, chronically ill and physically disabled people, and voluntary nursing homes contributed 15 000 places out of the total (including the private and statutory sectors) of 557 200 places.

Many voluntary homes were founded to cater for a particular section of older people. The Distressed Gentlefolks Aid Association Homelife, the Civil Service Benevolent Fund and the British Sailors' Society catered for retired professional and ex-service people. Some homes catered for religious groupings, e.g. Methodist Homes and Jewish Care, others for those belonging to certain trades, e.g. Licensed Victuallers' National Homes and Linen and Woollen Drapers' Cottage Homes. Many of these charitable activities started in the last 50–100 years, in response to perceived gaps in the types of homes available in the statutory sector, and in particular for those of their client group who had insufficient resources to pay for private residential and nursing care. This 'particularity' of many voluntary homes is increasingly under threat. The dilemma, for example for Methodist Homes, is whether to accept the local people assessed under the Community Care Act as needing their care most, or whether to keep some vacancies for life-long Methodists who wish to end their days among others with the same beliefs. In future (Forder and Knapp, 1993), there will be little room to manoeuvre if the local authorities, who are virtually monopoly purchasers, decide to impose tight contracts that ignore such considerations. Loss of variety between voluntary homes and others might be the consequence of such policies, for all except those who can pay for and choose for themselves.

CHANGES IN NUMBERS OF HOMES BEFORE AND AFTER 1993

The expansion of homes in both the voluntary and private sectors in the 1980s was driven by demographic changes in the population and fuelled by the ready availability of income support payments. Simultaneously, there was a decrease in the numbers of long-term hospital beds for geriatric and psychogeriatric patients and of Part III places, giving a further stimulus to the private and voluntary sectors. However, during the period of expansion, there was a far greater increase in private homes than in voluntary homes. Between 1970 and 1993 (Laing & Buisson, 1994), there was an increase of nearly 600% in the number of places in private residential homes in the UK (often in small owner-managed homes), while places in voluntary residential homes increased by just over 25%. From 1987 (when private and voluntary nursing homes were first counted separately) to 1993, places in private nursing homes increased by over 200% while those in voluntary nursing homes (a much smaller group) increased by 80%. A somewhat higher proportion of those in voluntary homes were self-funding, so the fact that income support was available was less of an incentive to prospective clients than the particular atmosphere in a home.

The combination of high interest rates and decreasing property values after 1990 brought a number of bankruptcies and repossessions of (mainly private) residential homes, but these were not as numerous as had been expected. The changes in the numbers of older people going into homes before and after April 1993 were distorted by the 'rush' of entrants before the Income Support rules changed, and the slowing of entrants after April as local authorities adapted to their responsibilities for assessment etc. and disbursed their money carefully. These initial changes mean that no clear trends can be discerned from the years 1993–1994.

Voluntary and private homes now need to survive in a rapidly changing environment. After 1993, many potential residents preferred to receive 'packages of care' in their own homes, and for frail older people these 'packages' will be complex. The greatest shift in funding has been towards such packages. However, there is a limit of dependency beyond which it becomes impractical and over-expensive to support very disabled people in their own homes, and residential or (more likely) nursing care will then be the only option. There may well be fewer new entrants into residential homes, and those who do choose to enter will be frailer and more disabled than in the past. From August 1992 to January 1994, there was only a small drop in occupancy rates from 91.7% to 91.2% in voluntary residential homes and from 93.7% to 89.1% in voluntary nursing homes. Similar falls occurred over the same period in private homes. Residential homes will increasingly want to keep their existing residents (from partly philanthropic and partly financial motives), even though they may begin to have nursing needs.

There is already a considerable overlap in level of incapacity between older people in residential and in nursing homes and this will be accentuated. A further factor is the alleged unwillingness of some social service departments to consider placing clients in the private sector (Forder and Knapp, 1993). Voluntary (not-for-profit) homes may be preferred by clients and carers as giving a well-differentiated service (e.g. with religious or occupational orientation). Their policy of ploughing any surplus revenue back may give rise to a greater degree of trust. For these reasons, voluntary homes have suffered less since 1993, but overall it is too early yet to evaluate the full effect on voluntary homes of the community care changes.

The demographic changes in the population continue, and Laing & Buisson (1994) estimate that we may require a further 68 000 residential and nursing home places by the turn of the century. Therefore, despite funding of complex home packages and possible re-provision of some hospital long-term care beds (NHSME, 1995), well-built and well-run homes can be cautiously optimistic about their prospects.

FACILITIES IN VOLUNTARY HOMES

It is not easy to establish what facilities are available in voluntary residential and nursing homes as many studies of private homes include only one or two voluntary homes. However, a report commissioned by Counsel and Care on privacy in residential care based on a survey of 114 registered homes in inner and outer London included 83 private and 24 voluntary homes (21 residential homes and three nursing homes) (Counsel and Care, 1991a). Eighty per cent of homes expected the residents to share rooms (85% of private homes and 59% of voluntary homes). Commonly residents had to move from single to shared rooms as their capital ran out. Overall 70% of homes expected residents to use commodes in shared rooms (77% of private homes and 48% of voluntary homes), and in nearly a quarter of the shared rooms there were no curtains or screens. Fourteen per cent of residential homes and 47% of nursing homes had no locks on the doors of bathrooms and lavatories (26% private residential and nursing homes; 15% voluntary residential and nursing homes).

Just under half of the homes had no locks on the doors of residents' rooms and home owners often didn't knock on entering, so finding the resident on a commode was all too common. Residents and their relatives had low expectations and were unlikely to protest about such invasions of their privacy. In 20% of the voluntary homes, there was no lockable storage space for residents' clothes and valuables and the same was true in 56% of private homes. Eighty-six per cent of the homes allowed residents to eat in their rooms (89% private homes, 71% voluntary homes). All the voluntary homes had a telephone available for residents' use in private but not all the private homes did. The layouts of communal rooms can enhance or restrict residents' privacy, but the majority of residential and nursing homes had chairs placed round the walls (with no choice of neighbours) and with the television as the central feature. Overall, the voluntary homes in this study scored better than the private ones for five of the six aspects investigated, but there was no room for complacency in either sector. Attitudes of staff were crucial and far more important than the layout of the buildings.

'Home Life', the publication from a working party sponsored by the Department of Health and Social Security and convened by the charitable Centre for Policy on Ageing (1984), set the standards by which aspects of quality of life for residents have been judged. It particularly emphasizes training of care workers. In nursing homes, concern for the safety of the most disabled residents sometimes led to practices that withdrew choice and independence from those who were less frail.

In general, nursing and residential homes provide a lower standard of amenity than the general public has come to expect, but there has been improvement. Between 1989 and 1994 (Laing & Buisson, 1994), the facilities in private care nursing and residential care homes improved with regard to single rooms (offered in 51% of nursing and 66% of residential homes), en suite toilets (in 23% and 26%), separate activity rooms (in 24% and 16%), and minibuses (in 26% and 21%). Eighty-one per cent of nursing homes and 68% of residential homes offered respite care and smaller percentages (19% and 28%) offered day care. There was a small increase in the percentages of nursing homes offering care for older mentally infirm people (supervised by a registered mental nurse), from 15% in 1989 to 18% in 1994.

Table 26.1   Survey of residential home and nursing home costs per bed per week (1990)

	(Number of units)	Staff costs	Total running costs (R)	R + capital costs = S	S + profits	Profit
Private residential home	(328)	56	111	142	155	13
Voluntary residential home	(182)	134	183	234	256	22
Private nursing home	(99)	126	186	238	260	22
Voluntary nursing home	(31)	252	334	427	468	41

Adapted from Price Waterhouse (1990)

STAFFING AND COSTS IN VOLUNTARY HOMES

A 1990 report by Price Waterhouse for the Department of Social Security contained information from 640 homes which were a representative sample of voluntary and private residential and nursing homes in the UK. The costs of running these homes were calculated assuming a 90% occupancy rate (Table 26.1). For all types of unit, capital costs (S minus R) amounted to about 28% of the running costs of the home. Voluntary residential and voluntary nursing homes cost more to run than private homes, due to higher staffing costs. Staff costs were 73–75% of the total running costs of voluntary homes and 50–68% of the costs of private homes. Profits were largest in voluntary nursing homes (a comparatively small sample), but the average profit throughout the care sector was only £25 per bed per week. In a similar study in 1991, profits for residential homes had dropped to £12 and those for nursing homes to £6 per week, despite a rise in average residential home fees from £185 to £203 per week and in nursing home fees from £256 to £293 per week.

A survey of 291 private and voluntary homes for older people in England and Wales (Darton and Wright, 1990) showed that, on average, the voluntary homes were 12 places larger than the equivalent private homes, and the nursing homes 8 places larger than the residential homes. Average length of stay was over two years longer in the voluntary homes (51 months versus 23 months). The highest levels of dependency were in the nursing homes (67% of patients highly dependent), but many highly dependent people (35% of residents) were being cared for in residential homes, both voluntary and private. The 1973 DHSS Building Note stating that 40–50% of beds should be in single rooms was largely achieved by homes in this study, as were the requirements for one bathroom per 15 residents and one toilet per four residents. About 50% of those in residential and nursing homes were receiving financial support.

Larder *et al.* (1986a) studied the geographical differences in running costs of nursing homes – from £104 per bed per week in Lancashire to £240 in outer London – and ascribed them largely to variations in the cost of the premises. There were large geographical variations in provisions of public, voluntary and private homes per thousand of the population over 75 years old (Larder *et al.*, 1986b). Local authority beds (in 1984) were more numerous in the north of England (53:30), whereas private residential homes (12:39) and voluntary residential homes (4:16) were more numerous in the south.

ASPECTS OF QUALITY

REGISTRATION

In the past, there has been ample evidence of poor long-term care in all sectors, with a series of scandals about individual establishments but little national data. As the numbers of independent homes increased during the 1980s, there was anxiety that rapid expansion might lead to a further fall in standards, and the responsibilities of local authorities for registering and inspecting residential homes and of the health authorities for nursing homes were redefined. Day and Klein (1985) studied registration procedures by postal questionnaire sent to all 201 health districts in England and Wales, asking about independent hospitals and nursing homes including voluntary nursing homes in each area (response rate 86%, relating to a total of 1259 nursing homes). Some 131 establishments in the independent sector had changed ownership or management in the preceding two years and had needed rechecking. Health districts had been given wide discretion in how to interpret DHSS regulations, and considerable local variation developed in the levels of staffing and the practices required of independent nursing homes. For instance, 76% of districts used NHS standards for keeping drug records, 69% for keeping patient records and 68% for hygiene requirements. In contrast, only 56% used NHS guidelines for staff/patient ratios, and only 53% used such guidelines for the ratio of state-registered nurses to other nursing staff. The registration system was flexible and dependent on the subjective impression made on the registration nurse. Extra visits were made by the registering nurse either to boost morale or to give advice, especially if there was concern about standards (Day and Klein, 1987). The main difficulty that emerged was that of recruiting adequately qualified staff, sometimes reflecting unwillingness to pay high enough salaries. The ultimate sanction of de-registering was carried out infrequently – over the two years of the survey, 37 nursing homes were considered for de-registering and only six of these were eventually struck off.

GUIDELINES

There is no lack of guidelines for long-term care based on registration and inspection bodies. Health authorities have often based their requirements on those of the National Association of Health Authorities (NAHA, 1985). Guidance on Standards for Residential Homes for Old People (SSI, 1990), 'Home Life' (Centre for Policy on Ageing, 1984), the Wagner report (NISW, 1988) and its sequel (NISW, 1993) all provide guidance on wide-ranging aspects of life in residential homes, including the voluntary sector. The booklet 'Working with Older People', jointly produced in 1993 by the British Geriatrics Society, the Royal College of Psychiatrists and the Royal College of Nursing, gives advice on aspects of care for frail older people in all forms of institutional care. The issue of quality services for old people in nursing and residential homes is discussed in 'A Scandal Waiting to Happen?' (RCN, 1992). All these documents may be useful in defining care standards for the health authorities, local authorities and fundholding general practitioners who purchase long-term care.

Considerable emphasis must be given to the number, grading and training of the staff employed. Basic care has often been left to the least trained, least skilled and least well-paid staff (Day and Klein, 1987). In addition, there has been a tendency towards fixed routines, batch treatment, and lack of autonomy and privacy, with inactivity and boredom for many residents. Clearly none of these contribute to good quality care and methods are being sought that are suitable to judge the quality of care of very frail and sometimes confused older people.

Efforts have been directed towards changing the model of care from the rigid institutional one which is said to be provider-led into one that is more social (consumer-led). In the latter, the patient's autonomy is predominant and every effort is made to allow choice, without undue loss of safety. One way of monitoring is to look at eight key indicators (domains) through the 'Continuous Assessment, Review and Evaluation' (CARE) scheme (RCP and BGS, 1992). This scheme was piloted in 1991–1992 by two voluntary nursing homes (Royal Surgical Aid Society and Brendon-care) along with 16 other long-term care establishments. They found that it was possible to audit one domain, e.g. 'preserving autonomy' or 'environment and equipment' in 6–12 months. Such self-monitoring schemes help to motivate staff by showing the improvements they have achieved. The atmosphere of the home improves and this helps to keep staff motivated and interested.

NATIONAL ASSOCIATIONS

Although each voluntary home wants to maintain its independence and flavour, there are many advantages in joining together into associations to address nationwide issues. In the residential sector, VOICES (Voluntary Organizations Involved in Caring in the Elderly Sector) now comprises 37 voluntary organizations providing residential and nursing homes. They range from the very large providers of homes (Abbeyfield, Anchor

Housing with Care, Methodist Homes for the Elderly) to small organizations serving only one locality. In total, the organizations forming VOICES are responsible for 10 600 places. Because of its nationwide experience, VOICES can see that care homes will have to adapt in order to look after the frailer and more confused older people who will be their residents in the future. Together with other voluntary assocations, for mentally and physically handicapped people, VOICES worked with local authorities to produce 'Guidance on Contracting for Residential and Nursing Care for Adults' in 1994. They hope to see quality care funded by local authorities at a realistic level.

The Registered Nursing Homes Association has 1600 members representing 60 000 beds. Through its 30 local branches around the UK, it can offer advice on staffing levels, pre-printed patient contracts, insurance advice etc. The staff of voluntary homes make up 6% of attenders at its national study days.

EXAMPLES OF GOOD PRACTICE

Although many voluntary homes publish their own in-house quality control manuals, few have ventured into print in national journals. At least two, the Royal Surgical Aid Society (RSAS) and Brendoncare, have run national symposia, as has Age Concern. The RSAS symposium in 1989 concentrated on the philosophy of providing care until the patient died. Removing the fear of being moved to another home (either through worsening illness or diminishing finances) is a great relief to older people in homes. However, offering this facility does entail costs in providing additional nursing help, or financial support 'top-ups' from the society's funds. Some other charities operate the same policy, and Methodist Homes for example spent £550 000 in 'top-up' payments in 1994 (Methodist Homes, 1994).

'Building and Designing for the Frail Elderly' was the subject of the RSAS symposium in 1990 and the award by the society that year was for the best home showing good architectural design and good care for the residents (Salmon et al., 1991). Of the 42 entries from public, independent and voluntary sectors, six were short-listed by a panel of doctors and architects, and were visited to judge the buildings and the caring and lively atmosphere of the homes. The best design (not the most expensive) showed a mixture of public and private spaces, bustling and quiet rooms, allowing variety and choice. It had good relationships with the neighbouring schools, churches etc. and a day area where those still managing in the community could receive day care and rehabilitation. The central feature was the concourse, a lively sitting and meeting place with a shop in one corner (Figure 26.1).

In 1992, the RSAS symposium was on 'Good Nutrition in Old Age' and

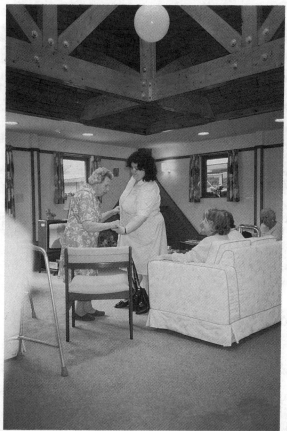

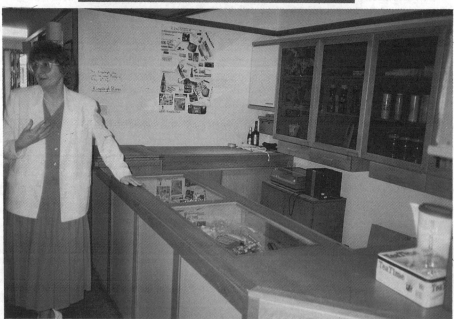

Figure 26.1 Features of an award-winning home

the same year the award was for cooking in public, private and voluntary homes. The panel visited 24 homes (usually at very short notice) and drew up a short-list of six cooks. The cooks subsequently competed against each other in London for the award.

The RSAS has just completed building a home with separate wings for older people with physical disability and for those with mental impairment, and its 1995 symposium was on 'Coping with the Problems of Dementia in Old Age'. The society has cooperated with the Royal College of Physicians and the Royal College of Psychiatrists to see whether two more 'domains' relevant to older people with dementia can be added to the eight 'domains' in the CARE scheme.

Brendoncare (a voluntary organization running homes in the South of England) held a national symposium in 1995 including a section on voluntary provision. This expanded the meaning of complete care to include the option of respite care, a centre for domiciliary care support and a resource centre for carers. The director of Brendoncare argued for a breakdown in the treble system of registration (residential home, dual-registered home and nursing home) and its replacement by a single registration. Research is being undertaken in conjunction with the Personal and Social Services Research Unit in Canterbury backed by VOICES and by the Rowntree Trust to see whether the weighting of fees could come from the mix of dependency in the residents in a particular home.

Brendoncare are fortunate in having a number of long-term contracts with health authorities, so they have some financial security in planning for future needs. Difficulties will arise with homes whose contracts are on a patient-by-patient basis (spot purchasing). Currently the system is working for the purchaser because of excess residential home capacity, but the provider homes do not know whether they will be able to continue from year to year. There is a danger of insecure residential homes taking more disabled residents than their staff can care for, and this will need to be watched. Both writing careful contracts and monitoring them will be expensive. The local authority will be unlikely to rescind a contract when a number of frail older people would then have to be found other placements. Despite these difficulties, monitoring must be made effective if quality is to be upheld.

Age Concern does not itself run homes but it organizes valuable national conferences such as the one in 1994 'Achieving High Quality Long-Term Care for Elderly People'. This concentrated on the needs of consumers and the responsibilities of purchasers, and included sections on quality and the role of training. The quality of care assessment tool Inside Quality Assurance emphasizes much the same topics as feature in, for example, 'Homes Are For Living In' (SSI, 1989) and 'Home Life' (Centre for Policy on Ageing, 1984). A representative from the Registered Nursing Homes Association argued for specific funding for staff training to be included in contracts – a sum of £2 per bed per day for this contribution to quality assurance was suggested. Such a sum would allow a clinical tutor to be employed who would work alongside new and established nursing and care staff, showing them and working out with them the best ways to do the work and relate to the residents. The very time-consuming work of assessment for national vocational qualifications could then be performed without detriment to clinical care, and the many motivated staff could develop their skills and qualifications.

Another aspect of good practice in the voluntary sector is the flexibility shown, for example, by Abbeyfield in moving towards 'extra care homes' and by Anchor Housing in moving towards residential homes. Methodist Homes has adapted its training towards the care of older people with dementia who will be its main residential group in the future. Small care groups consisting of a number of patients with dementia in a home and a staff member, stay together throughout the day, including at meal times, to provide familiarity and continuity. This voluntary organization is also cooperating with Dr Tom Kitwood of the Dementia Research Group in Bradford in research and drafting policy documents and a training strategy. A book about Methodist care homes gives details about care homes as a positive choice (Webb, 1995). It is also ensuring that every new home built (it currently has 37 residential and two nursing homes) should be under the wing of one of the local churches, and in touch with local schools and communities.

The needs of older people belonging to ethnic minorities have been noted by voluntary services. Counsel and Care have arranged to have their explanatory leaflets available in eight languages, and the Centre for Policy on Ageing has published a report detailing the difficulties of growing old in a second homeland (Norman, 1985).

One of the features that make voluntary homes different is the presence of volunteers within the homes, often befriending residents who have few visitors. They organize and join in a variety of activities, and act in numerous ways to support the head of the home and its staff and to co-operate with residents' relatives, if wanted. Suitable volunteers can act as advocates for residents, for example. Many charities have home committees that support the homes and can bring an independent outside view to bear on their activities. Volunteer trustees serve the organization of the charity, and oversee the policy of the homes. They can take responsibility alongside paid officials for the way the homes meet the needs of their residents. They may take part in the appeals by which most charities fund their new home building. Funding for such capital projects is more easily obtained than revenue support. Benefactors are attracted by homes that are trying to give quality care and those building to today's standards, for example with single rooms and *en suite* toilet facilities.

CHANGING ROLE OF THE VOLUNTARY SECTOR

The precise role and extent of the voluntary sector has not been defined and its role in residential care has often been a response to perceived local or national needs for identified groups. There has been increasing use of volunteer groups throughout the 1980s. The 'discovery' of the amount done by carers, as an essential part of care of older people (among others) at home, has come just at a time that the voluntary force (mainly older women) may be a decreasing resource. Many factors are involved – the greater number of women in paid work, their involvement at the same time in care of young people and of older relatives, family dispersal to find jobs, the effect of divorce on the likelihood of care for older in-laws and so on. At its best, volunteering allows people to use their gifts in caring for each other, and can be flexible and innovative, acting as a spur and source of competition to the statutory and private sectors. However, critics have attacked the 'particularity' of voluntary homes, and said that the sector serves those it chooses. It has been pointed out that voluntary homes are present in greatest number where the need for them is probably least (Larder *et al.*, 1986b). The 'amateurism' of voluntary bodies running homes has been recognized and people with relevant skills and experience are being recruited in a number of charities.

The statutory and voluntary sectors are not strictly in competition as they may work in different ways for good reasons. For example the volunteers in a Methodist home may befriend residents but not wash and dress them – nor do the volunteers think they should be relied upon as a substitute for properly resourced staffing levels.

Despite the growth in occupational pensions, a high proportion (estimated at 90%) of frail older people do not have enough money to pay for their care in nursing and residential homes without raising money on their own homes (Sinclair *et al.*, 1990). When this capital has diminished, these residents will need state funding, as will others with less than £16 000 capital. A particular difficulty arising from the purchaser/provider split is that voluntary associations that run homes become paid agents of the local authorities for the 50% or more of residents who receive state funding at any one time. As a result, they may lose their freedom to act as a constructive critic of local authorities or as advocate for particular client groups (Baker, 1992). However, the shift from grants to contracts may make funding for successful residential homes more secure after an initial period of turbulence. The issue is not whether there should be a 'mixed economy of care' but what balance there should be between the statutory, private and voluntary sectors and whether the necessary funding will be available to run homes of good quality.

PROBLEMS IN JUDGING QUALITY

There are special problems in measuring quality in care homes as the desired outcomes are hard to define. This is particularly true for older people who may have multiple diseases, variations in dependency and the presence or absence of dementia, all of which may interfere with 'resident satisfaction'. This has perhaps led to undue dependence on the processes of care (activities in care giving) and on structure (buildings, staffing etc.) in judging quality.

Advice is available for older people and their carers to help them to choose a good home (Counsel and Care, 1991b; Elderly Accommodation Council, 1994) and Which? Way to Health (Consumers' Association, 1993). The Which? publication resulted from incognito visits to 30 private and voluntary residential homes, when it was found that the most expensive homes were not necessarily the best. Checklists largely concerned structural matters such as lifts, availability of single rooms, *en suite* toilets, door-locks, telephones etc. Flexibility in meal times, or in times to get up and go to bed, are important to many residents, as is the opportunity to bring in personal possessions and some furniture, or to choose what to eat. A choice of social activities or the opportunity to sit in a quiet room might be appreciated. Staff numbers and training, and charges for 'extras' such as physiotherapy or chiropody, are very relevant. Eventually, the residents' own preferences might best be determined by planning ahead and spending a period in the chosen home in order to judge the atmosphere and so on. For non-demented older people, this advice is likely to give confidence in judgement, but carers of demented relatives may still be left in uncertainty. Some homes can be provisionally assessed as good and some as poor using these criteria, but little work has been done until recently on whether high-scoring homes are in fact delivering a higher quality of care.

In a cross-national study in eight homes in Florida and in nine homes in Israel, Fleishman *et al.* (1992) looked at a number of tracer conditions in residential homes. They compared them with the previous rating by an independent assessor of the homes as good or poor. Tracers were defined as frequently occurring well-defined problems with known treatments. They included medical and nursing aspects of care (such as poor vision, deafness or incontinence), nutrition, and measures of activities of daily living. Psychosocial factors included lack of autonomy and feelings of loneliness. The tracer approach combines structure (e.g. staffing ratios), process (procedures and activities in caregiving) and outcome (resident satisfaction etc). Data were collected by medical and paramedical staff who examined patients (who had consented), reviewed records, conducted observations and interviewed staff. Despite differences in culture and in organization in the two countries, the tracer method proved to be a feasible way of assessing quality of care, and showed that homes previously assessed as good consistently scored better than poor/mediocre units in quality of care.

At the 8th annual elderly care conference organized by Laing & Buisson in March 1995 attenders included those from statutory (NHS and social service departments), private and voluntary organizations. Dr Edward Dickinson, Senior Clinical Research Fellow of the Royal College of Physicians, assessed the merits and shortcomings of existing quality assurance schemes including CARE and Inside Quality Assurance and the management performance system BS5750. Despite difficulties, a paradigm seemed to be emerging, that of empowering staff to meet the needs of residents, including their autonomy. However, this autonomy depends on the numbers, accreditation, training and attitudes of staff, all of which are essential in practice if quality long-term care is to be achieved, in whatever sector.

The voluntary sector has distinctive qualities to bring into the mixed economy of care. It can use the best national guidelines and standards, while being flexible enough to attempt new local initiatives, and maintaining the 'differences' that are the reason for its existence.

ACKNOWLEDGEMENTS

I should like to thank the staff of the following charities who have given me valuable help and advice: Abbeyfield, Age Concern, Anchor Housing, Brendoncare, the Centre for Policy on Ageing, Counsel and Care for the Elderly, Distressed Gentlefolks Aid Association Homelife, Elderly Accommodation Counsel, Help the Aged, Methodist Homes for the Aged, the National Council for Voluntary Organisations, the Relatives' Association, the Royal Surgical Aid Society, RUKBA Friends of the Elderly, and VOICES.

REFERENCES

Baker, M. (1992), The role of the voluntary sector: pump primer or pit prop? *J. Neurol. Neurosurg. Psychiatry*, **55**(Suppl), 45–6.

British Geriatrics Society, Royal College of Psychiatrists and Royal College of Nursing (1993) *Working with Older People*, Royal College of Nursing, London.

Centre for Policy on Ageing (1984) *Home Life: a code of practice for residential care*, Centre for Policy on Ageing, London. (Updated 1996 as 'A Better Home Life'.)

Consumers' Association (1993) Choosing residential care. *Which? Way to Health*, **October**, 170–2.

Counsel and Care (1991a) *Not Such Private Places*, Counsel and Care, London.

Counsel and Care (1991b) *Fact Sheet 5. What to Look for in a Private or Voluntary Registered Home*, Counsel and Care, London.

Darton, R. and Wright, K. (1990) The characteristics of non-statutory residential and nursing homes, in *Privatisation* (ed. R. Perry), Kingsley, London, pp. 55–95.

Day, P. and Klein, R. (1985) Maintaining standards in the independent sector of health care. *BMJ*, **290**, 1020–2.

Day, P. and Klein, R. (1987) Quality of institutional care and the elderly; policy issues and options. BMJ, **294**, 384–7.

Elderly Accommodation Council (1994) *For You and Yours*, Elderly Accommodation Council, London.

Fleishman, R., Ross, N. and Feierstein, A. (1992) Quality of care in residential homes: a comparison between Israel and Florida. *Qual. Assurance Health Care* **4**, 225–44.

Forder, J. and Knapp, M.R.J. (1993) Social Care Markets: The Voluntary Sector and Residential Care for Elderly People in England, in *Researching the Voluntary Sector*, 1st edn (eds S. Saxon-Harrold and J. Kendall), Charities Aid Foundation, Tonbridge, pp. 129–42.

Laing & Buisson (1994) *Review of Private Healthcare*, Laing & Buisson, London.

Laing & Buisson (1995) *Longterm Care. Directory of Major Providers*, Laing and Buisson, London.

Larder, D., Day, P. and Klein, R. (1986) *Pricing the nursing home industry: capital and turnover. Bath Social Policy papers no. 9.* Bath University, Bath.

Larder, D., Day, P. and Klein, R. (1986) *Institutional care for the elderly: the geographical distribution of the public/private mix in England. Bath Social Policy papers no. 10.* Bath University, Bath.

Methodist Homes (1994) *Annual Review 1993–1994*, Methodist Homes, Derby, UK.

National Association of Health Authorities in England and Wales (1985) *Registration and Inspection of Nursing Homes*, NAHA, Birmingham.

National Institute for Social Work (1988) *Residential Care, a Positive Choice (Wagner Report)*, HMSO, London.

National Institute for Social Work (1993) *Positive Answers*, HMSO, London.

NHS Management Executive (1995) *Responsibilities for Meeting Continuing Health Care Needs*, NHS Management Executive, Leeds.

Norman, A. (1985) *Triple jeopardy: growing old in a second homeland*, Centre for Policy on Ageing, London.

Price Waterhouse (1990) *A survey of residential care and nursing home running costs: a report to the Department of Social Security*, Department of Social Security, London.

Price Waterhouse (1991) *Independent Health Care Association Survey of Residential and Nursing Home Costs*, Department of Social Security, London.

Royal College of Nursing (1992) *A Scandal Waiting to Happen? Elderly People and Nursing Care in Residential and Nursing Homes*, Royal College of Nursing, London.

Royal College of Physicians and the British Geriatrics Society (1992) *High Quality Long-Term Care for Elderly People. Guidelines and Audit Measures*, Royal College of Physicians, London.

Salmon, G., Hildick-Smith, M. and Wedgwood, J. (1991) Award-winning homes link design to 'complete care'. *Care of the Elderly*, **3**(7), 335–7.

Sinclair, I., Parker, R. and Leat, D. (eds) (1990) *The Kaleidoscope of Care. Part 3. Care and the Voluntary Sector*, HMSO, London.

Social Services Inspectorate (1989) *Homes are for Living In*, HMSO, London.

Social Services Inspectorate (1990) *Caring for Quality. Guidance on Standards for Residential Homes for Elderly People*, HMSO, London.

VOICES (1994) Guidance on contracting for residential and nursing care for adults. *This Caring Business*, **February**, 8.

Webb, P. (1995) *Facing Home Truths*, Methodist Homes, Derby, UK.

Improving quality of life 27

INTRODUCTION

In considering the topic of care for older people in the private sector, it is first necessary to outline the legislative approach and then consider the statutory quality controls on care that have been applied. Consideration is then given to the initiatives that the sector has taken to ensure that appropriate quality of care is delivered to patients and residents.

THE REGISTERED HOMES ACT 1984

The major legislative control on the quality of residential and nursing homes is the Registered Homes Act 1984. The Act also applies to the provision of qualified nursing staff from nursing agencies. Privately owned hospitals fall within the provisions of the Act, but not all voluntary sector facilities do. No legislation covers the provision of domiciliary care by unqualified staff.

The 1984 Act replaced several pieces of legislation, and has achieved a significant effect over the past ten years. Its purpose is to protect the public by ensuring minimum standards for all those who are cared for in these environments. It is not designed to control quality of care. The fundamental concept behind the Act is that of adequacy, defined as 'suitable and sufficient'. The facilities and features of the home are required by the Act & Regulations to be adequate with regard to the number, age and sex of the persons to be cared for.

THE NHS & COMMUNITY CARE ACT 1990

The NHS & Community Care Act 1990 was designed to control the financial expenditure on long-term care within the independent sector and therefore create a more competitive market within long-term care. As such, the Act does not directly address the quality of care but does require contracting by independent sector care providers with social service/work departments of local authorities. However, since resources are now rationed in the long-term care sector, competition is increasingly having an effect on the quality of care provided.

RATIONING

Fundamental to the distribution of resources in the long-term sector is the fact that health care as a market has an infinite size. In other words, the resources applied will always be used, however great. We will always be able to identify health needs that will benefit from the allocation of additional resources. Similarly, I contend that the social care market is infinite. The consequence is that we will always be in a position where we have to ration the supply of such services, however great the resources allocated to the sector.

NEEDS, WANTS AND REQUIREMENTS

A key concept that is very necessary in these days of rationing of health and social care is the difference between needs, wants and requirements. The recently implemented Community Care Act uses one key word relating to the user of services and that is need. But what is a need? An example of transport will illustrate the situation. We all **need** to travel to work each day. We have a need for daily transport. The **want** is to travel by the easiest, quickest, cheapest, most comfortable method. In other words, to travel to work in under five minutes, at a cost of less than £1, in the most luxurious surroundings possible, and without being inconvenienced in any way. The **requirement** is a balance between all these factors, which leads each of us to make a different decision as to the way we travel. So any requirement is between the need and the want.

To return to the healthcare sector, no individual wants health care, or for that matter social care. Health and social care are a distress purchase. They are something that we all want to believe we will never need. However, when we do need it, then we want our general practitioner, and no one but our general practitioner, to be able to prescribe a simple tablet that needs to be taken when we remember it, and for the symptoms to be removed.

There is a hierarchy in these three words: needs are those things we cannot do without, e.g. food, heat, shelter and life-saving health care. Wants are more demanding: we want to be comfortable, not to be exerted, to be healthy without effort, and all at no cost. Requirements are what in the end we provide in health and social care. They are the things that we can deliver when all the technology has been used, all the budget-balancing has been optimized, and the practicality of service delivery fully considered.

The key point about setting requirements, for they are the cornerstone of quality systems, is that it is an art and not a scientific process. If requirement-setting were a scientific process, then we could develop a fixed formula to define such requirements. However, the process is one of balancing competing demands for resources on the one hand and expectations of the product or service on the other. If the requirement for health care is set too close to the needs, and far away from the wants of the population, then customer dissatisfaction will result. The needs will be addressed, but the expectations of the population, expressed in the wants, will not receive any resources. If the wants for health care are set too close to the requirements, then resources will be significantly stretched, Treasury budgets will be exceeded and subsequently the requirement will have to be set nearer the needs.

WHO IS THE CUSTOMER?

It is also useful to consider what might appear to some as an obvious question: who is the customer? The patient or resident who is receiving care is obviously the customer (Figure 27.1). Is this correct? Often the care

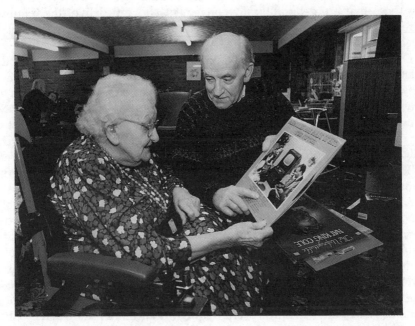

Figure 27.1   Who is the customer?

that the person receives is the subject of significant specification by relatives who take a keen interest in the care of their loved ones. On many occasions, this is positive and to be encouraged, but in some cases, the guilt of the relative can interfere to the detriment of the person being cared for. Many professionals have witnessed relatives who cannot, for whatever reason, accept that their loved ones are no longer fully independent and capable of making the day-to-day decisions of life. In such cases, the customer may be the relative or friend.

In the event of mental incapacity, then the relative or friend may need to undertake the role of advocate in order to ensure the best interests of the patient. In this case, the requirements for care need to be interpreted by the advocate in order to ensure that the care provided is appropriate to the history and character of the patient.

WHO IS THE PURCHASER?

The selection of long-term care is always dependent on the geographical location of the patient. Within that geography, the decision or at least a short list is frequently made by a relative or another person acting on the patient's behalf. The more highly dependent the patient becomes, the less they are able to participate in the decision. Who then is the purchaser? We frequently observe that the relatives of the potential patient are the ones required to visit potential long-term care establishments in order to shortlist those that are geographically convenient and can deliver the required care and to check that the accommodation is available at the time it is needed.

Differences in attitude and expectation between the patient and the relative are frequently apparent, particularly when there is a generation between the patient and the relative. Examples are the expectation of physical accommodation such as *en suite* facilities by those who have grown accustomed to equivalent hotel facilities, even though the patient to be cared for may not be able to use such facilities after admission. The private sector has for many years been improving facilities in order to satisfy such expectations, even though they are not strictly justified by patient need.

A secondary version of who is the purchaser occurs whenever public funding is involved in the purchase of long-term care. Social service/work departments are responsible for the purchasing of such care since the implementation of the Community Care Act and therefore they require their requirements to be satisfied. These requirements can become an issue for long-term care providers where there is conflict between the general intentions of the contracting authority and the specific requirements of a patient. Whilst such conflicts were frequent occurrences immediately after the implementation of the Act, subsequent experience is now ensuring that patient wants are being addressed even when they are in conflict with purchaser requirements.

WHAT IS QUALITY?

The private sector has increasingly adopted a strategy of implementing formal quality systems on a significant scale over recent years in order to ensure that the patients who are cared for receive a quality of care that is consistent and totally appropriate to the needs and wants of the individual patient. One such model that is highly relevant to the health and social care sector is the Crosby model (Crosby, 1984) which initially defines what are known as the four absolutes and then provides an implementation plan for quality. The four absolutes are summarized as follows: the definition of quality as conformance to requirements; a quality system aimed at prevention; a performance standard of 'zero defects'; and definition of the measurement of quality as the price of not conforming with requirements.

THE DEFINITION OF QUALITY

Conventional wisdom defines quality as goodness, or best, or even luxury. When discussing the quality of long-term care, it is frequently the building or furnishings that are uppermost in a relative's mind. Consider, by comparison, the purchase of a car. Jaguar or Rolls-Royce are perceived as quality products, but is a Mini also a quality car? A car owner who wants a car to drive five or ten miles a day to work through urban traffic and needs to park in small gaps by the roadside may well regard his Mini as a quality car. The fundamental problem with 'goodness' is that it is subjective and not measurable, and is therefore difficult to manage. Quality must be defined in a way that allows an accurate determination of whether the product or service meets the customer needs.

A quality service is therefore defined as one that 'conforms to the requirement', i.e. the product or service meets the requirements. To consider the car example again, if the requirement is for a small car that is easily parked and economical to purchase and run, then the Mini is a quality product, just as the Jaguar is a quality product if the requirement is for startling road performance.

In a long-term care context, the requirement is for some mixture of health and social care, and while the buildings and furnishings play a part in providing that care, it is the care that is fundamental to whether the provider is providing quality care or not. Therefore, it is as valid to provide a quality facility at cheaper rates in a city centre location as it is to run another quality home in the country at a much higher price, if those parameters are the ones that the respective groups of users consider to be their requirements. In other words, the requirements of the individual must be addressed in the areas of physical accommodation, location, price and the care that they receive. Quality must therefore be defined as conformance to the requirement and not as some ill-defined view of goodness.

THE SYSTEM FOR QUALITY

Conventional systems of quality are based on sorting the good from the bad. When someone starts looking for defects that have already occurred, they are carrying out appraisal (whether it is called checking, inspection or testing) and by so doing are encouraging the attitude that defects are inevitable and therefore unavoidable. In practice, the only system which produces quality is one which prevents these defects from occurring in the first place. Defects don't just happen, their cause can be traced either to a lack of knowledge or to a lack of attention. Adopting a system of prevention means that if we meet the user requirements in the first place, then we will not have to take action to remove the defects afterwards.

To apply this to long-term care, prevention of defects means fully understanding the requirements of the residents in our care, and the commitment of both ourselves and our staff to satisfy those requirements whenever they occur. Take the example of a resident who is asking for the toilet every half hour until the staff tell her that she will have to wait as they are busy and they have only just lifted her back into her chair from the last visit anyway. A requirement is to assist the resident whenever she needs the toilet, and since she has been refused we cannot claim to be giving quality care. Conventionally, we might approach the problem by checking how often this happens and how often we do not have enough staff to help residents to the toilet on request. By adopting a preventive approach, we would consider why the resident is asking for a toilet every half hour and probably discover that she has a urine infection.

The system for producing quality is prevention, not appraisal.

THE PERFORMANCE STANDARD

When considering a performance standard, we are faced with a range of potential targets that could be set as the performance standard. Especially when dealing with people, we are used to the concept that we are only human, we are not perfect, and therefore that we will all make mistakes. However, if we accept to begin with that we will make mistakes, the obvious consequence is that we will expect mistakes and that we will react when a mistake occurs as though it is a normal occurrence. In this event it is fair to ask whether we are prepared to accept the same level of mistakes in all spheres of our lives. Are we happy to accept that on only 99% of occasions our salary will go into the correct bank account, or to accept that on 97% of occasions we will correctly approach our own house when going home, and on the other 3% we will approach another home? If we do not accept these mistakes, then this must be a function of the importance that we place on the task we are undertaking. We must hold some tasks as being more important than others. If we accept a performance standard of 'that's close enough', then we have accepted before we start that we will not meet the requirement. Therefore, we must set ourselves the target of no defects or mistakes, known as zero defects.

Mistakes are caused by two factors: lack of knowledge and lack of attention. Knowledge can be measured and deficiencies corrected. Lack of attention must be corrected by the person, since it is an attitude problem. Zero defects is the expression of an attitude of preventing mistakes. It is the only performance standard that cannot be misunderstood and it will only be achieved by management determination to bring about the cultural change required.

CONTROL OF NON-CONFORMANCE

The cultural change that is needed can be illustrated using a common concept in quality systems, the control of non-conformance. What can be done after a mistake has occurred, given that we have failed to prevent the non-conformance in the first place?

The control of such situations is usually divided into a two-stage process: the quick-fix followed by a long-term corrective action to prevent recurrence. Any situation that results in a non-conformance or failure to meet the performance standard needs to be recorded and any action taken to remedy the immediate situation noted. However, if we are to adopt a system of prevention, we must consider the actions necessary to prevent that non-conformance occurring again, known as corrective action. This latter process does not need to be achieved immediately, but the incidence should be the starting point for a full investigation of all the circumstances surrounding the incident.

Consider the situation where a drug is out of stock for a particular patient. The immediate action would be to order a repeat prescription of that drug. However, the long-term corrective action needs also to be reviewed, e.g. has the general practitioner changed the dosage recently but failed to change the quantity prescribed, or is the recording of changes of drugs and how they are requested in need of amendment? Such actions may take several days or even weeks, but the key point is that the corrective action process is geared to ensuring that the particular non-conformance is prevented from happening again.

Attitude is a key parameter in managing quality, and never more so than in corrective action. Investigation of non-conformances can be seen as a negative activity if the entire staff of the organization are not committed to the concepts of quality. Therefore, it is vital to spend considerable time and effort communicating with all staff to ensure that they adopt a positive attitude and are fully involved with the goal of achieving total quality management.

The performance standard is, therefore, simply the answer to the question, 'how often do you want me to meet the requirement?' and the answer is 'all the time'. Hence the performance standard must be zero defects, not 'that's close enough'.

GET IT RIGHT FIRST TIME, EVERY TIME

The setting of a performance standard that requires a target of 100%, of zero defects, frequently causes discussion or even disbelief. In the context of caring, the target is often more acceptable to nursing staff than it is to administrative personnel. Nursing staff are used to the discipline of the theatre where sterile conditions must be maintained and an audit of all equipment made before the operation is complete. However, non-nursing staff have not before needed to adopt the attitude necessary to embrace such a demanding performance standard.

An example of a multi-stage process, such as four-hourly pressure area turns, that is accomplished to a 90% performance standard may be more compelling. While the process will result in 90% of patients being cared for to the standard after four hours, only 72% of patients will have been adequately cared for after 12 hours, and after two days, less than 35% of patients will have received quality care over the period. Hence, a 90% performance standard, being less than 100%, very quickly results in the majority of patients receiving care that is below the performance standard.

THE MEASUREMENT OF QUALITY

Once quality is defined and accepted as 'meeting the requirement', it has become a specific and measurable thing. However, as we traditionally thought of quality as goodness, we have always thought of quality in relative terms, as in degrees of goodness, when attempting to measure it. Because it was not related to money, quality has never been taken seriously by management. In order to ensure that everyone fully understands the impact that quality makes, the best measure is one that is stated in money terms. The measurement of quality, is therefore, defined as the price of not meeting the requirement or the price of non-conformance, and not as percentages or ratios.

THE OWNERSHIP OF QUALITY

We need to consider who 'owns' quality in an organization. Is it a staff function? Is it the nursing staff? Is it the managers of the facility? Is it the medical staff? The fundamental point is that it is the employers or providers who are responsible for the quality of care that is delivered. If the providers do not take that responsibility and accept that it applies throughout the line of management, then it simply will not happen. Placing the responsibility for staff competence in a staff function is merely to abdicate the responsibility. Expecting an external inspector to be able to inspect quality of care is to fly in the face of all experience, realism and logic.

Consider for a moment the experience of the car-manufacturing industry, when it placed the responsibility for quality on inspectors who performed a final inspection of a car at the end of the production line. When they found faults on the cars, they then had the task of going up the assembly line to find out what caused the problem. No single person on the production line felt responsible for quality. Imagine what would happen if, in an operating theatre environment, we were satisfied to leave quality to the post-operative nurses! The message is very clear. We are all responsible for the quality of care that our patients receive. To carry this example further in the nursing home sector, how can health authority inspectors, who are required to make two visits per year to a nursing home, take responsibility for the quality of nursing care that is delivered in that home? They simply cannot. Quality must be the responsibility of the managers and owners of that business, the provider of that care.

COMPONENTS OF A QUALITY SYSTEM

The next issue to consider is the mix of general components within a quality system (Figure 27.2). Then, the range of existing quality systems can be considered. Different quality systems should not be seen as being in competition with each other, i.e. ISO9002, the international standard for quality systems, is not in competition with the Department of Employment's initiative Investors In People (IIP). These systems are merely different arrangements of the components described earlier, and therefore, are complementary approaches to running quality systems rather than competing approaches. It is to be expected that, having implemented one quality system, a provider may well wish to enhance the system by offering another standard that will build on previous work and be a minor amendment to existing documentation and processes.

The other aspect that providers should consider is the existing documentation with the home. In many cases, this documentation can be used as a base point on which to build a quality system, even though it may require

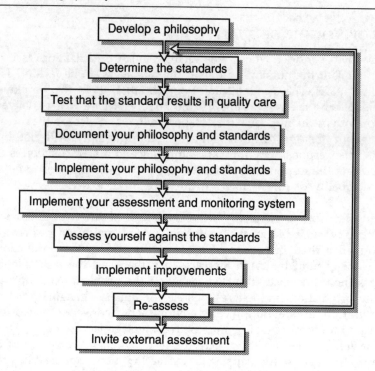

Figure 27.2   Components of a quality system.

modification or re-writing in order to comply with the standard(s) being used.

Also, it is necessary to separate performance standards from quality systems. Many people have perceived the implementation of charters as being a quality system. The charter presents performance standards and requires other elements of quality systems, for example a monitoring system, to be implemented in order to ensure that the standards are actually being achieved on a day-to-day, week-to-week basis.

THE DIVERSITY OF SYSTEMS

A wide diversity of quality systems is available to the healthcare sector, each of which have been tried and tested in many different settings. Each system takes different elements of general quality systems and arranges them to focus on a desired outcome. Within the private long-term care sector, common systems that have been implemented include the systems whose key components and objectives are described below.

KING'S FUND ORGANIZATIONAL AUDIT

The quality improvement programme developed in the early 1990s at the King's Fund Centre is a system to set and monitor organizational standards for acute units. This system is termed organizational audit. The work developed rapidly from an initial feasibility study involving nine hospitals to a programme that now includes well over 100 hospitals throughout the UK. In addition, the approach is being extended to include health centres, general practices and some long-term care establishments.

Organizational audit concerns those standards that relate to the systems and processes that need to be in place to promote organizational effectiveness. The logic of this approach is that, in meeting the standards, a facility is ensuring that an efficient and effective service is provided to users and there is a good working environment for the staff. Such an environment will contribute to the provision of high-quality patient/client care. The second and equally important part of the process, the assessment of a provider's progress towards meeting those standards, takes place by means of a survey, conducted by a team of trained senior healthcare professionals.

ISO9000 SERIES

The ISO9000 series of standards (British Standards Institution) tells healthcare organizations what is required of a quality-oriented system. The standards do not set out extra requirements that only a few organizations can, or need, comply with, but are practical standards for quality systems which can be used by all. The underlying philosophy of ISO9000 is that you cannot test the quality of every service delivered, so instead you test the system that produces the services. That way you can assure the consistency of the service that the system provides. While ISO9000 does not specify performance standards, it ensures that the standards of performance set by the organization and its users can be consistently delivered by the management of the organization. ISO9000 describes what must be included in the quality system; it is not prescriptive and allows managers freedom in how they implement the quality system such that it is appropriate to the size and character of the organization. The standard is a framework that consists of a range of tools and techniques such as management review, training needs analysis and patient assessment, as well as a requirement for the ongoing monitoring of the system by internal auditing. The documentation should ensure that the quality system is comprehensive, consistent and unambiguous and that the procedures adopted by the organization are compatible with each other and with the stated quality aims. Independent verification of compliance with the standard, known as 'certification', is available from bodies recognized by the National Accreditation Council for Certification Bodies; BSI Quality Assurance is one such body. The certification process consists of an initial assessment followed by regular checks to ensure continuing compliance with the standard. The implementation of a quality system is a long-term commitment spread over a number of years; the standard must not be seen as an end in itself but as a checkpoint on a road towards total quality management.

INVESTORS IN PEOPLE

The Investors in People system (Department of Employment via Local Training and Enterprise Councils in England and Wales and Local Enterprise Companies in Scotland) is based on a national standard for effective investment in people which is reproduced here.

- An Investor in People makes a public commitment from the top to develop all employees to achieve its business objectives.
- An Investor in People regularly reviews the training and development needs of all employees.
- An Investor in People takes action to train and develop individuals on recruitment and throughout their employment.
- An Investor in People evaluates the investment in training and development to assess achievement and improve future effectiveness.

Use of the Investor in People standard is therefore appropriate when management consider that to focus on people's skills and competence will improve the quality of care that is received by the patient being cared for. The lead agencies for the promotion and support of this system are Training and Enterprise Councils.

CONCEPT OF COMPETENCE

The last system described above, Investors in People, concentrates on the development of staff in order to ensure the competence of those staff when they undertake work. The proving of such competence is traditionally undertaken by training (Figure 27.3), but is that sufficient in a world where the knowledge, systems and techniques of any profession are changing not in a lifetime, but over a decade, or even shorter period of time? If we consider the computer industry in the early 1970s, staff required retraining every seven years because of the technological changes. By the mid-1980s, that rate of change had resulted in retraining being necessary every 18 months. The technology was changing at the rate measured in months: not a lifetime, or even decades, but months. Now the rate of change in the health and social care sector is not quite as quick as

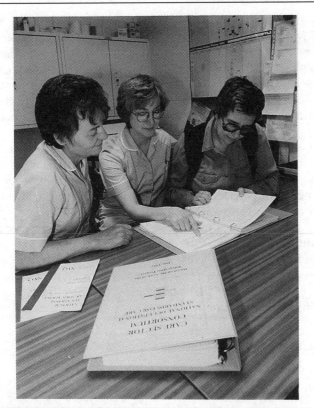

Figure 27.3   The need for training.

in the computer sector, but it is certainly changing significantly more quickly than in the recent past.

A further point is that retraining in techniques or factual research is, relatively speaking, easy. What is significantly more difficult, but much more necessary as our society becomes ever more complex, is change in our attitudes. However, attitudinal change is much more difficult, and takes more time, since our resistance to change increases as our age increases. The crux of the issue is that we must attempt to remove the resistance to change and be prepared to demonstrate our competence on an ongoing basis. We must not perceive training as something that we return to the classroom or lecture theatre to receive, but undertake to review our knowledge, skills and understanding on a continuous basis, using whatever techniques are relevant and practical to the situation and the resources available to us.

The result of training therefore needs to be perceived as the demonstration of competence on a continuous basis, which may well be in the workplace by assessment against nationally set standards. The private sector has embraced occupational standards, national vocational qualifications and post-registration programmes in order to prove competence, or to identify specific training needs which, when addressed, can result in competence across a particular area of expertise. That takes us to the point where we have proved, either by formal examination or by the use of an assessment tool, the competence of our staff to perform the tasks required by our patients.

Now, how do we prove that those staff actually use that competence every day of their working lives, and with every patient whom they are required to care for? The point is that the two cannot be separated. Training and quality systems are needed to prove, not just to an assessor, not just to our managers or peers, not just to those who may undertake our clinical audit, and not just to the courts when we are accused of bad practice, but to ourselves when we go home at night, that the care we have provided to our patients has been that which we would have wanted for ourselves, if we were the patient. In short, we are aiming to provide the care that our patients require, the first time they require it, and every time they require it.

REFERENCE

Crosby, P.B. (1984) *Quality Without Tears*, McGraw-Hill, New York.

Conclusion

'In 1942, Winston Churchill stated: 'This is not the end, it is not even the beginning of the end, but it is perhaps the end of the beginning.' The quotation could perhaps be applied to a person now requiring continuing care. Within the last few years, the range and quality of continuing care accomodation has improved considerably. The challenge facing all health professionals is to ensure that new residents are properly assessed, and provided with appropriate support to ensure that their quality of life, whether at home or in a continuing care home, is of the best, i.e. to use the well-known phrase, 'the aim is to add life to years, not years to life'. With enlightened attitudes, good quality staff and managers applying proper standards of audit, it should be possible. Case studies prove it. The challenge for us is to ensure the features of institutionalization described so well by Dr Marjorie Warren do not re-emerge (Warren, 1946).

REFERENCE

Warren, M.W. (1946) Care of the chronic aged sick. *Lancet*, **i**, 841–3.

Index